Intelligent Systems Reference Library

Volume 228

AF768700

Series Editors

Janusz Kacprzyk, Polish Academy of Sciences, Warsaw, Poland

Lakhmi C. Jain, KES International, Shoreham-by-Sea, UK

The aim of this series is to publish a Reference Library, including novel advances and developments in all aspects of Intelligent Systems in an easily accessible and well structured form. The series includes reference works, handbooks, compendia, textbooks, well-structured monographs, dictionaries, and encyclopedias. It contains well integrated knowledge and current information in the field of Intelligent Systems. The series covers the theory, applications, and design methods of Intelligent Systems. Virtually all disciplines such as engineering, computer science, avionics, business, e-commerce, environment, healthcare, physics and life science are included. The list of topics spans all the areas of modern intelligent systems such as: Ambient intelligence, Computational intelligence, Social intelligence, Computational neuroscience, Artificial life, Virtual society, Cognitive systems, DNA and immunity-based systems, e-Learning and teaching, Human-centred computing and Machine ethics, Intelligent control, Intelligent data analysis, Knowledge-based paradigms, Knowledge management, Intelligent agents, Intelligent decision making, Intelligent network security, Interactive entertainment, Learning paradigms, Recommender systems, Robotics and Mechatronics including human-machine teaming, Self-organizing and adaptive systems, Soft computing including Neural systems, Fuzzy systems, Evolutionary computing and the Fusion of these paradigms, Perception and Vision, Web intelligence and Multimedia.

Indexed by SCOPUS, DBLP, zbMATH, SCImago.

All books published in the series are submitted for consideration in Web of Science.

Chee-Peng Lim · Ashlesha Vaidya ·
Yen-Wei Chen · Tejasvi Jain · Lakhmi C. Jain
Editors

Artificial Intelligence and Machine Learning for Healthcare

Vol. 1: Image and Data Analytics

Springer

Editors
Chee-Peng Lim
Institute for Intelligent Systems Research and Innovation
Deakin University
Waurn Ponds, VIC, Australia

Yen-Wei Chen
College of Information Science and Engineering
Ritsumeikan University
Kusatsu, Shiga, Japan

Lakhmi C. Jain
KES International
Shoreham-by-Sea, UK

Ashlesha Vaidya
Department of Geriatric and Rehabilitation Medicine
Royal Adelaide Hospital
Adelaide, SA, Australia

Tejasvi Jain
HCL Technologies Limited
Noida, India

ISSN 1868-4394 ISSN 1868-4408 (electronic)
Intelligent Systems Reference Library
ISBN 978-3-031-11156-3 ISBN 978-3-031-11154-9 (eBook)
https://doi.org/10.1007/978-3-031-11154-9

© The Editor(s) (if applicable) and The Author(s), under exclusive license to Springer Nature Switzerland AG 2023
This work is subject to copyright. All rights are solely and exclusively licensed by the Publisher, whether the whole or part of the material is concerned, specifically the rights of translation, reprinting, reuse of illustrations, recitation, broadcasting, reproduction on microfilms or in any other physical way, and transmission or information storage and retrieval, electronic adaptation, computer software, or by similar or dissimilar methodology now known or hereafter developed.
The use of general descriptive names, registered names, trademarks, service marks, etc. in this publication does not imply, even in the absence of a specific statement, that such names are exempt from the relevant protective laws and regulations and therefore free for general use.
The publisher, the authors, and the editors are safe to assume that the advice and information in this book are believed to be true and accurate at the date of publication. Neither the publisher nor the authors or the editors give a warranty, expressed or implied, with respect to the material contained herein or for any errors or omissions that may have been made. The publisher remains neutral with regard to jurisdictional claims in published maps and institutional affiliations.

This Springer imprint is published by the registered company Springer Nature Switzerland AG
The registered company address is: Gewerbestrasse 11, 6330 Cham, Switzerland

Preface

Advances in digital and computing technologies have driven a rapid growth in artificial intelligence (AI) and machine learning (ML) and their applications to a variety of sectors, including the medical and healthcare domains. Nowadays, electronic medical records and diagnostic imaging of patients can be readily collected and analysed by utilising AI and ML systems to derive insights and assist medical professionals in making accurate clinical decisions. As a result, effective and efficient services pertaining to diseases diagnosis and prognosis, treatments, rehabilitation, and other patient-care tasks can be realised for improving healthcare delivery.

In this edition on "Artificial Intelligence and Machine Learning for Healthcare", a total of 21 chapters from researchers and practitioners around the world are presented. Divided into two volumes, the first covers selected AL/ML-based image and data analytic solutions to address a variety of medical and healthcare problems, while the second presents several current methodologies and future trends in advancement of AL/ML for healthcare.

There are 11 chapters in this first volume. A general overview of AI/ML is given in the first chapter. Other selected chapters describe various AL/ML models, e.g. support vector machine, convolutional neural networks, decision trees, graph-based models, for healthcare research, development, and applications from the image and data analytic perspectives. A summary of each chapter in this volume is as follows.

Belciug provided an overview of AI in healthcare. The importance of AI in medicine is first elucidated. A number of commonly used AI and ML models are described, which include the decision tree, random forest, Bayesian classifier, multilayer perceptron, and convolutional neural networks. The advantages and limitations of AI for healthcare are explained, and several successful AI-based applications are described. Useful resources pertaining to AI and ML for healthcare and related domains are also presented.

Precision medicine, a concept that focuses on customisation of healthcare, e.g. diagnosis, treatment and follow-up, for individual patients, is a recent topic of interest. Jin et al. developed a radiogenomics method to discover imaging biomarkers related to breast cancer. Based on magnetic resonance imaging (MRI), a sequential forward floating selection technique coupled with a support vector machine (SVM) is developed for predicting genetic test results with respect to breast cancer. Good results are reported and discussed.

Data-driven techniques are useful for processing MRI to improve image quality and temporal resolution. Placidi et al presented a GReedy Adaptive Data-driven Environment (GRADE) for intelligent radial sampling. It uses the power spectrum of a reconstructed image and AI-based super-resolution strategies in an iterative acquisition/reconstruction process to reduce data redundancy. The method leads to high-quality images as compared with those from other under-sampling radial modalities.

To facilitate automatic and accurate liver tumour detection in multi-phase computed tomography (CT) images, Jain et al. proposed a domain adaptation-based method to overcome the lack of annotated data issue in training deep learning models. The domain shift problem in different phases of liver CT images is discussed. To address the associated domain gap, adversarial learning scheme with an anchor-free object detector is employed. In addition, a maximum square loss function for mid-level output feature maps is formulated to improve the performance. The proposed domain adaptation method outperforms other models trained with normal settings in several experimental studies.

On the other hand, to tackle the similar issue on unavailability of large sets of labelled data for supervised learning, Andreini et al. developed a new approach to generate synthetic images. The method can be applied to semantic segmentation, where the generated images can be used to augment real data sets for model training. A multi-stage approach is designed, whereby the generation procedure is carried out in multiple steps, in order to simplify the overall generation task. Based on retinal fundus and chest X-ray images, the multi-stage approach is effective and computationally economic in generating high resolution, realistic images to be used for training deep learning models.

Arrhythmia is a fatal cardiovascular disease with the symptoms of fast heartbeat, slow heartbeat, or irregular heartbeat rhythms. Siao and Ramli investigated the convolutional neural network (CNN) for arrhythmia classification based on electrocardiogram (ECG) signals and improved its performance by leveraging the long short-term memory (LSTM) model. ECG signals are pre-processed with filtering, segmentation, and median wave selection. The results indicate that the CNN-based solution is useful for atrial fibrillation diagnosis, contributing towards healthcare advancement.

Colorectal cancer is a leading cause of mortality, and early and accurate detection of polys in colonoscopies plays a significant role in increasing the survival rate of patients. Automatic polyp detection systems are useful tools for assisting medical decision-making. Nanni et al. devised an ensemble of CNN models and data augmentation methods for polyp segmentation. The results from five benchmark problems indicate efficacy of the developed ensemble approach for segmenting polys in colonoscopy images.

To help patients with Autism Spectrum Disorder (ASD) in communication, de Luise et al. analysed head bouncing actions recorded in diverse circumstances. A short tracking and lightweight processing approach is applied to a video test set concerning autistic individuals. A workflow for processing stimming and collecting relevant metadata is devised. ML models are adopted for tuning the tracking process. The results indicate good precision in detecting specific individual's autistic verbal behaviours.

Patients in medical wards exhibit multiple pathologies, which lead to burdens in terms of activities, risks, and costs for the health system. Landa et al. investigated the use of AI-based modelling methodologies pertaining to medical wards in a medium hospital setting. Unsupervised methodologies combining the self-organising map (SOM) and K-means clustering are exploited. Patients are organised in specific diagnosis-related groups, and the SOM is leveraged to identify the underlying cluster features. The developed data-driven solution offers an effective methodology to study resource utilisation in hospital environments.

Priday et al. conducted a study to create person-centred care measures for hearing rehabilitation. A dashboard, which is an AI-based infrastructure, is designed and developed to bring together the relevant data sources for analysis and interpretation with respect to defined goals. The process to ensure the right patient data samples which are collected and fed into the system to achieve meaningful care measures is described, while the barriers faced when collating and interpreting the measures of the dashboard in practice are explained. Implications on the implementation of AI for improving person-centred care are discussed.

Graphs offer a ubiquitous and expressive form of data representation, which is useful for elucidating information on entities and their interrelationships. Bongini et al. exploited the properties of Graph Neural Networks (GNNs) in processing data with minimal loss of structural information to tackle three biological problems. Specifically, graph-based models for the prediction of protein–protein interfaces, prediction of drug side effects, and generation of molecular graphs are developed. The findings are in line with theoretical expectations on the expressive capabilities of GNNs, which indicate many possible future directions for research and application of new and existing graph-based models for solving biological problems.

The editors would like to thank all authors and reviewers for their contributions and the Springer editorial team for their help in this publication. The chapters presented in this volume are just a small selection to cover the rapidly changing AI and ML paradigms in the healthcare domain, aiming to inspire researchers and practitioners to further advance AI and ML technologies for advancing the healthcare sector.

Waurn Ponds, Australia — Chee-Peng Lim
Adelaide, Australia — Ashlesha Vaidya
Kusatsu, Japan — Yen-Wei Chen
Noida, India — Tejasvi Jain
Shoreham-by-Sea, UK — Lakhmi C. Jain
May 2022

Contents

1 An Introduction to Artificial Intelligence in Healthcare 1
Smaranda Belciug
1.1 Introduction to Artificial Intelligence 2
1.2 Artificial Intelligence in Healthcare 3
1.2.1 Natural Language Processing (NLP) Technology 5
1.2.2 Machine Learning (ML) Algorithms 5
1.2.3 Artificial Neural Networks 6
1.2.4 Bayesian Classifier 6
1.2.5 Classification/Decision Trees. Random Forest 7
1.2.6 Survival Regression Models 8
1.2.7 Cluster Analysis 8
1.3 Advantages of Artificial Intelligence in Healthcare 9
1.4 Limitations of Artificial Intelligence in Healthcare 11
1.5 Successful Applications of Artificial Intelligence in Healthcare 12
1.6 Conclusions 13
Appendix 13
References 15

2 Radiomics: Approach to Precision Medicine 17
Ze Jin, Taiguang Yuan, Yukiko Tokuda, Yasuto Naoi, Noriyuki Tomiyama, and Kenji Suzuki
2.1 Introduction 18
2.2 Materials and Methods 19
2.2.1 Building of a Database 20
2.2.2 Segmentation of Target Volume 21
2.2.3 Extraction and Selection of Useful Radiomics Features 22
2.2.4 Model Building Based on Machine Learning Technologies 25
2.3 Results and Discussion 25

2.4 Conclusions 26
References 28

3 Artificial Intelligence Based Strategies for Data-Driven Radial MRI 31
Giuseppe Placidi, Luigi Cinque, Filippo Mignosi, Matteo Polsinelli, and Alessandro Sciarra
3.1 Introduction 32
3.2 Related Work 34
3.2.1 Sparse Sampling Strategies 34
3.2.2 Contribution of the Manuscript 37
3.3 Problem Statement and Framework Description 38
3.3.1 Relationship Between Radial Projections and Image 38
3.3.2 Image Reconstruction, Resolution and Noise 41
3.3.3 Super-Resolution 44
3.3.4 Framework Details 46
3.3.5 Noise Threshold *T* 49
3.4 Results and Discussion 50
3.5 Conclusion 53
References 55

4 Unsupervised Domain Adaptation Approach for Liver Tumor Detection in Multi-phase CT Images 61
Rahul Kumar Jain, Takahiro Sato, Taro Watasue, Tomohiro Nakagawa, Yutaro Iwamoto, Xianhua Han, Lanfen Lin, Hongjie Hu, Xiang Ruan, and Yen-Wei Chen
4.1 Introduction 63
4.1.1 Domain-Shift Problem 63
4.1.2 Domain Adaptation 65
4.2 Domain Adaptation Using Adversarial Learning 66
4.2.1 Anchor-free Detector 66
4.2.2 Proposed Multi-phase Domain Adaptation Framework Using Adversarial Domain Classification Loss 67
4.3 Proposed Multi-phase Domain Adaptation Framework Using Adversarial Learning with Maximum Square Loss 69
4.3.1 Maximum Square Loss 70
4.3.2 Overall Framework with Adversarial Domain Classification and Maximum Square Loss 70
4.4 Experiments 71
4.4.1 Implementation Details 71
4.4.2 Dataset 71
4.4.3 Evaluation 72
4.4.4 Results 73

4.5 Conclusions 77
References 78

5 **Multi-stage Synthetic Image Generation for the Semantic Segmentation of Medical Images** 79
Paolo Andreini, Simone Bonechi, Giorgio Ciano, Caterina Graziani, Veronica Lachi, Natalia Nikoloulopoulou, Monica Bianchini, and Franco Scarselli
5.1 Introduction 80
5.2 Related Works 82
5.2.1 Synthetic Image Generation 82
5.2.2 Image-to-Image Translation 83
5.2.3 Retinal Image Synthesis and Segmentation 83
5.2.4 Chest X-ray Image Synthesis and Segmentation 84
5.3 Multi-stage Image Synthesis 85
5.3.1 Image Generation 85
5.4 Evaluation of Multi-stage Methods 88
5.4.1 Datasets 89
5.4.2 Segmentation Network 90
5.4.3 Experimental Setup 90
5.4.4 Two-Stage Method Evaluation 91
5.4.5 Three-Stage Method Evaluation 95
5.5 Conclusions 98
References 99

6 **Classification of Arrhythmia Signals Using Hybrid Convolutional Neural Network (CNN) Model** 105
Evelyn Siao Yung Ern and Dzati Athiar Ramli
6.1 Introduction 106
6.2 Literature Review 108
6.3 Methodology 113
6.4 Results and Discussion 120
6.5 Conclusions 126
Appendix 1 128
Appendix 2 128
Appendix 3 130
References 130

7 **Polyp Segmentation with Deep Ensembles and Data Augmentation** 133
Loris Nanni, Daniela Cuza, Alessandra Lumini, Andrea Loreggia, and Sheryl Brahman
7.1 Introduction 134
7.2 Related Methods 136
7.2.1 Overview of the Propose System 138
7.2.2 Loss Functions 139

7.3 Data Augmentation 143
7.3.1 Shadows 143
7.3.2 Contrast and Motion Blur 143
7.3.3 Color Mapping 144
7.4 Experimental Results 145
7.4.1 Data and Testing Protocol 145
7.4.2 Experiments 146
7.5 Conclusions 150
References 150

8 Autistic Verbal Behavior Parameters 155
Daniela López De Luise, Federico Hertzulis, Jesica Peralta, Pablo Pescio, Ben Raúl Saad, and Tiago Ibacache
8.1 Introduction 156
8.2 Estate of the Art 157
8.3 Proposal, Materials and Methods 158
8.4 Testing Protocol 161
8.5 Analysis of Tests 165
8.6 Conclusions and Future Work 167
References 168

9 Advances in Modelling Hospital Medical Wards 171
P. Landa, M. Resta, E. Tànfani, and A. Testi
9.1 Introduction and Problem Addressed 172
9.2 Case Study and Data Analysis 173
9.3 Methodology and Results 176
9.4 Conclusion 181
References 182

10 Tracking Person-Centred Care Experiences Alongside Other Success Measures in Hearing Rehabilitation 185
Gareth Priday, Sonja Pedell, Jessica Vitkovic, and Lauren Story
10.1 Person-Centred Care in Research and Practice 186
10.1.1 Situated Action—Understanding the Context as a Basis for Meaningful Measures 187
10.1.2 Situated AI for Achieving High-Quality Person-Centred Care 188
10.2 Co-design for Person-Centred Care Measures 189
10.2.1 Co-design of Evaluation Instruments 191
10.2.2 Artificial Intelligence and PCC 191
10.3 Case Study: Co-creation of PCC Measures and Dashboard with Hearing Rehabilitation Provider 192
10.3.1 Method 192
10.4 Results 195
10.4.1 Stakeholder Workshops—Development of Tools 195
10.4.2 Stakeholder Feedback 196
10.4.3 Piloting the Dashboard 200

10.5 Discussion 203
10.5.1 Summary of Case Study 203
10.5.2 Discussion on Opportunities and Challenges for AI 203
10.5.3 Quality of Data 206
10.6 Conclusions 207
References 208

11 BioGNN: How Graph Neural Networks Can Solve Biological Problems 211
Pietro Bongini, Niccolò Pancino, Franco Scarselli, and Monica Bianchini
11.1 Overview of the Research Area 212
11.1.1 Biological Problems on Graphs 212
11.1.2 Deep Learning Models for Biological Graphs 213
11.2 Graph Neural Networks 214
11.2.1 The Graph Neural Network Model 214
11.2.2 Composite Graph Neural Networks 216
11.2.3 Layered Graph Neural Networks 216
11.2.4 Approximation Power of Graph Neural Networks 217
11.2.5 Software Implementation 218
11.3 Biological Applications 218
11.3.1 Prediction of Protein-Protein Interfaces 218
11.3.2 Drug Side-Effect Prediction 220
11.3.3 Molecular Graph Generation 223
11.4 Conclusions and Future Perspectives 226
References 227

Chapter 1
An Introduction to Artificial Intelligence in Healthcare

Smaranda Belciug

Abstract The chapter presents a brief overview of Artificial Intelligence (AI) in healthcare. We start with the why and the how of AI in medicine. The most known and commonly used AI algorithms are presented. We continued the chapter with the pros and cons of AI, highlighting the main advantages and disadvantages it has. The chapter finishes with some of the newest real-life applications of AI in different healthcare sectors from diagnostic, drug development to administrative work.

Keywords Artificial Intelligence · Healthcare · Natural language processing · Machine learning · Statistics

Abbreviations

AI	Artificial Intelligence
ANN	Artificial Neural Networks
CNN	Convolutional Neural Networks
CT/DT	Classification/Decision trees
DL	Deep Learning
EHR	Electronic Health Record
ICU	Intensive Care Unit
ML	Machine Learning
MLP	Multilayer Perceptron
NLP	Natural Language Processing
RF	Random Forests

S. Belciug (✉)
Faculty of Sciences, Department of Computer Science, University of Craiova, Craiova, Romania
e-mail: sbelciug@inf.ucv.ro

© The Author(s), under exclusive license to Springer Nature Switzerland AG 2023
C.-P. Lim et al. (eds.), *Artificial Intelligence and Machine Learning for Healthcare*, Intelligent Systems Reference Library 228,
https://doi.org/10.1007/978-3-031-11154-9_1

1.1 Introduction to Artificial Intelligence

There is a quote from a famous 1990s movie, Forrest Gump: *"life is like a box of chocolate, you never know what you're going to get"*. The line is true if you think about it. But what if we push things even further. What if we want to get the praline chocolate one, and not the hazelnut one? How can we tell from just looking at them? How do we make that choice? Nevertheless, in this case, unless we are allergic to hazelnuts, it is not a tragic situation if we make the wrong choice. But what if we are not making a choice regarding which chocolate to eat? What if our decision evolves someone's life? What if our decisions are health related?

At any moment in time, someone out there is making a decision which regards someone's health. We are talking about physicians, hospital managers, nurses, etc. In triage, they choose you will they attend first; they decide if they admit a patient or not; they choose which tests to order, they interpret the test results; they choose which treatment fits best the patient and the disease. You think that this is all? Of course not. How many beds should be purchased? How many nurses should be hired? Should the patient be discharged? Will the patient make a full recovery at home, or will she/he be readmitted? Sometimes their best course of action is the Occam's razor principle, or if you wish, Dr. Theodore Woodward's idea: *"when you hear hoofbeats, think of horses not zebras"*. Until now. Now they are no longer alone. They have the help of a true power: Artificial Intelligence (AI).

Obviously, things are never that easy. Many people fear of the 'doctorless hospitals', which we believe is never going to happen. AI is not voodoo, is not magic. It is just mathematics with a high computation power. We should look at AI as a friend that is there for us to offer its help, support, and advice. We have the power to make the final choice.

How did it all start? How did we get to this point? In 1977, in Holsapple dissertation appeared the definition of the Intelligent Decision Support System, [1]. As time passed more and more intelligent decision support systems appeared. The ultimate goal was to develop computer programs that could gather and analyze data, identify a problem, and suggest a solution. Hence, the *expert systems* were introduced by Edward Feigenbaum in the 1970s, during the Stanford Heuristic Programming Project [2]. The expert system had a knowledge base that contained facts and rules, and an inference engine that applied the rules and deduced facts. The program worked with if–then rules. If the decision parameters are known and the dataset is small, an expert system works ok. But nowadays there is a massive amount of data produced on a regular basis. We need methods that can search for hidden patterns in huge datasets. Hence, the if–then rules fail us. We need a super merger between Statistics and Artificial Intelligence, that is able to *"find the needle in the haystack"*. Today, more than ever, the 1597 phrase *"scientia potential est"*, or *"knowledge is power"* stands out.

Our lives are out there. We post our photos on Facebook and Instagram. We tweet. We use our phone to count our daily steps. We scan our fidelity cards when we buy almost anything. We upload videos on YouTube or TikTok. 10 million photos are uploaded per hour on Facebook. 95 million photos and videos are shared daily on Instagram. Everyday over 12 terabytes of tweets are analyzed. This is Big Data.

accessed March 28, 2022—the researchers from the Department of Zoology, University of Graz, Austria, developed robot fish that monitor, search, explore, harvest, and maintain underwater habitats. Ever wanted to stay in a hotel where the staff isn't human? Well, go pay a visit to the Weird Hotel or Henn na Hotel—http://www.h-n-h.jp/en/—accessed March 28—in Japan. The staff is made up of robots with AI. You do not have an electronic key; you check-in using facial recognition. And yes, don't be alarmed, but the reception clerk is a dinosaur.

Some people are still trapped in the past when optical character recognition was considered AI. AI means 'thinking' machines. Machines that make decisions taking into account the possible consequences of their actions. For instance, autonomous self-driving cars are controlled by a neural network that takes into account all the possible variables (e.g. traffic, moving objects, weather conditions, road conditions, pedestrians) and drive in such a manner that collision are prevented. Another example of AI is the industrial robot that is able to assemble a STEFAN chair from IKEA [4]. The robot has a 3D camera as eyes, arms with six-axis motion, and sensors for each finger that decide the strength of the grip. The robot deciphers the instructions in 11 min, leaving 9 min for actually assembling the chair. It can even create Chinese poetry from Images, [5].

AI will have a major impact on future jobs. Machines will perform some tasks that are currently jobs for many people. Using a machine instead of a person is cheaper. You do not have to pay a salary, there is no need for medical insurance, no retirement plan, no holidays. Besides these reasons, the process is smoother: no mistakes from fatigue, etc. Even if this is could be an issue, we still need to remember that we have something that machines will never have: empathy. We, humans, use our emotional intelligence when taking a decision. At least one important domain takes more than mathematical precision: healthcare. So, let us see how we use AI in healthcare in the next subsection.

1.2 Artificial Intelligence in Healthcare

The healthcare system is complex. It covers the diagnostic, treatment, prevention of diseases and injuries, to hospital and patient management. It generates massive amount of data from image scans to electronic medical records, different administrative reports, etc. A lot of industries are connected to the healthcare sector:

- The *Pharma* industry which covers drug development, production, and marketing.
- *Biotechnology* industry which uses gene engineering technology to develop novel patented medicines.
- *Healthcare equipment industry* which develops medical devices, instruments, etc.
- *Healthcare distribution industry* which consists of all the wholesalers of healthcare products.

- *Healthcare facilities* which include hospitals, clinics, birthing centers, psychiatric care centers, outpatient care centers, nursing homes, dental clinics, home healthcare agencies, healthcare laboratories, etc.
- *Healthcare management* which deals with activities as reducing the costs, improving the healthcare quality, health insurance etc.

The first AI system that was ever created is the MYCIN. It was developed by Edward Shortliffe in 1972 as his doctoral dissertation for Stanford Medical School [6]. MYCIN was derived from the DENDRAL project, [7], and was a clinical expert system which was able to select antibiotics for patients with blood infections. Even if MYCIN had a consultation, explanation and rule acquisition system, it was never used in clinical practice.

Over the years many AI systems have been developed for healthcare [8]. Here we shall mention some of the most-well known applications: AAPHelp developed by researchers from Leeds Universitty, UK, for helping doctor diagnose acute abdominal pain, [9]; INTERNIST-I developed at the University of Pittsburg for diagnosing cases relate to general internal medicine, [10]; CASNET glaucoma was developed at Rutgers University for the diagnosis and treatment of glaucoma, [11]; ONCOCIN developed at Stanford University School of Medicine for cancer patients, [12].

Did you ever ask yourself why would be need AI in healthcare? The answer is quite simple. If you look at the relationship between the doctor and the patient, you can see that it is a very complex one. It includes information management, expertise, empathy, unpredictable response to treatment (e.g. in surgery or intensive care unit (ICU), etc. According to a study, a physician spends only 27% of her/his total time face to face with the patient, 49.2% of the time on Electronic Health Record (EHR) and desk, [13]. Obviously, this situation must be changed. When does a doctor have time to practice medicine, do research, master new skills, or improve older ones? Therefore, we need AI in healthcare. It is important for doctors, as well as patients, to understand and embrace the automation in medicine through AI, because it is a safe way to optimize patient care. The healthcare landscape will change. Actually, it is changing as we speak. Future doctors will have news skills like robotics and computer skills. Indeed, this may be seen as a bold visionary opinion of the future, but take into account the fact that on November 6, 2018, Xiaoyi, a Chinese AI-powered robot successfully passed a medical examen—http://techthelead.com/robot-chinas-medical-exam/—accessed March 29, 2022.

Now that we have seen why, we must see how. There are two approaches for AI in healthcare: *natural language processing* algorithms for extracting knowledge from unstructured data (e.g. clinical notes), and cutting edge *machine learning* algorithms which can be applied on structured data. Briefly, we shall browse through some approaches.

1.2.1 Natural Language Processing (NLP) Technology

NPL technology remains a hot topic today, even if it started a long time ago with Turing's test. In NLP applied in healthcare we are interested in transforming unstructured data into structured data. By unstructured information we understand any data that does not come in a predefined model, or it cannot fit well into tables. Some examples of unstructured data are: health records, clinical opinions, audio/video files, analog data, sentiments, images, etc. If we want to apply AI in healthcare we need data, or data about data, also known as metadata. Metadata is for instance the syntax of a language. We have structured languages like C or Java, and unstructured languages like English or French, but all of them have a syntax or a grammar, that clarifies the relationship between words. If we are interested in the interpretation of words, for instance to understand the explanations of patients, we need to understand, not the syntax, but the *semantics*. We can use NPL methods to extract data from observations and thoughts, obtained during the patient-doctor dialogue, [14]. A well-known example of such an AI system is Watson Oncology, which is used since 2013 at the Memorial Sloan Kettering Cancer Center, New York City. The system supports the oncology community of doctors when deciding the treatment options (https://www.mskcc.org/about/innovative-collaborations/watson-oncology). Another example is the Google Cloud Natural Language—https://cloud.google.com/natural-language/.

1.2.2 Machine Learning (ML) Algorithms

Machine learning algorithms use structured data to accomplish different tasks. They are divided into two types of algorithms depending on the learning paradigm, which can be *supervised* or *unsupervised*. *Supervised learning* is also known as *learning with a teacher*, and relies on past experience, that is previously labeled data, that establishes a link between the input and the output. The algorithm trains under supervision, tunes its parameters, and afterwards it is able to make predictions. *Unsupervised learning* is known as *learning without a teacher* because there is no one to monitor the learning process. This category is split further into *reinforcement learning* that connects situations to actions through a reward (reinforcement) signal. Practically, the learning is done by a repeated interaction with the environment. The second split is *self-organized learning*, such as clustering and outlier detection. In this case, the model adapts to the observations, without any a priori input, that is only questions, no answers.

Supervised models are used for *classification* or *regression* tasks. Classification means class prediction, pattern recognition, or discriminant analysis. Given a set of features, the model guesses the class label. Briefly, we are going to present the most popular classification models in use today.

1.2.3 Artificial Neural Networks

Artificial Neural Networks or ANN are adaptive processing systems, that is they learn from examples and behave similar to the human brain. ANN learn by adapting their synaptic weights, that quantify the intensity of the connection between neurons. Oncc the training process is over, and the synaptic weights are tuned, the ANN is ready to classify new objects. An ANN has a large number of artificial neurons that are interconnected, and work in parallel. The neurons are mapped onto three types of layers: the input layer, the hidden layer, and the output layer. The most known ANNs are the *multi-layered perceptron* (MLP) and *convolutional neural networks* (CNN) or *deep learning*. Both networks have multiple hidden layers that are interconnected in a feed-forward way. Each neuron from one layer is connected to the neurons in the subsequent layer. An activation function (e.g. ReLU, hyperbolic tangent, sigmoid, etc.) is used for firing a neuron. The classical manner of training an ANN implies finding out the error, (i.e. difference between the ground truth and the predicted label) and propagating it backwards throughout the network in order to fine tune the synaptic weights. This is the backpropagation algorithm. Other learning paradigms can be found in [15–20].

Deep learning (DL) is an extension of the classical ANNs. In a simple way we can consider CNNs as an NN with many hidden layers. DLs perform very well on medical images such as MRIs, CT scans, X-rays or ultrasounds. Besides CNNs, DL algorithms include recurrent NNs and deep belief networks. 'Fed' with images, the CNN transfers the input pixel values with the use of the synaptic weights through multiple convolutional layers and pooling layers. Just like in the classical ANN's case, the weights are tuned so that the network minimizes the average error between the ground truth and the predicted value, [21]. CNNs are implemented in TensorFlow, Keras, Caffe, or CNTK.

1.2.4 Bayesian Classifier

The Bayesian classifier is based on Thomas Bayes famous theorem, [22]. The theorem computes the probability of an event, taking into account prior knowledge of other conditions that might be related to that event. Bayes' formula can be written non-mathematically that following way:

$$\text{Posterior probability} = \frac{\text{Likelihood } \times \text{Prior probability}}{\text{Evidence}}.$$

A more technical equation is the following:

$$P(H|E) = \frac{P(E|H) \cdot P(H)}{P(E)},$$

where H is the hypothesis and E is the corresponding evidence.

The Bayesian classifier makes the decision that minimizes the expected risk. The classification or decision rule can be formulated as such: let D_k be the decision rule that regards A_k, and $P(error|x) = 1 - P(A_k|x)$ be the error that is related to A_k, given x. The Bayesian classifier tries to minimize $P(error|x)$, by making the choice D_k.

There should be noted that this classifier presumes that all attributes A_k are independent.

1.2.5 Classification/Decision Trees. Random Forest

Classification/Decision Trees (CT/DT) are a simple and efficient way to use when we are dealing with small datasets. The idea behind this method is that we want to divide the data space into distinct classes using classification rules. Let us suppose we have $A_i, i = 1, \ldots, m$ attributes and j decision classes. A classification rule has the following form: **if** the value of A_1 is lower than a_1, **then if** the value of A_2 is lower than a_2, and so on, **then** the object belongs to class C_j. Practically, we compare the values of the attributes with the thresholds $a_1, a_2, \ldots, a_m$. We built the classification rules during the *tree induction* or *tree learning process*, meaning that we are finding the thresholds' optimal values, that divide the initial data space into subspaces that are as homogeneous as possible. The training process respects the following rules:

- The leaf nodes represent the decision classes.
- Each non-leaf node is a test based on a certain attribute
- Each branch represents the test result.

We split each node using a metrics that measure the node's *impurity*. The most common used metrics are the entropy, the information gain, GINI index, misclassification measure, chi-square error, G-square, variance reduction, etc.

Multiple CT/DT can be used, forming a random forest (RF). We built multiple trees using random objects from the training dataset. Using RF lets us manage a dataset with a large number of attributes. We can use sensitivity analysis to rank the variables based on what impact they have on the class variable. Other advantages include: no overfitting, detecting correlations and interactions between variables, handling missing values, etc. To classify a new object, we simply assign that object to all the trees in the forest. Afterwards, each tree votes for a certain class, and the RF chooses the class that has the most votes in that forest, [23].

We have briefly passed through some classification methods. Before we move onto the next subsection, we shall discuss other types of ML algorithms such as survival regression methods and cluster analysis.

1.2.6 Survival Regression Models

An important role that AI plays in the healthcare systems related to survival analysis. In many clinical investigations there are different circumstances that might affect the outcome of a patient. Through AI, we can analyze the survival taking into account different factors at the same time, specifying the effect size of each factor. We are interested in seeing whether different independent features are correlated with the survival or failure times. Some believe that this issue can be resolved through applying a multilinear regression, when in fact by applying this method we ca only achieve two major issues. The first one is the fact that the variable of interest, the survival or failure time, is most like not governed by the Gaussian distribution. The second one is that we might encounter *censored data.* Hence, the most known and used AI model is the *Cox proportional hazard model.* This model does not make assumptions regarding the nature and shape of the hazard function. The *Cox* mode is extended through the *Cox's proportional hazard model with time-dependent covariates.*

1.2.7 Cluster Analysis

This type of exploratory data analysis model is also known under the names of segmentation or taxonomy analysis. Its goal is to identify different structures within the data. It is an unsupervised ML technique. Using it we divide the data into several groups called *clusters*. The division is made taking into account predetermined similarities. Please note that classification techniques are different from clustering techniques, because with clustering we do not assign labels to the objects, we group them so that the objects from one cluster are similar to each other than to those from other clusters. We have two major approaches when it comes to clustering:

- *Hierarchical* clustering in which the clusters are organized in the shape of a tree.
- *Partitional* or *flat* clustering which divides the data into distinct clusters. Each object belongs to only one cluster (*hard* clustering). If an object has fractional membership to multiple clusters, then we are dealing with soft clustering.

When we perform clustering analysis, we need to undertake the following steps:

1. Define a similarity metric.
2. Define which criteria to take into account into the clustering building process.
3. Choose a clustering algorithm that fits your data the best.

The most used clustering algorithm are the *k*-means and the *hierarchical* clustering (bottom-up, top-down, and conceptual). More details can be found in [24, 25].

Before we finish this subsection, we must cover another important aspect of AI in healthcare: comparing algorithms. The majority of papers that cover AI in healthcare lack of rigor regarding the assessment of their performance. Most authors limit the statistical analysis to reporting the classification accuracy, precision, or F1-score.

The more evolved report some performance metrics such as the confusion matrix, sensitivity, specificity, positive and negative predictive values, or area under the ROC curve.

Since AI algorithms have a stochastic nature, we need to run them multiple times to obtain a reliable result regarding their performance and robustness. Consider the accuracy recorded after multiple computer runs a sample of decision performance. We can assess the benchmarking process through:

- *Data screening* which involves checking whether we can apply different statistical tests to our sample data. Data screening involves tests for checking the normality (e.g.Kolmogorov–Smirnov, Lilliefors, Shapiro Wilk) and the equality of variances (e.g. Levene's test).
- *Hypothesis testing*
- which deals with the comparison between the obtained performances: e.g. *t*-test for independent samples, Mann–Whitney U test, one-way ANOVA together with post-hoc Tukey, Bonferroni or Scheffe, Cohen's kappa test,
- *Over-learning control* which involves the analysis of the training/testing performances correlation. We are interested to see if the model is able to generalize well given new cases.

Before starting the statistical analysis it is recommended to perform an a priori statistical power analysis (*two-tailed* type of null hypothesis) to determine the proper sample size (e.g. how many computer runs are needed so that we can achieve and adequate statistical power).

1.3 Advantages of Artificial Intelligence in Healthcare

Whether we want it or not, the AI revolution in healthcare has begun and it is here to stay. This does not mean that we are going to have doctorless hospitals, but it doesn't mean that medicine will ever be the same as it was a decade ago. AI methods will never replace human's sixth sense. Recall the famous saying: *medicine is not mathematics*. The sad part of the story is that even if we are going to have an "intelligent" healthcare system, this does not mean that we are going to have 100% accuracy in diagnosis, treatment, or patient management. This is just an impossible dream, because we cannot foresee what will happen to a person even if we do everything by the book. There will always a chance factor which we will never be able to control with or without AI. AI and Statistic play with numbers, but when applied to the healthcare system, those numbers become someone's father, mother, brother, sister, wife, husband, or child. We cannot tell for sure what will happen, but AI and statistic can give a probability.

The major advantage of AI in healthcare is the huge computational power. Without AI we could have never been able to dream about personalized medicine that gathers huge amount of intel about a person so that tailored treatment could be developed for that individual. Without AI we could not monitor and predict with a certain probability the patient's response to treatment.

Let's see some of the benefits of AI in healthcare:

1. *Management of medical records.* Using an AI system to manage the medical records will increase the face time doctor-patient. The system can collect, store, search, modify the information regarding the patient at a faster pace.
2. *Virtual nurses.* In the last years different AI apps have been developed to monitor patient's condition and follow up (e.g. Molly—http://www.sensely.com—accessed March 31, 2022). Other apps help parents decide whether they should take their child to see a doctor, or if it is ok to stay at home.
3. *Digital consult.* There is an app named Babylon. It uses speech recognition and compares the reported symptoms to the symptoms it has stored in its database. Babylon can recommend treatments as well. Another symptom checker can be found at https://symptoms.webmd.com/#info—accessed March 31, 2022.
4. *Reading medical image scans or ultrasound movies.* Using deep learning, we can read more precisely and even faster different medical scans. This speeds up the process, and leaves the doctor attend to other medical issues.
5. *Drug development.* Besides actually creating new drugs with the help of AI, there are other apps such as https://www.atomwise.com/—accessed March 31, 2022—that can check whether existing drugs can be applied successfully to other conditions. In 24 h, the program was able to find two drugs that can reduce Ebola infectivity.
6. *Treatment management.* The National Institutes of Health developed an app, AICure—https://aicure.com/—accessed March 31, 2022—that is able to monitor how and if the patient takes it medication treatment. Using the smartphone's camera, the AI system checks whether indeed the patient has taken his medication.
7. *Health monitoring.* All the wearable health trackers that monitor somebody's health can alert the user's possible health issues and even share that intel with the patient's doctor.
8. *Precision medicine.* Through AI personalized treatment can be tailored taking into account the patient's genetics, lifestyle, workplace, etc.
9. *Robot-assisted surgery.* In many surgeries the precision of a robot could increase the chances of survival and also may lead to a faster recovery.
10. *Fraud detection.* Using AI the insurance companies can easier detect insurance fraud.
11. *Cybersecurity.* The amount of medical data needs to be secured before being used.

Let us look at the impact of the top 10 applications of AI in healthcare, [26] (Table 1.1):

Before we end our discussion regarding the benefits of AI in healthcare, we would like to make you aware of the fact that the WHO claims that the uneven access to health services leads to an 18.1-year gap in the life expectancy between the

Table 1.1 Top 10 AI applications in healthcare and their value

Application	Value—potential benefits by 2026
Robot-assisted surgery	$ 40 billions
Virtual nursing assistants	$ 20 billions
Administrative workflow assistance	$ 18 billions
Fraud detection	$ 17 billions
Connected machines	$ 14 billions
Clinical trial participant identifier	$ 13 billions
Preliminary diagnosis	$ 5 billions
Automated image diagnosis	$ 3 billions
Cybersecurity	$ 2 billions

poorest and the richest countries—https://www.who.int/news/item/04-04-2019-uneven-access-to-health-services-drives-life-expectancy-gaps-who—accessed April 1, 2022. AI could and is making a difference in this area. We shall leave only one example the Ada App, —https://ada.com—accessed April 1, 2022—which is available in 140 countries, and provides access to medical care for the people in undeveloped countries.

So much for the advantages. Let us see now whether AI in healthcare is only a ray of sunshine, or if there's also a dark side to it.

1.4 Limitations of Artificial Intelligence in Healthcare

First stop: AI lacks empathy and sixth sense. When a robot performs a surgery, it is completely mathematical, logical. Robots do not have any feelings towards the patients. Some see this as an advantage, recall you are never supposed to operate on a member of your family or on a friend, others view this as a disadvantage. Why is that? Because a robot will follow the rules, will follow protocol. A doctor having feelings may violate a rule or two that might lead to saving their patient's life.

Second stop: due to AI in healthcare, the unemployment rates might go up. Because chatbots and robots can predict and analyze a patient's health, or can inject the correct dosage of a drug, automatically change the ventilation parameters, etc., many healthcare workers may lose their work.

Third stop: the diagnosis/treatment etc. is dependent on the training set that the AI system has been trained on. Hence, if we use small dataset, or biased datasets, or unbalanced datasets, the AI system will give a wrong diagnosis.

Forth stop: because of the lack of sympathy, an AI system will not take into consideration all the aspects of a person's life. For instance, it might recommend a treatment/surgery/healthcare facility without taking into account factors such as the patient's income. This will make that person stop the treatment/surgery etc. A human doctor can decide the optimum treatment taking into account other factors, that might not be in the training dataset.

Last stop: privacy issues. Black-hat hackers are always trying to get access at all costs. If Google has privacy issues, it is clear that no one is safe.

1.5 Successful Applications of Artificial Intelligence in Healthcare

We shall end this chapter with some success of AI applications in healthcare.

AI can assess a person's risk of developing a heart disease before this actually happens. In order to achieve this prediction, the data scientists from GOOGLE and Verily apply a deep learning algorithm that uses the scans taken from the back of a patient's eye together with the patient's age, blood pressure, and the smoking status [27]. The dataset contained 300 000 patients. Another AI algorithm is able to foresee heart failure in early stages using EHR. This leads to the possibility of developing a tailored prevention plan, [28].

"Deep-patient" is another AI system that uses EHR to predict the future of patients for 78 diseases that include amongst others diabetes, schizophrenia, and various types of cancer, [29]. Another study developed an AI system that automatically controls the mechanical ventilation for acute respiratory distress syndrome. The system is based on the open lung concept and AI, [30].

The COVID-19 pandemic boosted AI in healthcare. Image scans and clinical data of patients with COVID-19 have been analyzed with an AI system at Mount Sinai. PathAI—https://www.pathai.com/—accessed April 1, 2022—is a ML technology that assists pathologists in setting the diagnosis. PathAI has been working with drug developers like Bristol-Meyrs Squibb and with Bill & Melinda Gates Foundation to increase the use of AI in healthcare. Buoy Health—https://www.buoyhealth.com—accessed April 1, 2022—is a symptom and cure checker. A chatbot listens to the patient's symptoms and other worries and then provides a correct treatment based on the diagnosis it had set. This chatbot is used at Harvard Medical School.

The 5th smartest AI company in the world is Enlitic—https://enlitic.com—accessed April 1, 2022. Enlitic ranks above Meta or Microsoft. It develops deep learning tool that analyze unstructured medical data to help the doctors diagnose and treat patients faster and more accurate. Freenome—https://www.freenime.com—accessed April 1, 2022—diagnosis cancer through an AI system that analyzes screenings, diagnostic test and blood work. Their aim is to detect cancer in the early stages and develop quickly new treatments.

At Beth Israel Deaconess Medical Center—https://www.bidmc.org—accessed April 1, 2022—the doctors use AI to diagnose deadly blood disease at a very early stage. They use AI to scan blood samples for harmful bacteria. The accuracy is 95%.

Regarding drug development, here are some companies that use AI to develop next wave of drugs: BioXcel Therapeutics—https://www.bioxceltherapeutics.com—accessed April 1, 2022—used AI to develop new drugs for immune-oncology and neuroscience; BERG—https://berghealth.com—accessed April 1, 2022—is combining interrogative biology with traditional research and development to find new drug that combat diseases like Parkinson; Atomwise—https://www.atomwise.com—accessed April 1, 2022—uses neural networks to identify patient characteristics and predict bioactivity for clinical trials; Deep-Genomic—https://www.deepgenomics.com—accessed April 1, 2022—uses AI to find developmental drugs for neuromuscular or neurodegenerative disorders.

AI technology is also used in streamlining patient's experiences. AI can help healthcare managers manage patient flow better. Here are some examples: Babylon Health—https://babylonhealth.com—accessed April 1, 2022—is trying to prevent sickness through an interactive symptom checker and a health monitoring system; Spring Health—https://springhealth.com—accessed April 1, 2022—is using AI to match patients with the right specialist for mental health problems; One Drop—https://onedrop.today—accessed April 1, 2022—is an app for the management of diabetes, heart health, blood pressure and weight management.

And the list could go on. Everyday new apps are being developed. Who knows what the future might bring? What we do know is that researchers such the authors from this book are working every day to develop new AI technologies for the healthcare sector. So, what better way to see what the future might bring, but further reading this wonderful book?

1.6 Conclusions

The chapter provides a briefly overview of AI in the healthcare sector. We have discussed the need for AI in medicine and some of the most known and used AI algorithms. In this day of age, we believe that AI might be the 'holy grail' in healthcare. Obviously, AI in healthcare has benefits as well as disadvantages, which we have browsed in this chapter. We ended our introduction with some real-life AI applications in healthcare, that we hope to have risen your interest on this chapter. Eager to learn more about AI in healthcare? Then just continue reading this book and find out what we might see in the neared future!

Appendix

The following resources may prove useful for exploring the "Artificial Intelligence in Healthcare" further. This list is neither complete, nor exclusive. It can be seen as a starting point to explore this field of research further.

Books

1. Lim, C.P., et al. (eds.): Handbook of Artificial Intelligence in Healthcare, vol. 2. Springer, Heidelberg (2022)
2. Lim, C.P., et al. (eds.): Handbook of Artificial Intelligence in Healthcare, vol. 1, Springer, Heidelberg (2021)
3. Brooks, A., et al. (eds.): Recent Advances in Technologies for Inclusive Well-Being: Virtual Patients, Gamification and Simulation. Springer, Heidelberg (2021)
4. Woodcock, A., et al. (eds.): Design of Assistive Technology for Ageing Populations. Springer, Germany (2020)
5. Belciug, S., Gorunescu, F.: Intelligent Decision Support System—A Journey to Smarter Healthcare. Springer, Heidelberg (2020)
6. Belciug, S.: Artificial Intelligence in Cancer: Diagnostic to Tailored Treatment. Elsevier, Academic Press (2020)
7. Agrawal, B., et al. (eds.): Deep Learning Techniques for Biomedical and Health Informatics. Academic Press, UK (2020)
8. Chen, Y.-W., Jain, L.C. (eds.): Deep Learning in Healthcare: Paradigms and Applications. Springer, Germany (2020)
9. I. Maglogiannis, et al. (eds.): Advanced Computational Intelligence Paradigms in Healthcare 7: Biomedical Informatics. Springer, Heidelberg (2020)
10. Holmes, D.E., Jain, L.C. (eds.): Advances in Biomedical Informatics. Springer, Germany (2018)
11. Brooks, A.L., et al. (eds.): Technologies of Inclusive Well-Being. Springer, Germany (2014)
12. Ma, M., et al. (eds.): Virtual, Augmented Reality and Serious Games for Healthcare 1. Springer, Germany (2014)
13. Brahnam, S., Jain, L.C. (eds.): Advanced Computational Intelligence Paradigms in Healthcare 6: Virtual Reality in Psychotherapy, Rehabilitation, and Assessment. Springer, Heidelberg (2011)
14. Bichindaritz, I.S., et al. (eds.): Advanced Computational Intelligence Paradigms in Healthcare 4: Advanced Methodologies. Springer, Heidelberg (2010)
15. Brahnam, S., Jain, L.C. (eds.): Advanced Computational Intelligence Paradigms in Healthcare 5: Intelligent Decision Support Systems. Springer, Heidelberg (2010)
16. Vaidya, S., et al. (eds.): Advanced Computational Intelligence Paradigms in Healthcare 2. Springer, Heidelberg (2008)
17. Sardo, M., et al. (eds.): Advanced Computational Intelligence Paradigms in Healthcare 3. Springer, Heidelberg (2008)
18. Yoshida, H., et al. (eds.): Advanced Computational Intelligence Paradigms in Healthcare 1. Springer, Heidelberg (2007)
19. Ichalkaranje, N., et al. (eds.): Intelligent Paradigms for Assistive and Preventive Healthcare. Springer, Heidelberg (2006)
20. Silverman, B., et al. (eds.): Intelligent Paradigms in Healthcare Enterprises. Springer, Heidelberg (2005)
21. Teodorescu, H.-N., Jain, L.C. (eds.): Intelligent Systems and Technologies in Rehabilitation Engineering. CRC Press, USA (2001)
22. Jain, A., et al. (eds.): Artificial Intelligence Techniques in Breast Cancer Diagnosis and Prognosis. World Scientific (2000)
23. Teodorescu, H.-N., et al. (eds.): Soft Computing in Human Related Sciences. CRC Press, USA (1999)

Conference Proceedings

1. Chen, Y., et al. (eds.): Innovation in medicine and healthcare 2021. In: Proceedings of the KES-InMed 2021 Conference. Springer, Germany (2021)
2. Chen, Y., et al. (eds.): Innovation in medicine and healthcare 2022. In: Proceedings of the KES-InMed 2022 Conference. Springer, Germany (2022)
3. Chen, Y.-W., et al. (eds.): Innovations in medicine and healthcare systems, and multimedia, KES-InMed-19 and KES-IIMSS-19. Springer, Germany (2019)
4. Chen, et al. (eds.): Innovation in medicine and healthcare 2017. In: Proceedings of the KES-InMed 2017 Conference. Springer, Germany (2017)
5. Chen, Y., et al. (eds.): Innovation in medicine and healthcare 2016. In: Proceedings of the KES-InMed 2016 Conference. Springer, Germany (2016)
6. Chen, Y., et al. (eds.): Innovation in medicine and healthcare 2015. In Proceedings of the KES-InMed 2015 Conference. Springer, Germany (2015)
7. Grana, M., et al. (eds.): Innovation in Medicine and Healthcare. IOS Press (2014)

References

1. Holsapple, C., Whinston, A., Whinston, A.: Bussiness Expert Systems. McGraw-Hill (1987)
2. Leondes, C.T.: Expert Systems: The Technology of Knowledge Management and Decision Making for the 21st Century, pp. 1–22 (2002)
3. Mohler, G.O., Short, M.B., Malinowski, S., Johnson, M., Tita, G.E., Bertozzi, A.L., Brantigham, P.J.: Randomized controlled filed trials of predictive policing. J. Am. Stati. Assoc. **110**(512), 1399–1411 (2016)
4. Suarez-Ruiz, F., Zhou, X., Pham, Q.C.: Can robots assemble an IKEA chair? Sci. Robot. **3**, 17 (2018). https://doi.org/10.1126/scirobotics.aat6385
5. Xu, L., Jiang, L., Qin, C., Wang, Z., Du, D.: How images inspire poems: generating classical Chinese poetry from images with memory networks. In: Proceedings of the Thirty-Second AAAI Conference on Artificial Intelligence and Thirtieth Innovative Applications of Artificial Intelligence Conference and Eight AAAI Symposium on Educational Advances in Artificial Intelligence, vol. 689, pp. 5618–5625 (2018)
6. Shortliffe, E.: Computer-Based Medical Consultations: MYCIN. Elsevier (1976)
7. Feigenbaum, E., Buchanan, B.: DENDRAL and Meta-DENDRAL roots of knowledge systems and expert systems applications. Artif. Intell **59**, 233–240 (1993)
8. Belciug, S., Gorunescu, F.: Era of intelligent systems in healthcare. In: Belciug, S., Gorunescu, F. (eds.) Intelligent Decision Support Systems: A Journey to Smarter Healthcare. Springer, Heidelberg (2020)
9. Sim, I., Gorman, P., Greenes, R.A., et al.: Clinical decision support systems for the practice of evidence-based medicine. J. Am. Med. Inform, Assoc. **8**(6), 527–534 (2001)
10. Miller, R.A., Pople, H.E., Jr., Myers, J.D.: Internist-1, an experimental computer-based diagnostic consultant for general internal medicine. N. Engl. H. Med. **307**(8), 468–476 (1982). https://doi.org/10.1056/NEJM19820818=93070803
11. Weiss, S., Kulikowski, C.A., Safir, A.: Glaucoma consultation by computer. Comput. Med. Biol. **8**(1), 25–40 (1978)
12. Shortliffe, E.H., Scott, A.C., Bischoff, M.B., Campbell, A.B., Van Melle, W., Jacobs, C.D.: ONCOCIN: an expert system for oncology protocol management. In: IJCAI'81: Proceedings of the 7th International Joint Conference on Artificial Intelligence, vol. 2, pp. 876–881 (1981)
13. Sinsky, C., Colligan, L., Li, L., Prgomet, M., Reynolds, S., Goeders, L., Westbrook, J., Tutty, M., Blike, G.: Allocation of physician time in ambulatory practice: a time and motion study in 4 specialties. Ann. Intern. Med **165**(11), 753–760 (2016). https://doi.org/10.7326/,160961

14. Townsedn, A.: Smart Cities: Big Data, Civic Hackers, and the Quest for a New Utopia. W.W. Norton & Company (2013)
15. Haykin, S.: Neural Networks, A Comprehensive Foundation, 2nd edn. Prentice Hall (1999)
16. Belciug, S.: Artificial Intelligence in Cancer: Diagnostic to Tailored Treatment. Elsevier (2020)
17. Belciug, S.: Parallel versus cascaded logistic regression trained single-hidden feedforward neural network for medical da. Exp Sys App **170**, 114538 (2021)
18. Belciug, S.: Logistic regression paradigm for training a single-hidden layer feedforward neural network. Application to gene expression datasets for cancer research. J. Biomed. Inf. **102**. https://doi.org/10.1016/j.jbi.2019.103373 (2020)
19. Belciug, S., Gorunescu, F.: Learning a single-hidden layer feedforward neural network using rank correlation based strategy with application to high dimensional gene expression and proteomic spectra datasets in cancer detection. J. Biomed. Inf. **83**, 159–166. https://doi.org/10.1016/j.jbi.2018.06.003 (2018)
20. Gorunescu, F., Belciug, S.: Boosting backpropagation algorithm by stimulus-sampling: application in computer-aided medical diagnosis. J. Biomed. Inf. **64**, 74–81 (2016). https://doi.org/10.1016/j.jbi.2016.08.004
21. Bayes, T.: An essay towards solving a problem in the doctrine of chance. Phil. Trans. **53**, 370–418. https://doi.org/10.1098/rrstl.17963.0053 (1763)
22. Jiang, F., Jiang, Y., Zhi, H., Dong, Y., Li, H., Wang, Y., Dong, Q., Shen H., Wang, Y.: Artificial intelligence in healthcare: past, present and future. BMJ Stroke Vasc. Neurol. 1–14. https://doi.org/10.1136/svn-2017-000101 (2017)
23. Yang, Z.R.: Machine Learning Approaches to Bioinformatics. World Scientific (2010)
24. Rokach, L., Maimon, O.: Clustering methods. In: Maimon, O., Rokach, L. (eds.) Data Mining and Knowledge Discovery Handbook. Springer, Boston (2005)
25. Mirkin, B.: Clustering, A Data Recovery Approach, 2nd edn. Chapman & Hall, CRC Press (2013)
26. Accenture. https://accenture.com/au-en/insights/health/artificial-intelligence-healtchare (2022)
27. Poplin, R., Varadarajan, A., Blumer, K., Liu, Y., McConnell, M.V., Corrado, G.S., Peng, L., Webster, D.R.: Prediction of cardiovascular risk factors from retinal fundus photographs via deep learning. Nat. Biomed. Eng. **2**, 158–164. https://doi.org/10.10138/s41551-018-0195-0 (2018)
28. Sun, J., McNaughton, C., Zhang, P., Perer, A., Gkoulalas-Divanis, A., Denny, J.C., Kirby, J., Lasko, T., Saip, A., Malin, B.A.: Predicting changes in hypertension control using electronic heart records from a chronic disease management program. J. Am. Med. Inform. Assoc. **21**(2), 337–344 (2013)
29. Miotto, R., Li, L., Kidd, B.A., Dudley, J.T.: Deep patient: an unsupervised representation to predict the future of patients from electronic health records. Sci. Rep. **6**. https://doi.org/10.1018/srep26094 (2016)
30. Poprapa, A., Muanghong, D., Kony, M., Leonhardt, S., Pickerodt, P., Tjarks, O., Schwaiberger, D., Lachmann, B.: Artificial intelligence for closed-loop ventilation therapy with hemodynamic control using the open lung concept. Int. J. Intelli. Comput. Cybern. **8**(1), 50–68 (2015). https://doi.org/10.1108/IJICC-05-2014-0025

Chapter 2
Radiomics: Approach to Precision Medicine

Ze Jin, Taiguang Yuan, Yukiko Tokuda, Yasuto Naoi, Noriyuki Tomiyama, and Kenji Suzuki

Abstract Precision medicine, as a concept of customization of healthcare for individual patients with diagnosis, treatments, and follow-up, has been a hot topic in recent years. Large-scale molecular-biology-level information, such as genome, proteome, and metabolome, is collected from patients for analyzing biomarkers for subpopulation of a particular disease. This is import for the targeted therapy, which is expected to be more effective and less harmful to normal cells than traditional chemotherapy. Meanwhile, due to the rapid development in medical imaging and machine learning technology, we are able to extract more and more "unseen" disease characteristics from medical images. Radiomics, a method that extracts a large number of features from medical images, has been established for a variety of purposes such as a prediction of risks for a particular disease, classification of lesions, a prediction of outcome of patients, etc. Genetic tests can provide prognostic information in breast cancer for both diagnosis and treatment planning. In this study, we developed a radiogenomics method to discover imaging biomarkers on breast MRI for prediction of genetic test results for breast cancer by means of our original sequential forward floating selection (SFFS) coupled with a support vector machine (SVM) classifier that maximizes the area under the receiver-operating-characteristic curve (AUC). Our proposed method aimed at predicting the results of the 95-gene classifier (95-GC) and immune-related 23-gene signature (IRSN-23), which consists of a feature extraction from a tumor region, discovery of biomarkers based on our SFFS feature selection method, and an SVM classifier operated on the discovered

Z. Jin · T. Yuan · K. Suzuki (✉)
Biomedical Artificial Intelligence Research Unit, Institute of Innovative Research, Tokyo Institute of Technology, Tokyo, Japan
e-mail: suzuki.k.di@m.titech.ac.jp

Z. Jin
e-mail: jin.z.ab@m.titech.ac.jp

Y. Tokuda · N. Tomiyama
Department of Radiology, School of Medicine, Osaka University, Osaka, Japan

Y. Naoi
Department of Endocrine and Breast Surgery, Kyoto Prefectural University of Medicine, Kyoto, Japan

© The Author(s), under exclusive license to Springer Nature Switzerland AG 2023
C.-P. Lim et al. (eds.), *Artificial Intelligence and Machine Learning for Healthcare*, Intelligent Systems Reference Library 228,
https://doi.org/10.1007/978-3-031-11154-9_2

imaging biomarkers. Our database contained 118 dynamic contrast-enhanced (DCE) breast MRI studies from 118 patients. We extracted 318 morphological and texture features from each segmented tumor region on DCE MRI in three phases (i.e., pre-contrast, early phase, and delayed phase). We achieved an AUC value of 0.97 with 22 discovered imaging biomarkers in predicting the results of 95-GC and that of 0.96 with 24 imaging biomarkers in predicting the results of IRSN-23 in a five-fold cross-validation test.

Keywords Radiomics · Personalized medicine · Medical image analysis · Machine learning · Radiogenomics · Imaging biomarker

Abbreviations

Acronym	Meaning
AUC	Area under the receiver-operating-characteristic curve
DCE	Dynamic contrast enhanced
Gp-R	Genomically predicted responders
Gp-NR	Genomically predicted non-responders
IRSN-23	Immune-related 23-gene signature
MRI	Magnetic resonance imaging
pCR	Pathological complete response
ROC	Receiver operating characteristic
SFFS	Sequential forward floating selection
SVM	Support vector machine
2D/3D	Two dimensional/three-dimensional
95-GC	95-Gene classifier

2.1 Introduction

Over past several decades, medical imaging has been rapidly expanded from a primarily tool as reference for diagnosis of certain diseases, to a more central role of providing general and essential information of a patient as basis for diagnosis. The state-of-the-art medical images can provide tremendous detailed information compared with other non-image methods. The improvement of imaging allows advanced evaluation methods developed from analyzing simple features such as intensity, size, shape, to large number of complicated features such as heterogeneity, texture [1, 2]. By these large scale of features, medical images could be used for not only showing anatomical structures with or without abnormalities, but also for mining the "unseen" characteristics that related to individual patient traits, leading a better personalized diagnosis, treatments, and follow-up, i.e. the precision medicine [3].

Radiomics is from neologism -omics originally refer to a field of study in biology such as genomics, proteomics, etc. Radiogenomics is an emerging field that links cancer genotypes with non-invasive imaging phenotype biomarkers [4]. Omics in biology aims at the collective characterization and quantification of pools in molecular level that translate into the structure, function. Meanwhile, in radiomics methods, a huge number of image-level features are extracted from a variety of medical images with different modalities. A radiogenomics approach employs a machine-learning technique for the discovery of imaging biomarkers [5] from medical images to identify the relationship among imaging phenotypes and a specific genotype of the cancer. Recent radiogenomics studies have demonstrated that molecular markers and clinical variables of interest correlate with magnetic resonance imaging (MRI) features of tumors in breast cancer [6, 7].

Breast cancer is a complex disease caused by multiple factors, major one of which is progressive accumulation of gene mutations combined with epigenetic dysregulation of critical genes and protein pathways [8]. A number of studies have shown that gene expression analysis (genetic test) can provide prognostic information on breast cancer. For example, a 95-gene classifier (95-GC) and an immune-related 23-gene signature (IRSN-23) recently developed by Naoi, Y., et al., were able to predict the risk of recurrence and the pathological complete response (pCR) to neoadjuvant chemotherapy for breast cancer, respectively [9, 10]. However, the cost of a genetic test is still high; for example, $3400 for the first genetic test. Therefore, we have an assumption that advanced dynamic contrast-enhanced (DCE) breast MRI images may already implied information related to genetic test results that could be extracted from the radiomics features.

The purpose of this study was to develop a radiogenomics method to discover imaging biomarkers on breast MRI for predicting the genetic test results for breast cancer by means of our original sequential forward floating selection (SFFS) method coupled with a support vector machine (SVM) classifier that would maximize the area under the receiver-operating-characteristic curve (AUC) [11].

2.2 Materials and Methods

Radiomics are normally consists of four major steps:

1. Building of a database
2. Segmentation of target volume
3. Extraction and selection of useful radiomics features
4. Model building based on machine learning technologies.

Figure 2.1 illustrates the block diagram of our proposed radiogenomics method. The proposed method is composed of three major components: feature extraction from a manually segmented tumor region, discovery of biomarkers based on our original

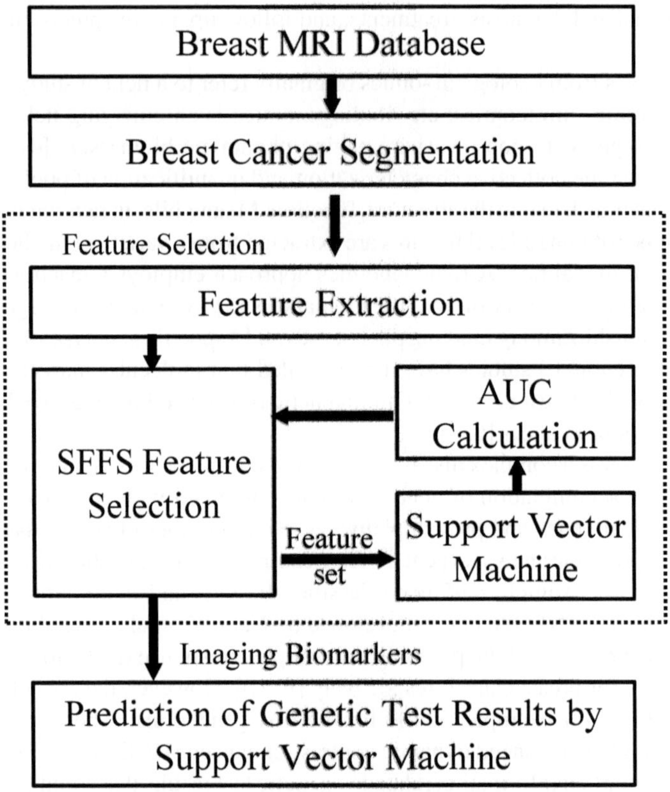

Fig. 2.1 Illustration of the block diagram of our proposed radiogenomics method

SFFS feature selection method, and an SVM classifier for predicting genetic test results. Image features including 318 morphological, gray-level-based, and texture features were extracted from each segmented tumor region. The maximal AUC SFFS feature selection method was applied on these 318 features to discover the most effective imaging biomarkers for predicting genetic test results of 95-GC as a high risk or low risk for recurrence of breast cancer, and of IRSN-23 as a Gp-R or Gp-NR, respectively. Once the most effective combination of imaging biomarkers was discovered, the prediction system could be established with the imaging biomarkers and an SVM classifier with the discovered biomarkers as input.

2.2.1 Building of a Database

For reducing the influence of imaging parameter and/or reconstruction parameter setting, images taken with same protocol are highly recommended. Especially for

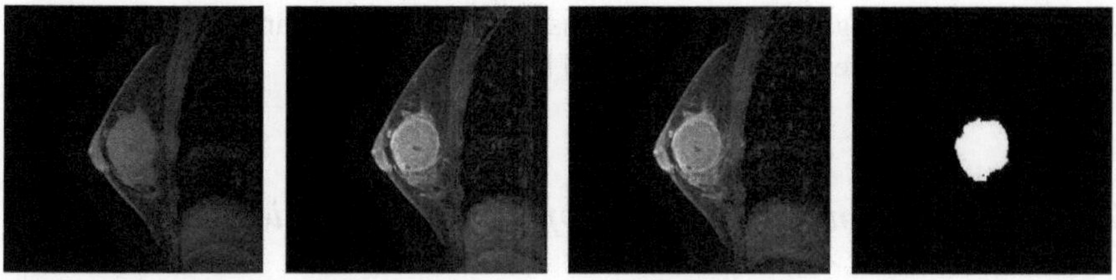

Fig. 2.2 Example images of a dataset of dynamic contrast-enhanced breast MRI: **a** Pre-contrast MR image, **b** early-phase MR image, **c** delayed-phase MR image and **d** "Gold-standard" manual segmentation by a radiologist

MR images, even for the same protocol, different machines may have variety of signal strength due to the diversity in the design of machines [12].

In this study, our database contained 118 dynamic contrast-enhanced (DCE) breast MRI studies from 118 patients, acquired at the Osaka University Hospital. Each DCE MRI study consists of three phases (i.e., pre-contrast, early phase, and delayed phase). Each MR image has a matrix size of 256 × 256 pixels with pixel sizes of 0.7–0.9 mm in transverse planes with 2.0–3.0 mm slice thicknesses. "Gold-standard" breast tumor regions were determined manually by an experienced breast radiologist. Figure 2.2 shows example images of a dataset of dynamic contrast-enhanced breast MRI: (a) Pre-contrast MR image, (b) Early-phase MR image, (c) Delayed-phase MR image and (d) "Gold-standard" manual segmentation by a radiologist. All images were showing the same slice that with the largest diameter of tumor region.

Genetic tests of 95-GC were performed on 76 patients, which classified the patients into 43 high-risk patients and 33 low-risk patients for the recurrence of breast cancer. Genetic tests of IRSN-23 were performed on all 118 patients, which classified the patients into 45 patients as genomically predicted responders (Gp-R) who are likely to achieve pCR and 73 patients as genomically predicted non-responders (Gp-NR) who are unlikely to achieve pCR.

2.2.2 Segmentation of Target Volume

In order to extract features of tumor regions, precise segmentation should be done in advance of feature extraction. Tumor segmentation is usually tedious and time-consuming. Due to high inter- and intra-observer variability, manual segmentation also suffers from inaccuracy and imprecision. The limitation was addressed in numerous studies [13–15], and lots of methods have been proposed to overcome these limitations by automatic segmentation of tumor regions [16–19]. However, to make features calculated from tumor regions meaningful and discriminant, the delineation of the candidates is required to correspond closely to the real object boundaries. In this study, to ensure the requirements, the tumor regions were segmented by one experienced radiologist. Figure 2.2d illustrates the "Gold-standard" breast tumor regions that delineated by an experienced breast radiologist.

2.2.3 *Extraction and Selection of Useful Radiomics Features*

Given the manually segmented breast tumor regions, 106 two-dimensional (2D) and three-dimensional (3D) features including 42 morphological and gray-level-based feature, 36 margin and peak-related features [20], and 28 texture features [21] were extracted from each segmented tumor region per phase in DCE breast MRI to form an initial feature set of 318 features in total. For each tumor, 2D features were calculated in a slice with the largest area of a segmented tumor region; and 3D features were computed in the overall segmented volume. Intensity information of tumors and surrounding regions were characterized in gray-level features. Shape information such as diameter and roundness indices of the tumors a were computed as shape-related features. Histogram-based features were extracted to specify the range, distribution, and overlap of the voxel values in gray-level and edge-enhanced images to provide information about homogeneity and heterogeneity of intensity distribution within tumor region. These features aimed at serving as imaging biomarkers to prediction of genetic test results. All radiomics feature values were converted to z-scores, as shown in Fig. 2.3.

Maximal AUC SFFS Feature Selection

Not all of the features would be useful for the prediction of genetic testing results. Overfitting might happen if all the radiomics feature were directly input to the discriminator, ending with a low generalized model. It is necessary to perform feature selection in order to construct a robust prediction model. To discover the most effective imaging biomarkers, we used our original maximal AUC SFFS feature selection method to remove ineffective features.

We used SVM as the classifier in our prediction system because of its excellent performance in many tasks. Given a set of N training samples $\{(x_i, y)\}_{i=1}^{N}$ where x_i is the feature vector with $x_i \in \Re^L$ and y_i represents the genetic test results (i.e., 95-GC, IRSN-23) with a binary range of $y_i \in \{-1, 1\}$. The decision function for the SVM classifier is defined as:

$$f(x) = \sum_{i=1}^{N} \alpha_i y_i K(x_i, x) + \alpha_0 \tag{2.1}$$

where $\alpha_i \geq 0$ are Lagrange multipliers optimized through quadratic programming. $K(x_i, x_j)$ is a symmetric nonnegative inner-product kernel, where (x_i, x_j) is the selected feature vector. In this paper, we focused on the linear kernel function and the radial basis function (RBF) kernel function that are defined as:

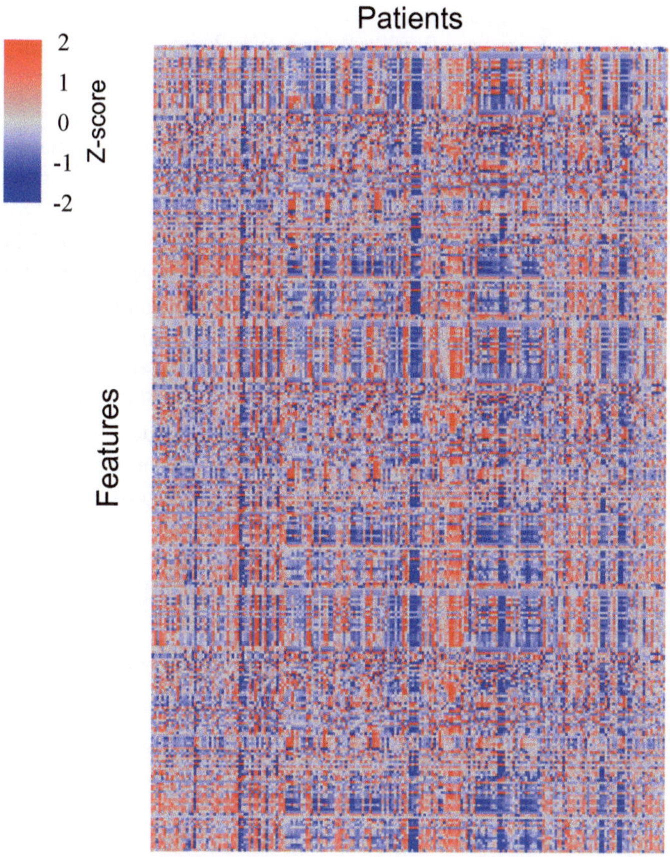

Fig. 2.3 Radiomics features for 118 patients

$$\text{Linear kernel function: } K\left(x_i, x_j\right) = x_i^T x_j \tag{2.2}$$

$$\text{RBF kernel function: } K\left(x_i, x_j\right) = \exp\left(-x_i - x_j^2/2\sigma^2\right) \tag{2.3}$$

The optimal Lagrange multipliers $\alpha_i \geq 0$ in the optimal decision boundary (2.1) is computed through the maximization of the following objective function:

$$\max_{\alpha_i} \sum_{i=1}^{N} \alpha_i - \frac{1}{2} \sum_{i=1}^{N} \sum_{j=1}^{N} \alpha_i \alpha_j y_i y_j K\left(x_i, x_j\right) \tag{2.4}$$

subject to the following constraints:

$$\sum_{i=1}^{N} \alpha_i y_i = 0, \alpha_i \geq 0 \text{ for } i = 1, 2, \ldots, N.$$

As the SVM can be reformulated through the regularized function estimation problem with a hinge loss criterion [22], it can be shown that the SVM classifier has property of large margin and is robust against outliers.

Table 2.1 shows the main procedures of our SFFS feature selection. The selected feature set starts with an empty set F0. Then in optimization procedure of the feature set, add one feature {x} at a time while monitoring the change of AUC, which is calculated by the SVM classifier, until a maximal AUC value was achieved. This is given in Eq. 2.5 where the criterion $J(Fk + \{x\})$ is the AUC value of the SVM classification with the selected feature set $(Fk + \{x\})$. Thus, Eq. (2.1) guarantees that the selected feature set would achieve the maximal AUC value with the combination of the existing features in the subset. This step, however, is only considering adding features without removing any existing ones. It might be possible to improve the

Table 2.1 Procedures of maximal AUC SFFS feature selection method

Initialization:

Full feature set from MR images *X*, selected feature set at step 0 $F_0=\{\emptyset\}$, predefined feature number $l=318$, $k=0$.

while $k<=l$

$$x^+ = \underset{x \in X - F_k}{\arg\max} J(F_k + \{x\}) \quad (2.5)$$

$F_{k+1} = F_k + \{x^+\}$

$k=k+1$

if $k>2$

$$x^- = \underset{x \in F_k}{\arg\max} J(F_k - \{x\}) \quad (2.6)$$

while $J(F_k-\{x\})>\max J(F_k)$ **and** $k>2$

$F_{k-1}= F_k - x^-$

$k=k-1$

if $k>2$

$$x^- = \underset{x \in F_k}{\arg\max} J(F_k - \{x\})$$

end

end

end

end

Output:

Selected feature set Y_l

performance (the AUC value) by removing some features from the selected subset. A removing procedure was implemented by Eq. 2.6. One feature was removed from the selected feature set at a time if the remaining feature subset performs better than the previous maximal AUC value. Inclusion or exclusion of a particular feature is judged by the difference of two AUC values, regardless of whether the difference is statistically significant or not. The procedure continued until all necessary combination of features in the subset were tested. The feature subset with the maximal AUC value would be selected as the final output of the procedure.

2.2.4 *Model Building Based on Machine Learning Technologies*

A five-fold "nested" cross-validation method was used to select hyperparameters of the SVM classifier including the optimal kernel function and other hyperparameters. With the "nested" cross-validation, the hyperparameters were selected in a cross-validation manner so that the performance evaluation was not biased. In this study, we only focused on the linear kernel and the RBF kernel. Table 2 presents the AUC values indicating the performance of the SVM classifier with different kernels and parameters.

With our maximal AUC SFFS feature selection and the optimized SVM classifier, 22 and 24 effective imaging biomarkers, e.g., Radial gradient index, Tangential gradient index, Histogram contrast, Inverse difference moment, minimum pixel value, etc. have been selected respectively in predicting the genetic test results of 95-GC and IRSN-23 in a five-fold cross-validation test.

2.3 Results and Discussion

To evaluate statistical difference of two AUC values, a binormal model was used to estimate the AUC value from the outputs of the SVM classifier [23]. Given the null hypothesis that the two outputs from the SVM classifier with two different selected feature subsets arose from ROC curves with equal areas beneath them, we calculated the z-score statistic [24]. The z-score statistic is then referred to tables of the standard normal distribution. The value of z above a threshold, e.g., $z > 1.96$, is considered as evidence that the null hypothesis has to be rejected, and hence the difference between two AUC values is statistically significant (two-tailed p-value < 0.05).

We compared the proposed method with the SVM with a popular stepwise feature selection based on Wilks' lambda coupled with an LDA classifier [25] in a five-fold cross-validation test in the prediction of the genetic test results of 95-GC and IRSN-23. We used the Wilks' lambda method, because it is optimal for a linear classifier. Figure 2.4 plots the ROC curves for both methods. The proposed method achieved

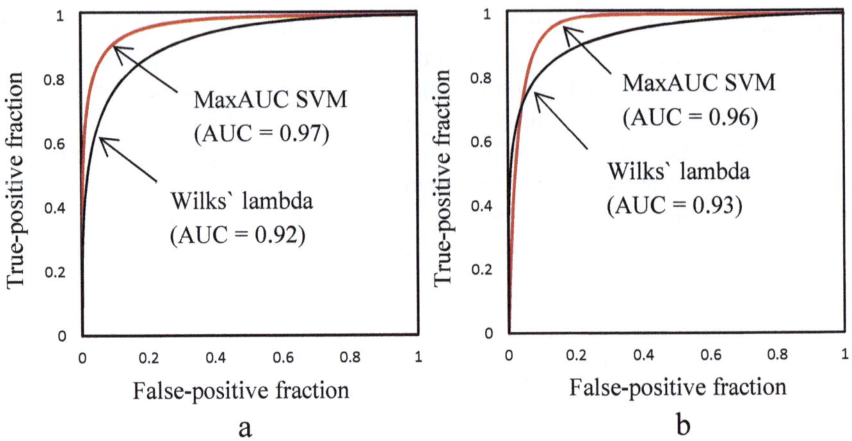

Fig. 2.4 ROC curves of **a** 95-GC test result prediction and **b** IRSN-23 test result prediction. Our method is compared with a conventional Wilks's lambda method

AUC values of 0.97 and 0.96 in predicting the genetic test results of 95-GC and IRSN-23, respectively, whereas the stepwise feature selection based on Wilks' lambda achieved AUC values of 0.92 and 0.93. We performed a statistical significance test. The differences in AUC values between two methods were not statistically significant with two-tailed p-values of 0.13 and 0.31 in predicting the results of 95-GC and IRSN-23, respectively. The statistical significance was not obtained probably because of a smaller number of samples in the study.

The most useful features for predicting 95-GC and IRSN-23 test results are shown in Fig. 2.5. Texture features are most selected features. Our technique presented a consistent, principled manner for feature selection and classification such that the selected features are indeed optimal for the final classifier used in predicting the genetic test results. Though it is very hard to explain how the texture features related to genetic types, the results show reasonable comparing with other studies [26, 27], in which complex and distinct imaging patterns were found demonstrated biological mechanisms.

2.4 Conclusions

In this study, we developed a radiogenomics method to discover imaging biomarkers on DCE breast MRI for predicting genetic test results for breast cancer by means of our original maximal AUC SFFS feature selection method coupled with an SVM classifier. The proposed method discovered the most effective features as imaging biomarkers that maximized the AUC value of the ROC curve. Our results indicated that MR imaging biomarkers would be alternatives to genetic tests in evaluation of

95-GC	IRSN-23
(Delayed phase) Radio gradient index (RGI) inside the largest 2D lesion	(Pre-contrast) Texture feature: Histogram contrast
(Pre-contrast) Full width at half maximum of the histogram in Sobel image	(Pre-contrast) Line amplitude average value inside the lesion
(Delayed phase) Bhattacharyya coefficient	(Pre-contrast) Full width at half maximum of the histogram in Sobel image
(Early phase) Lowest intensity value on perimeter	(Pre-contrast) Tangential gradient index (TGI) inside the largest 2D lesion
(Pre-contrast) Voxel separation	(Pre-contrast) TGI outside the lesion
(Early phase) Standard deviation of intensity values	(Pre-contrast) Texture feature: Inverse difference moment
(Delayed phase) Texture: Maximal correlation coefficient	(Pre-contrast) X-axis of maximum value of histogram of in Sobel image
(Pre-contrast) Voxel separation in Sobel image	(Pre-contrast) Average Sobel power value
(Delayed phase) Lowest intensity value on perimeter	(Pre-contrast) RGI outside the largest 2D lesion
(Pre-contrast) Matsusita distance of normalized histograms in Sobel image	(Early phase) Standard deviation of histograms inside the lesion
(Pre-contrast) Full width at half maximum of the histogram in gray scale image	(Pre-contrast) Relative standard deviation in gray scale image
(Pre-contrast) Ratio of the overlapping volume between the lesion and a sphere to the overall volume	(Pre-contrast) Full width at 10% maximum of the histogram in Sobel image
(Delayed phase) Full width at half maximum of the histogram in Sobel image	(Pre-contrast) Highest intensity values inside the lesion
(Early phase) Texture feature: Difference variance	(Pre-contrast) Texture feature: Difference variance outside the lesion
(Delayed phase) Texture feature: Variance outside the lesion	(Pre-contrast) Line amplitude average value outside the lesion
(Delayed phase) Matsusita distance of normalized histograms in Sobel image	(Delayed phase) TGI inside the largest 2D lesion
(Early phase) Voxel separation in Sobel image	(Pre-contrast) Standard deviation of gray levels in Sobel image outside the lesion
(Early phase) Line amplitude average value	(Pre-contrast) TGI inside the largest 2D lesion
(Early phase) Shannon entropy of normalized histograms in Sobel image	(Delayed phase) Bhattacharyya coefficient of normalized histograms
(Early phase) Standard deviation of intensity values inside the largest 2D lesion	(Delayed phase) Texture feature: Inverse difference moment outside the lesion
(Delayed phase) Maximum value of the histogram in Sobel images outside the lesion	(Delayed phase) Lowest intensity values on perimeter
(Pre-contrast) Bhattacharyya coefficient of normalized histograms	(Delayed phase) Lowest intensity values inside the lesion
	(Pre-contrast) Texture feature: Correlation outside the lesion
	(Pre-contrast) Texture feature: Energy outside the lesion

Fig. 2.5 Most useful features for predicting 95-GC and IRSN-23 test prediction

breast cancer treatment. Note that genetic tests are still very useful in diagnosis and prediction of risks in the development of breast cancer.

References

1. Van Meter, T., Dumur, C., Hafez, N., Garrett, C., Fillmore, H., Broaddus, W.C.: Microarray analysis of MRI-defined tissue samples in glioblastoma reveals differences in regional expression of therapeutic targets. Diagn. Mol. Pathol. **15**(4), 195–205 (2006)
2. Lambin, P., Leijenaar, R.T., Deist, T.M., Peerlings, J., De Jong, E.E., Van Timmeren, J., Sanduleanu, S., Larue, R.T., Even, A.J., Jochems, A., van Wijk, Y.: Radiomics: the bridge between medical imaging and personalized medicine. Nat. Rev. Clin. Oncol. **14**(12), 749–762 (2017)
3. Gillies, R.J., Kinahan, P.E., Hricak, H.: Radiomics: Images are more than picture, they are data. Radiology **278**, 563–577 (2016)
4. Badic, B., Hatt, M., Durand, S., Jossic-Corcos, C.L., Simon, B., Visvikis, D., Corcos, L.: Radiogenomics-based cancer prognosis in colorectal cancer. Sci. Rep. **9**(1), 9743 (2019)
5. O'Connor, J.P., Aboagye, E.O., Adams, J.E., Aerts, H.J., Barrington, S.F., Beer, A.J., Boellaard, R., Bohndiek, S.E., Brady, M., Brown, G., Buckley, D.L.: Imaging biomarker roadmap for cancer studies. Nat. Rev. Clin. Oncol. **14**(3), 169–186 (2017)
6. Rutman, A.M., Kuo, M.D.: Radiogenomics: creating a link between molecular diagnostics and diagnostic imaging. Eur. J. Radiol. **70**(2), 232–241 (2009)
7. Mazurowski, M.A., Zhang, J., Grimm, L.J., Yoon, S.C., Silber, J.I.: Radiogenomic analysis of breast cancer: luminal B molecular subtype is associated with enhancement dynamics at MR imaging. Radiology **273**(2), 365–372 (2014)
8. Olopade, O.I., Grushko, T.A., Nanda, R., Huo, D.: Advances in breast cancer: pathways to personalized medicine. Clin. Cancer Res. **14**(24), 7988–7999 (2008)
9. Naoi, Y., Kishi, K., Tanei, T., Tsunashima, R., Tominaga, N., Baba, Y., Kim, S.J., Taguchi, T., Tamaki, Y., Noguchi, S.: Development of 95-gene classifier as a powerful predictor of recurrences in node-negative and ER-positive breast cancer patients. Breast Cancer Res. Treat. **128**(3), 633–641 (2010)
10. Sota, Y., Naoi, Y., Tsunashima, R., Kagara, N., Shimazu, K., Maruyama, N., Shimomura, A., Shimoda, M., Kishi, K., Baba, Y., Kim, S.J.: Construction of novel immune-related signature for prediction of pathological complete response to neoadjuvant chemotherapy in human breast cancer. Ann. Oncol. **25**(1), 100–106 (2014)
11. Xu, J.W., Suzuki, K.: Max-AUC feature selection in computer-aided detection of polyps in CT colonography. IEEE J. Biomed. Health Inform. **18**(2), 585–593 (2014)
12. Shah, M., Xiao, Y., Subbanna, N., Francis, S., Arnold, D.L., Collins, D.L., Arbel, T.: Evaluating intensity normalization on MRIs of human brain with multiple sclerosis. Med. Image Anal. **15**(2), 267–282 (2011)
13. Tanner, C., Khazen, M., Kessar, P., Leach, M.O., Hawkes, D.J.: Classification improvement by segmentation refinement: application to contrast-enhanced MR-mammography. In: International Conference on Medical Image Computing and Computer-Assisted Intervention, pp. 184–191. Springer, Heidelberg (2004)
14. Meinel, L.A., Stolpen, A.H., Berbaum, K.S., Fajardo, L.L., Reinhardt, J.M.: Breast MRI lesion classification: Improved performance of human readers with a backpropagation neural network computer-aided diagnosis (CAD) system. J. Magnetic Resonance Imaging: Official J. Int. Soc. Magnetic Resonance Med. **25**(1), 89–95 (2007)
15. Wismüller, A., Meyer-Bäse, A., Lange, O., Schlossbauer, T., Kallergi, M., Reiser, M., Leinsinger, G.: Segmentation and classification of dynamic breast magnetic resonance image data. J. Electron. Imaging **15**(1), 013020 (2006)
16. Jin, Z., Arimura, H., Shioyama, Y., Nakamura, K., Kuwazuru, J., Magome, T., Yabu-Uchi, H., Honda, H., Hirata, H., Sasaki, M.: Computer-assisted delineation of lung tumor regions in treatment planning CT images with PET/CT image sets based on an optimum contour selection method. J. Radiat. Res. **55**(6), 1153–1162 (2014)
17. Hussain, R., Arif, S., Sikander, M.A., Memon, A.R.: Fuzzy clustering based malignant areas detection in noisy breast Magnetic Resonant (MR) images. Int. J. Acad. Res. **3**(2) (2011)
18. Kannan, S.R., Sathya, A., Ramathilagam, S.: Effective fuzzy clustering techniques for segmentation of breast MRI. Soft. Comput. **15**(3), 483–491 (2011)

19. Noor, N.M., Khalid, N.E., Hassan, R., Ibrahim, S., Yassin, I.M.: Adaptive neuro-fuzzy inference system for brain abnormality segmentation. In: IEEE Control and System Graduate Research Colloquium (ICSGRC 2010), pp. 68–70 (2010)
20. Brake, G.M., Karssemeijer, N., Hendriks, J.H.: An automatic method to discriminate malignant masses from normal tissue in digital mammograms1. Phys. Med. Biol. **45**(10), 2843–2857 (2000)
21. Haralick, R.M., Shanmugam, K., Dinstein, I.H.: Textural features for image classification. IEEE Trans. Syst. Man Cybern. **SMC-3**(6), 610–621 (1973)
22. Vapnik, V.: The Nature of Statistical Learning Theory. Springer Science & Business Media (1999)
23. Metz, C.E., Herman, B.A., Shen, J.H.: Maximum likelihood estimation of receiver operating characteristic (ROC) curves from continuously-distributed data. Stat. Med. **17**(9), 1033–1053 (1998)
24. Hanley, J.A., McNeil, B.J.: The meaning and use of the area under a receiver operating characteristic (ROC) curve. Radiology **143**(1), 29–36 (1982)
25. Suzuki, K., Kohlbrenner, R., Grelewicz, Z., Ng, E., Hori, M., Baron, R.L.: Computer-aided early detection of hepatocellular carcinoma in contrast-enhanced hepatic CT by use of watershed segmentation and morphologic and texture analysis. In: Proceedings 95th Meeting of Radiological Soc. of North America (RSNA), p. 334 (2009)
26. Lambin, P., Rios-Velazquez, E., Leijenaar, R., Carvalho, S., Van Stiphout, R.G., Granton, P., Zegers, C.M., Gillies, R., Boellard, R., Dekker, A., Aerts, H.J.: Radiomics: extracting more information from medical images using advanced feature analysis. Eur. J. Cancer **48**, 441–446 (2012)
27. Yip, S.S., Kim, J., Coroller, T.P., Parmar, C., Velazquez, E.R., Huynh, E., Mak, R.H., Aerts, H.J.: Associations between somatic mutations and metabolic imaging phenotypes in non–small cell lung cancer. J. Nucl. Med. **58**(4), 569–576 (2017)

Chapter 3
Artificial Intelligence Based Strategies for Data-Driven Radial MRI

Giuseppe Placidi, Luigi Cinque, Filippo Mignosi, Matteo Polsinelli, and Alessandro Sciarra

Abstract Magnetic Resonance Imaging (MRI) represents one of the major imaging modalities for its low invasiveness and versatility. Functional MRI (fMRI) need rapid acquisition to follow dynamic processes. Radial directions, due to their quality of overfitting the k-space center, are particularly suitable to average the effects of movements and are hence often used in fMRI. The acquisition of a complete dataset could be too slow to follow dynamic processes and undersampling is required to improve temporal resolution. Undersampling is accomplished randomly, basing on Compressed Sensing (CS) constraints to reduce aliasing and structured artifacts after reconstruction. However, reconstruction could be improved and/or data can be further reduced if a-priori information is collected regarding the underlying image under reconstruction and Artificial Intelligence (AI)-based strategies are used to drive the process. As an example of the effective synergy between AI and data-driven acquisition/reconstruction in radial MRI, we present a GReedy Adaptive Data-driven Environment (GRADE) for intelligent radial sampling that uses the power spectrum of the reconstructed image and AI-based superresolution strategies in an iterative acqui-

G. Placidi (✉) · M. Polsinelli
A2VI-Lab c/o Department of MeSVA, University of L'Aquila, Via Vetoio Coppito, 67100 L'aquila, Italy
e-mail: giuseppe.placidi@univaq.it

M. Polsinelli
e-mail: matteo.polsinelli@graduate.univaq.it

L. Cinque
Department of Computer Science, Sapienza University of Rome, Via Salaria 113, 00138 Rome, Italy

F. Mignosi
Department of DISIM, University of L'Aquila, Via Vetoio Coppito, 67100 L'aquila, Italy
e-mail: filippo.mignosi@univaq.it

A. Sciarra
Medicine and Digitalization–MedDigit, Department of Biomedical Magnetic Resonance, Otto von Guericke University, Leipziger Str. 44, 39120 Magdeburg, Germany
e-mail: alessandro.sciarra@med.ovgu.de
URL: http://www.giuseppeplacidi.org

© The Author(s), under exclusive license to Springer Nature Switzerland AG 2023
C.-P. Lim et al. (eds.), *Artificial Intelligence and Machine Learning for Healthcare*, Intelligent Systems Reference Library 228,
https://doi.org/10.1007/978-3-031-11154-9_3

sition/reconstruction process. A detailed description of the method is furnished and experimental results are reported. Results demonstrate that GRADE reduces data redundancy and converges first to high quality images with respect to other under-sampling radial modalities, such as regular sampling and golden angle (GA).

Keywords Magnetic resonance imaging · Artificial intelligence · Radial acquisition · Data-drive acquisition · Sparse sampling · Super-resolution · Iterative acquisition/reconstruction

3.1 Introduction

MRI, by measuring the spatial distribution of specific nuclear spins in the body, is notable for its low invasiveness and versatility. Low invasiveness, because ionizing radiations are unnecessary. Versatility because, thanks to different combinations of imaging parameters, MRI gives rise to a huge set of different imaging sequences to produce images of even more informative content and contrast. Besides spatial and temporal resolution, MRI allow tremendous flexibility of orientations. A single image involves the acquisition of a set of sequential trajectories with different pathways (parallel lines, spirals, radial lines) either in 2D or in 3D. Each trajectory represents a time-varying signal in a complex domain, referred as k-space, whose values roughly correspond to spatial frequencies. The signal produced by a combination of magnetic field gradients along a given direction (we consider a planar configuration, since the extension to 3D is straightforward) is, in the k-space, the following:

$$s(t) = c \int \int f(x_1, x_2) e^{2\pi i (x_1 k_{x_1}(t) + x_2 k_{x_2}(t))} dxdy \tag{3.1}$$

where c is a constant which takes into account for imaging settings and represents the proton density in the plane and k_{x_1} and k_{x_2} are the components in the k-space [1]. This complex signal is collected, in its real and imaginary components, by orthogonal receivers. Equation (3.1) reveals that the MRI signal corresponds to the Fourier transform (FT) of the proton density along the defined direction. By collecting $s(t)$ at enough k-space locations by a sequence of directions, it is possible to completely cover the k-space and to obtain the unknown image by Inverse Fourier Transform. Hence, MRI is a Fourier imaging technique which, with its trajectories, traverses the frequency space of the image and collects frequency points and most of the MR images characteristics can be deduced from the mathematical properties of the Fourier transform. The coordinates in Fourier space and the shape of the traveled trajectories are identified by $s(t)$, sampled along time t and are given by the k-space position $k(t)$ obtained thanks to the appropriate choice of imaging parameters. As far as in other imaging modalities, the number of collected data is determined by spatial/temporal resolution requirements. In the last years MRI has developed toward dynamic imaging opening up to several new applications such as monitoring of contrast agent dynamics [2], mapping of brain activity [3], driving biopsies [4, 5], monitoring of ablations or guidance of intravascular procedures [6–8] and real-time cardiac monitoring and visualization [9, 10]. In dynamic MRI, radial trajectories are often used because of their capacity to oversample the k-space center (low frequencies), to reduce motion artifacts and to improve signal to noise ratio (SNR) [11–13].

Since the acquisition process is sequential and time consuming (parallel imaging allows time reduction with the use of parallel receivers [14–19] but it still remains sequential in each receiver), a compromise is necessary regarding the number of collected trajectories to obtain a trade-off between spatial and temporal resolution. In fact, the requirements of improving temporal resolution would imply the reduction of trajectories collected per image, that is to use "undersampling". Undersampling means that the Nyquist's criterion is violated, at least in some regions of the sampling domain, and images are reconstructed from a dataset of trajectories which is poorer than that theoretically required for fully-sampled images whose shape is unknown [20]. The gain, both in motion artifacts reduction and in temporal resolution gain (finer description of dynamic processes), is proportional to the time saved for acquisition. This makes undersampling necessary, since artifacts and structured noise are present in a quantity which is roughly proportional to the ratio between the speed of the observed dynamic process and that for data acquisition [21–28]. Artifacts and structured noise also depend on the combination of undersampling pattern, reconstruction procedure and shape of the underlying image [29–34]. In fact, an undersampling scheme could perform very well with one image and really bad with another and this is also true for reconstruction. In this scenario, it is fundamental to introduce the informative contribution offered by AI to the iterative radial MRI pipeline: (1) acquisition, (2) reconstruction, (3) stopping criteria (exit if true), (4) future informative directions estimation, (5) go to 1. The role of AI is particulalry important for steps 2 and 4.

To show the contribution of AI in the pipeline, we present GRADE, Greedy Radial Adaptive Data-driven Environment, for intelligent acquisition of radial sparse sampling in MRI that, by including iterative AI-based super-resolution and reconstruction, is capable to obtain high quality images by measuring just the highest power set of radial directions (considered to be those that maximize image energy). With respect to other adaptive strategies which apply to the current image similarities with previously collected images [20, 35–45] and to other undersampling strategies which distribute undersampling blindly [26, 27, 46–51], GRADE uses information collected by the image under examination with the following advantages: (1) undersampling is image-dependent; (2) image sparsity is estimated; (3) acquisition is terminated when no more informative directions are present; (4) image energy is maximized; (5) image quality is improved with respect to other blind undersampling schemes. Results are reported and their quality calculated on the reconstructed images and compared with those obtained by other methods.

The manuscript is organized as follows: Sect. 3.2 presents the related work in the field of sparse sampling and reconstruction, also by using AI-based models, and highlights the main contributions of the manuscript; Sect. 3.3 defines the problem and describes and justifies the proposed framework; Sect. 3.4 presents and discuss numerical and experimental results also by comparing them with other radial sampling strategies, including GA; Sect. 3.5 concludes the paper and suggests future investigations for which AI could play a central role.

3.2 Related Work

3.2.1 Sparse Sampling Strategies

During the last years, compressed sensing (CS) [20, 46, 47, 49–52] has offered great insight into both when and how an image may be recovered to high accuracy (or, for some instances, exactly) even when sampling space is significantly below the Nyquist rate. The key idea of CS is that an image, sparse in some domain, can be efficiently recovered by random samples (iid) and sparsity-promoting convex optimization. CS requires the measurement of a relatively small number of "random" samples, much smaller than the number of samples nominally defining it at a given resolution. In fact, because the underlying image is compressible, the nominal number of samples is a gross overestimate of the "effective" number of "degrees of freedom" of the image itself. As a result, the image can be reconstructed with good accuracy from relatively few measurements by convex constrained optimization. Besides depending on a non-linear reconstruction method, the quality of image in CS also depends both on the sparsifying transform and on sampling trajectories. The original paper by Candès et al. [46] was effectively applied to the practical situation of MRI [49, 50].

Despite its innovation, CS can be effectively used if the number of collected samples is not too far from the number of pixels (the unknowns). This is for two reasons. First, the sparsity of the image is unknown and it varies for different images. Second, CS, especially within medical imaging, is based on L1-minimization because the corresponding L0-minimization is intractable [42]. CS theory itself has been adjusted to increase the number of samples collected at low frequencies (k-space center, corresponding to high power) and to reduce samples at high frequencies, where the power decreases [53]. That has allowed a great improvement of the image quality by introducing an adaptation to power distribution [43, 48, 53–55].

Besides using prior information on data distribution, a data-driven sampling adaptive scheme, by reducing redundancy, would contribute to restrict the acquisition exactly to data that are effectively necessary to the optimal image reconstruction, that is to estimate the sparsity of the current underlying image (necessary conditions become also sufficient). This is very important because the sparsity of an image depends on its shape, symmetries and contrast that can variate from one image to another (particularly in MRI, where two images of the same body region could differ each other due to a different modulation of imaging parameters). Obviously, by increasing the collected data, asymptotically CS and any data-driven sensing scheme converge to the same result [56], though data-driven schemes converge faster than "blind" ones and, further, allow to define a termination criterion for the acquisition [53].

Several approaches are based on driving the acquisition process to adapt the collected signals to the sample shape, including data-driven modifications of CS [44]. However, they are based on similarity of previously collected data to drive future acquisition of the unknown sample. This methodology demonstrates that the adaptation to the sample is recommended to reduce acquisition time and improve reconstruction but is sub-optimal for the sample under examination because it does not represent the specific image but just a similar one.

In [29, 30], for the first time adaptive undersampling, data-driven, acquisition was introduced and used in magnetic resonance. In fact, the Authors presented adaptive acquisition techniques for radial sampling, defined first in the image space [29] and then in the k-space [30], to collect just the "most informative" trajectories using the information on the structured shape of the image collected during the acquisition process. An entropy function was used to estimate the information content of each trajectory, to discover internal symmetries, smoothness or shape regularity during the acquisition process and to avoid sampling where information was redundant. In the method applied in the k-space [30], the entropy function was defined on the power spectrum of the radial trajectories. A simple restoration/reconstruction strategy, based on FT [57] and nearest neighbor interpolation, was used to reconstruct the complete image by sparsely sampled data [31]. Nearest neighbor interpolation was justified by the fact that close projections should have had very similar shape, having them been selected by an adaptive method. A similar coding method was also used as a compression strategy for medical images [32] which demonstrates the good compression quality of the proposed strategy.

However, the previous data-driven acquisition strategies have the following limitations: some important trajectories could be excluded in the proximity of sharp variations of the entropy function; they are sub-optimal in estimating the image sparsity since some redundant trajectories could be collected in correspondence of maxima and minima of the entropy function; different projections could have the same entropy value. More recently, adaptive modifications to pure CS, with the inclusion of selective sampling strategies, have been presented [48, 54, 58–61]. In [48], the Authors proposed a selective sampling procedure, a distilled sensing (DS), for the association with the purification occurring during the process of distillation, which was demonstrated to be effective for restoring sparse noisy signals. The sequential process DS consists in a refinement of the observations of a sparse vector which iteratively allocates more sensing resources to most promising locations while ignoring those that are unlikely to contain significant signal components. The method uses the fact that it is highly improbable that the signal (assumed to be positive) is present where the observations are negative. The algorithm terminates after the final observation and its output is composed both by the final observations and by the set of locations measured in the last step. DS could allow a significant improvement in SNR [54] compared to traditional CS, though it is applicable just for positive signals, not the case of oscillating complex signals in MRI and for inversion recovery imaging. An interesting paper [58] demonstrates that, by using an adaptive recovery strategy of wavelets transform coefficients by modelling their statistical dependencies through Hidden Markov Trees, the sparsity pattern of structured sparse signals helps in improving results both with respect to traditional CS and with respect to adaptive CS and its findings fully support data-driven methods. The exploration of adaptive sparse sampling strategies was also supported in [59], where a Compressive Adaptive Sense and Search (CASS) algorithm was presented. CASS operates by dividing the signal into partitions and by using compressive measurements to test the presence of one or more significant (non-zero) elements in each partition. The procedure continues its search by bisecting the most promising partitions, with the goal of returning the largest s components of the vector, being s the sparsity of the signal. An analogous active search greedy algorithm was proposed in [60] where it was also shown that the proposed adaptive technique could substantially outperform classic CS when the measurements are subject to the physically constraints of region sensing, especially if the physical space has low dimensions. In [61], performance lower bounds regarding adaptive sensing for noisy sparse signal detection and support estimation were defined. Moreover, the necessary conditions for the minimum amplitude for non-zero components were settled on. Finally, the Authors showed that adaptive sensing strategies are essentially optimal and cannot be substantially improved. Though relevant to support data-driven acquisition strategies with respect to blind methods, the adaptive variations of CS [48, 53, 54] are not directly applicable in MRI. In fact, they are 1D techniques and, most important, are incompatible with MRI sampling trajectories and requirements (some of them require that the signal is non-negative). For the specificities of MRI, slightly different adaptive techniques have been proposed. The possibility of using hybrid, adaptive-CS, sampling strategies for MRI was proposed in [55], where it was also shown that adaptively, radially collected, samples satisfy CS constraints and a L1-norm based non-linear reconstruction could be used to obtain very accurate image reconstruction. In [62] an alternative adaptive-CS method was presented to combine random sampling of Cartesian trajectories with adaptive 2D acquisition of radial projections. It is based on the evaluation of the information content of a small percentage of the k-space data situated in the central region of the sampling space, collected along random Cartesian directions, to identify radial blades of coefficients having maximum information content. The information content of each direction is evaluated by calculating an entropy function defined on the power spectrum of the projections. The images were obtained by using a non linear reconstruction strategy based on the homotopic L0-norm [42], more effective than L1-norm in image reconstruction. The limitations of this method are that it wastes several directions to define the starting dataset, it could require specialized hardware and, finally, it always used entropy which can assume the same value for different directions. An iterative, CS-variant, Adaptive Acquisition Method (AAM) for radial sampling/reconstruction MRI was presented in [33]. AAM studies the inherent sparse structured pattern of the underlying image by analyzing the data collected during the sequential acquisition to gather useful information regarding the next "most informative" directions. Information about new directions are obtained by the high-frequency power spectrum analysis of an up-sampled image whose wavelets coefficients are extrapolated by those of an approximated image reconstructed by an starting subset of directions. Wavelet are justified because they sparsily represent images and for their good properties of multiresolution and locality. Both intermediate images and the final image are reconstructed by non-linear homotopic L0-norm optimization. Though AAM is data and reconstruction-guided, it is based on several parameters which make it difficult to tune and, hence, difficult to use. A data-driven sampling scheme, to be effective and near-optimal, should be adaptable to the specific image at hand (the reconstructed image should improve at each step), simple and simply tunable, efficient enough to be applied during acquisition and effective to capture only effectively relevant directions. These are the proposal of the present framework.

3.2.2 Contribution of the Manuscript

The idea is to design a smart subsampling strategy, adapted to the shape of the object under investigation, being driven by the partial data collected during the acquisition process. We adopt a different viewpoint with respect to CS; rather than placing general structural assumptions (e.g., sparsity) on the underlying image, we simply collect new data until new relevant information are present. Similar to modified CS, which uses information on data power distribution, we propose a method for the near-maximum power collection. We adopt a learning method that automatically extracts the structure of the inherent power spectrum, translates it in the signals to be collected and performs the process of acquisition/reconstruction/superresolution to gather information regarding the position of new trajectories for the next step where relevant is the power spectrum. We focus on the application of data-driven sparse MRI with substantial differences over previous approaches [33, 55, 62], in particular with respect to [33] of which GRADE is an improvement:

- Completely new strategies for reconstruction, super-resolution (AI-based approach) and missing projections evaluation have been adopted;
- A parameter-free procedure is used (no tuning is required);
- A general purpose method to be used alongside existing or future reconstruction methods is proposed;
- A direct optimization of the power spectrum, as opposed to less direct measures such as mutual information derived by data entropy, is performed;
- A direct optimization of underlying costs (e.g. acquisition time proportional to the number of trajectories), rather than auxiliary cost measures (e.g. number of samples), is used.
- A complete design description, extensive treatment of mage quality and resolution effects are presented and discussed.

3.3 Problem Statement and Framework Description

The acquisition process for sparse MRI can be modeled by the following underdetermined linear system [63]:

$$P = Af(x) + z \tag{3.2}$$

where P are the linear measurements of an m-dimensional unknown spin density image (in the following we call it I for simplicity) in the k-space, A is an $h \cdot m$ matrix of $h < m$ directions, and z represents the experimental additive Gaussian noise. The idea behind GRADE is to start with a low dataset of radial projections P (also called spokes) and to reconstruct a low resolution image I, the resolution R being compatible with the available P, and then to make a super-resolution of I from which we collect information regarding new projections to be added to P. The process is iterated until the maximum desired resolution is reached. GRADE consists on the following steps (Fig. 3.1): (1) acquisition of a regular dataset of P; (2) image reconstruction I of resolution R proportional to the cardinality of P (to avoid undersampling artifacts) (3) super-resolution SR of I; (4) calculation of the most informative directions; (5) inclusion in P of the collected most "powerful" projections and its completion, in less relevant directions, with projections estimated by SR; (6) repetition of steps 2–5 until the final resolution is reached. In the process, crucial steps are: the relationships between projections and image, the relationship between reconstruction process, image resolution and noise amplification, the super-resolution scheme, and the calculation of the most informative projections. In what follows, we define the essential concepts, describe the reconstruction method and the resolution as a function of the angular distance between consecutive projections, the super-resolution scheme used to gather information above the reconstructed bandwidth and, finally, explain the details of GRADE.

3.3.1 *Relationship Between Radial Projections and Image*

Equation (3.1) determines the MR signal model and its relationship with the resulting image. In what follows we discuss the acquisition and reconstruction used in MRI from parallel projections, on which GRADE is based. Imaging from parallel projections was first used by Lauterbur when invented MRI [1], deriving it by Computer Tomography. A projection from parallel lines of the two dimensional function calculated at an orientation angle with respect with the positive axis of is given by the following equation (Fig. 3.2):

$$p_{\phi}(u_1) = \int_{-\infty}^{\infty} f(u_1, u_2) du_2 \tag{3.3}$$

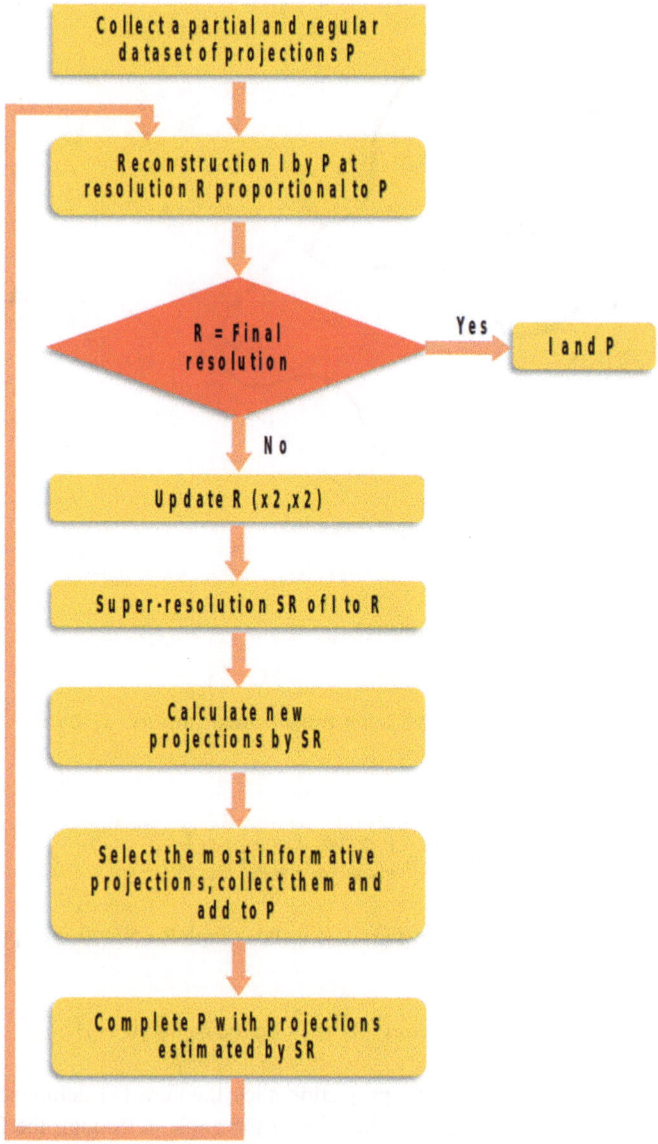

Fig. 3.1 General pipeline of GRADE. Output are the final reconstructed image (I) and the collected undersampled dataset (P) at the final resolution

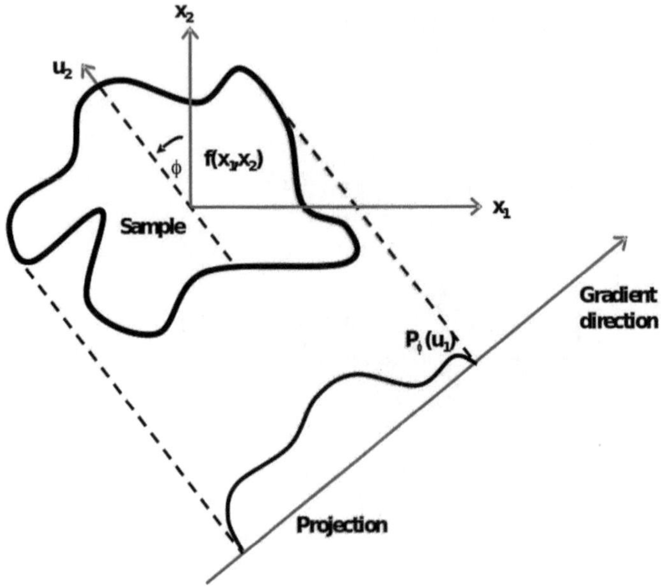

Fig. 3.2 Projection definition with orientation

in which the variables x_1, x_2 have been transformed into u_1, u_2 by the following rotation angle ϕ:

$$\begin{bmatrix} u_1 \\ u_2 \end{bmatrix} = \begin{bmatrix} cos\phi & sin\phi \\ -sin\phi & cos\phi \end{bmatrix} \begin{bmatrix} x_1 \\ x_2 \end{bmatrix} \tag{3.4}$$

The Radon transform of the image $f(x_1, x_2)$ is the complete collection of projections ($\phi \in [0, \pi)$):

$$f \leftrightarrow \text{Radon}\{p_\phi(u_1) : u_1 \in (-\infty, \infty), \phi \in [0, \pi)\} \tag{3.5}$$

and we often write $\mathbf{P} = \mathbf{A}f$. The projection-slice theorem [1] demonstrates that the FT of a projection $p_\phi(\cdot)$ equals the slice at the angle ϕ through the 2D FT of $f(x_1, x_2)$.

In fact, we can write the FT of a projection as:

$$
\begin{aligned}
P_{\phi}(v_{u_1}) &= \int_{-\infty}^{\infty} p_{\phi}(u_1) e^{-2\pi i v_{u_1} u_1} du_1 \\
&= \int_{-\infty}^{\infty}\int_{-\infty}^{\infty} f(x_1, x_2) e^{-2\pi i v_{u_1} u_1} du_1 du_2 \\
&= \int_{-\infty}^{\infty}\int_{-\infty}^{\infty} f(x_1, x_2) e^{-2\pi i (x_1 cos\phi + x_2 sin\phi) v_{u_1}} du_1 du_2 \\
&= F(v_{u_1} cos\phi, v_{u_1} sin\phi)
\end{aligned}
\tag{3.6}
$$

and the FT of the whole image $f(x_1, x_2)$ as:

$$
F(v_{x_1}, v_{x_2}) = \int_{-\infty}^{\infty}\int_{-\infty}^{\infty} f(x_1, x_2) e^{-2\pi i (x_1 v_{x_1} + x_2 v_{x_2})} dx_1 dx_2 \tag{3.7}
$$

Since:

$$
\begin{bmatrix} v_{x_1} \\ v_{x_2} \end{bmatrix} = \begin{bmatrix} cos\phi & -sin\phi \\ sin\phi & cos\phi \end{bmatrix} \begin{bmatrix} v_{u_1} \\ v_{u_2} \end{bmatrix} \tag{3.8}
$$

we can use 3.8 to write 3.7 as:

$$
P_{\phi}(v_{u_1}) = F(v_{x_1}, v_{x_2})|_{v_{u_2}=0} \tag{3.9}
$$

that is the Fourier coefficients of the image along the direction u_1. The Projection-slice theorem demonstrates that the Radon transform in Eq. 3.5 describes completely the image $f(x_1, x_2)$ through its 1D projections, because it defines a one-to-one correspondence between the Radon transform and the FT of the image.

3.3.2 Image Reconstruction, Resolution and Noise

In MRI the image is recovered by a direct inverse Fourier transform, since the collected signals are representations of the Fourier terms of the image $f(x_1, x_2)$ along the radial directions, as in Eq. (3.1), and a low number of computations are required. However, Radon inversion requires that the reconstruction is calculated by an infinite number of projections and, very important, without noise. Experimental conditions imply both a finite number of projections and the presence of noise. Starting by considering just the effects of discretization (noise contribution is included below), the direct Fourier reconstruction (FR) method with a discrete number of projections, each composed by a discrete number of samples, consists on the following steps:

1. Create a polar representation $F_*(u_1, \phi)$ of the 2D FT $F(v_{x_1}, v_{x_2})$ such that $F_*(u_1, \phi) = p_\phi(u_1)$, by using the set of collected projections;
2. Convert from polar representation $F_*(u_1, \phi)$ to Cartesian coordinates $F(v_{x_1}, v_{x_2})$ through gridding [64–66];
3. Perform the inverse discrete 2D FT of $F(v_{x_1}, v_{x_2})$ to get $f(x_1, x_2)$.

Step 2 is necessary due to the discrete number of projections and could be also performed after step 3, on the image reconstructed in polar coordinates $f(\rho, \phi)$, if polar FT is applied on data from Step 1 [66, 67]. When the number of projections is overestimated, gridding is irrelevant and a simple interpolation method yields good results [31]. Besides angular sampling, each projection is measured on discrete points and, hence, is band limited. Besides that, MRI receivers are band-limited, thus also limiting the bandwidth of the image. However, the image is reconstructed and digitized on discrete pixels and the fact that the number of projections and their bandwidth are limited does not necessarily imply limitations and/or artifacts in the reconstructed image if specific resolution constraints are satisfied. An important parameter is represented by the field of view (FOV), the spatial region occupied by the image. Along a given direction, say x_1, the FOV extension (Fig. 3.3) is determined by the sampling rate and it is related to the strength of the magnetic field gradients [55]. The signal bandwidth, indicated as $2B_v$ ($\pm B_v$) is related to the distance in time Δt ($\Delta t \approx \Delta k_{x_1}$in the k-space) between consecutive samples by the following relationship:

$$2B_v = \frac{1}{\Delta t} \approx \frac{1}{\Delta k_{x_1}} \approx FOV \tag{3.10}$$

The spatial extension of the image is determined by the bandwidth of the collected signal. The sampling rate is chosen to define the FOV to be just above D, the region of interest (see Fig. 3.3), also considering the gradient value (we can change the FOV both by variating the sampling rate or by changing the gradient value). The reason of choosing the FOV as close as possible to D is due to the necessity of including as much useful information as possible in the image (the frame outside D is irrelevant also if the examined object extends above D). If we collect N_{x_1} points of the signal,

$$N_{x_1} \Delta k_{x_1} \approx \frac{N_{x_1}}{FOV} \approx \frac{1}{\Delta x_1} \tag{3.11}$$

we obtain that:

$$\Delta x_1 \approx \frac{1}{N_{x_1} \Delta k_{x_1}} \tag{3.12}$$

Equation (3.12) represents the resolution along the direction x_1: it is inversely proportional to the length of the signal collected in the k-space. Equation (3.12) suggests that in principle we could obtain infinite resolution but this is obviously impossible due to the presence of experimental noise (infinite time would be required to obtain noise-free data). In MRI, noise is a Gaussian white noise with zero mean

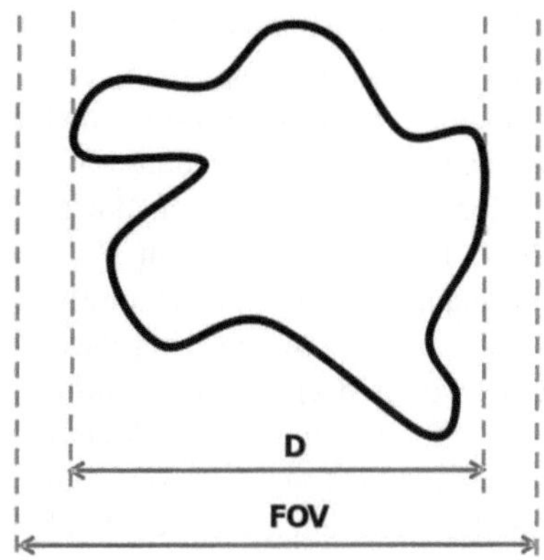

Fig. 3.3 Region of interest (D) and field of view (FOV). The FOV is always greater than D. The sample often exceeds the FOV but hardware limitations (transmitter/receiver sensitivity) attenuate or cancel external regions

and standard deviation σ. Being the signal a decaying signal in the k-space, its high frequency components get attenuated while noise power remain unchanged: there exists a cut-off point, $N_{x_{1T}} \Delta k_{x_1}$, above which the signal falls below the noise level [68]. The effective resolution along the direction x_1 is the following

$$\Delta x_{1T} \approx \frac{1}{N_{x_1 T} \Delta k_{x_1}} \tag{3.13}$$

Though the cut-off frequency could be different for different directions, usually it is chosen the same for all the directions (the maximum) to avoid loss of resolution. Hence, noise implies that the collected signal has to be low-pass filtered to attenuate high frequencies where the noise overcomes the signal:

$$s_c(t) = s(t) \star h(t) \tag{3.14}$$

being $s(t)$ the signal defined in Eq. (3.1), h(t) the low-pass filter and $\star$ the symbol for convolution. Besides the improvement of SNR, the shape of the filter (Hamming, Hanning, Gaussian, etc.) also serves to minimize the effects of data truncation (Gibbs artifacts) [64].

The noise level, function of its standard deviation σ, is estimated by the decaying signal $s(t)$ (from those points in which useful signal is absent). In radial sampling, besides the resolution term defined along each projection (1D), another resolution index (also 1D) concurs to the definition of the image resolution (2D): the angular distance among consecutive projections is strictly related to the radial resolution term defined in Eq. (3.13). In fact, to reconstruct a homogeneous image, radial and angular resolutions should be the same in the external arch of the circle inscribed in the image support (worst case) for regularly sampled projections (Fig. 3.4), that is:

$$\frac{1}{N_p \Delta s} = \frac{1}{N_{x_{1T}} \Delta k_{x_1}} \tag{3.15}$$

where N_p is the number of projections and Δs is the maximum arch distance between them. By assuming $\Delta s = \Delta k_{x_1}$, it is necessary to ensure that $N_p = N_{x_{1T}}$ for a uniform resolution. If this condition is met, the number of unknown variables (the pixels) is lower than or equal to data collected, thus ensuring that image reconstruction is performed without artifacts due to undersampling. When the number of projections N_p is fixed and lower than $N_{x_{1T}}$ (also greatly lower), it is possible to reconstruct an image with uniform resolution and without artifacts: it is sufficient to ensure $\Delta s_{N_{x_{1T}}} = \Delta k_{x_1}$ by lowering the radial resolution, that is by reducing $N_{x_{1T}}$. In this case, we can decrease $N_{x_{1T}}$ until $\Delta s = \Delta k_{x_1}$ and, hence, until we reach a limit value $N_{x_{1Tlim}}$ for which $N_{x_{1Tlim}} = N_p$ (we can get a smaller support in the Fourier space, as shown in Fig. 3.4). The result is that the FOV of the image is maintained unchanged but the resolution is reduced. Each projection involved in the reconstruction process must be filtered by a low-pass filter with cut-off frequency of $N_{x_{1Tlim}} \Delta k_{x_1}$ to avoid truncation artifacts. This strategy is the core of the reconstruction used by GRADE and discussed below.

3.3.3 Super-Resolution

The process of super-resolution (SR) corresponds to the reconstruction of a high-resolution (HR) image from its corresponding low-resolution version (LR) and this operation can be performed, between others, by producing an estimate of the wavelet coefficients of the image which has to be super-resolved.

Wavelet estimation has been used with success by interpolation strategies [69] and by other adaptive acquisition methods [33] since wavelet sub-bands are often sparse and particularly effective for sparse coding in medical imaging [34] but also for estimating image details and for significantly improving image resolution. Recently, deep learning has proposed an efficient method for SR [70] (to date, one of the best known method for SR regarding image quality improvement and artifacts limitation) based on a convolutional neural network acting on the reconstruction of the residuals of the wavelet coefficients details of the HR image with respect to the LR one.

The used neural network, whose scheme is reported in Fig. 3.5, has two input and output layers each composed by 4 channels. The input channels are composed by the wavelet transform (Haar wavelet is used to simplify the details estimation process) to provide the approximation, LA, vertical, LV, horizontal, LH, and diagonal, LD, details of the low resolution image. The output channels provide the difference residuals of the approximation, ΔA, vertical, ΔV horizontal, ΔH, and diagonal, ΔD, details which are summed to the input details to reconstruct the wavelet coefficients of the SR image. The inverse wavelet transform of the SR details gives the SR image. 64 filters of size $4 \times 3 \times 3$ in the first layer and 4 filters of size $64 \times 3 \times 3$ in the last layer are used. The deep structure of the network contains 10 convolutional hidden layers with $64 \times 3 \times 3 \times 64$ filters each. The method has proven to improve the image quality in terms of resolution gain with respect to other competitive SR methods, with reduced artifacts (higher SNR with respect to the others). It is important to note that,

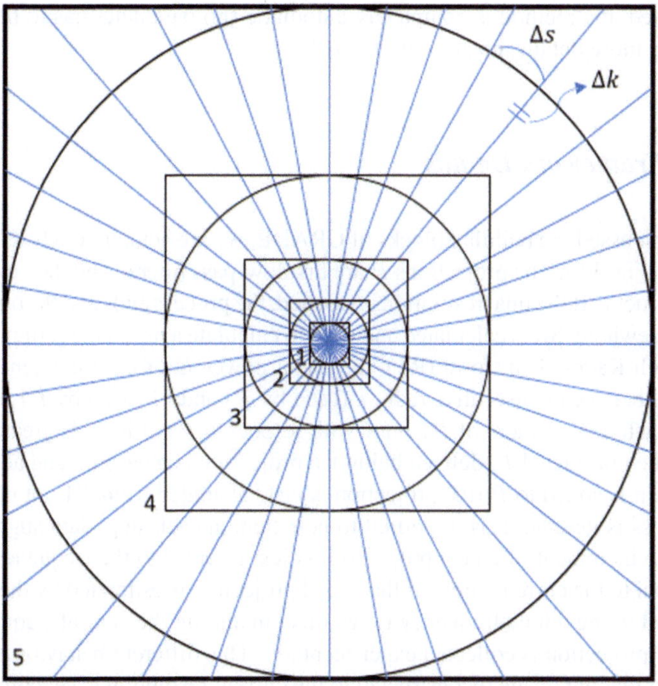

Fig. 3.4 Regular set of radial directions in the k-space (blue). Concentric squares indicate successive acquisition/reconstruction steps (low-pass filter sets to zero what is outside the current square). The most internal square (1) is the starting support: complete sampling is ensured by the condition that the maximum arch is equal to radial sampling. After each 2×2 SR step, a complete dataset is obtained, the bandwidth of the low-pass filter extended to the following circle and the image reconstructed (complete sampling continues to hold). For graphical purposes, just a reduced number of directions is shown. The resolution terms, Δk (fixed) and Δs (different in different circles), are represented

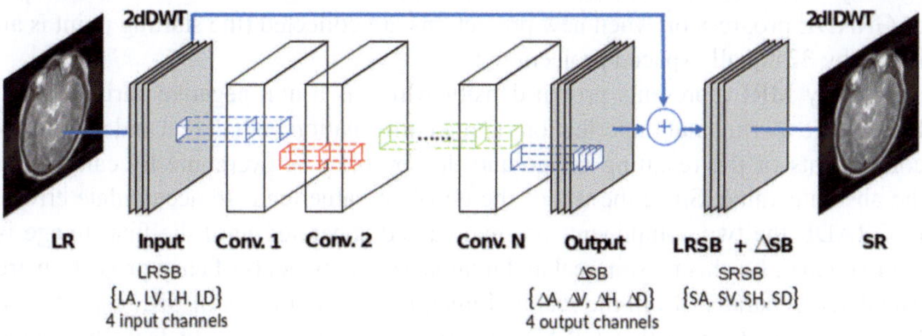

Fig. 3.5 CNN structure used to perform image super-resolution [70]

once trained, the method is completely automatic (no parameter has to be tuned at hand). For more details, please refer to [70].

3.3.4 Framework Details

Having discussed the building blocks of GRADE, we are actually ready to present it in details (Fig. 3.6). The projections P are first low-pass filtered and then used by FR to reconstruct I. If the final resolution is reached, the process ends and the output are I and P. Elsewhere, SR is calculated and used to calculate a new dataset of projections $P1$ through Radon Transform (RT), the mean power E of each element of $P1$ is calculated between consecutive radii, r (used by P) and $r1$ (used by $P1$, $r1 = 2r$), and, for each new element of $P1$ (new with respect to P), if its E is greater than or equal to the noise level T (defined below), a projection is measured and added to P, elsewhere it is added to P (the projection is just calculated from $P1$ not measured). The process is iterated. It is important to note that, at each step, data augmentation (that is the increment of a new projection) is just referred to the frequencies which are external to the current circle, if the added projection is estimated by the previous image, and to the whole frequency range (also including the central frequencies) if the added projection is collected experimentally. This different behavior is justified by the fact that the image reconstructed to the current resolution is yet complete and correctly sampled: experimentally collected low frequencies are added to increase SNR, elsewhere (numerically estimated) low frequencies are leaved out to avoid that data estimation errors could affect the central region of the k-space. The image at each step is reconstructed and, being its resolution reduced, it is free from undersampling artifacts. At each step, the image is super-resolved by a factor 2×2 ($r1 = 2r$) and, from it, the projections are calculated by IR, doubling the previous set. GRADE is "greedy" in the sense that it searches highest power. Figure 3.7 shows an example of GRADE progression when new projections are collected (the starting point is an image by 32 equally spaced projections).

Usually MRI represents proton density which is a non negative variable [55]. However, experimental imperfections spread information both in real and imaginary components of the resulting image and this problem is overcome by calculating the absolute value. Since the use of the absolute value tends to accumulate errors, in GRADE the two components are maintained separated until the final image is obtained and, for this reason, real and imaginary components of each projection are calculated separately from the real and imaginary components of SR, respectively. It is important to note that GRADE is completely automatic. In fact, the image resolution, at each step, is defined by the angular distance between the regularly collected (or calculated) projections, and this is also the case of the low-pass filter (we used an Hamming filter) for projections. FR takes P as only input, composed by experimentally collected projections and completed with those calculated by SR_I. Regarding the SR algorithm, it is completely parameter-free. We used the trained version of the algorithm [70] written in Python (http://signal.ee.psu.edu/research/

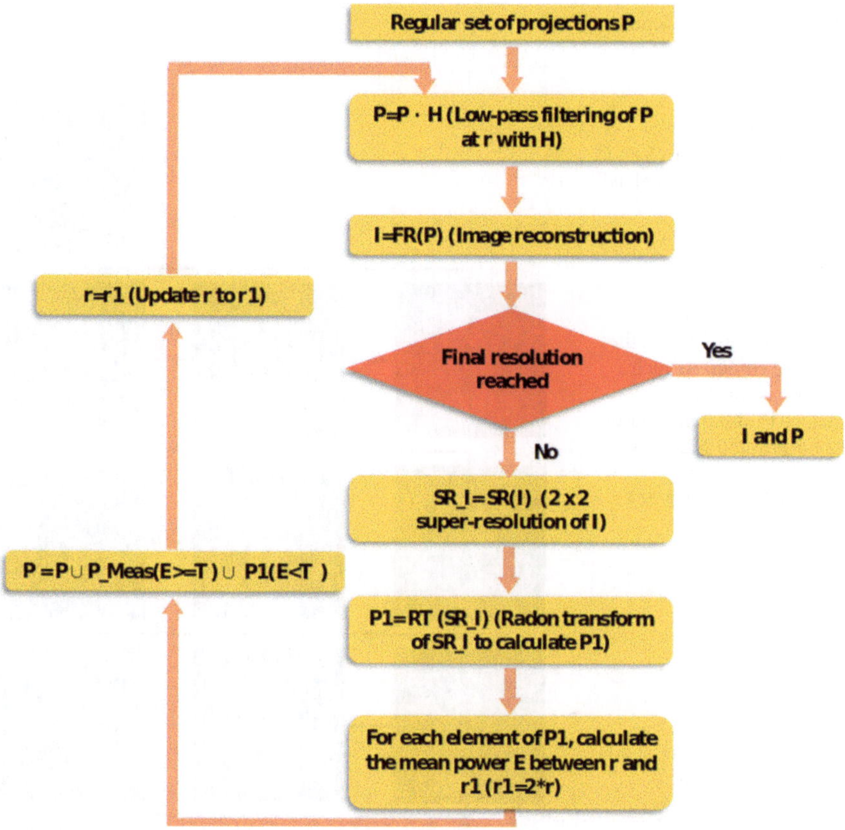

Fig. 3.6 Flow-chart of GRADE. The process is iterated until the final image dimension is reached. The final *I* and *P* are composed by the final image and by the projections selected by GRADE, respectively

DWSR.html) that we linked to our Matlab (https://mathworks.com/) implementation of GRADE. Regarding the calculation of projections from the SR image, we used the numerical Radon transform that takes in input the image to be used for calculating the projections (SR_I) and the number of regularly projections to be calculated: these are both well defined at each step of the algorithm. This also holds for the power spectrum calculation. The only parameter that needs to be explained is the noise level (or threshold), though it can be simply calculated and included into the calculation process, as described below.

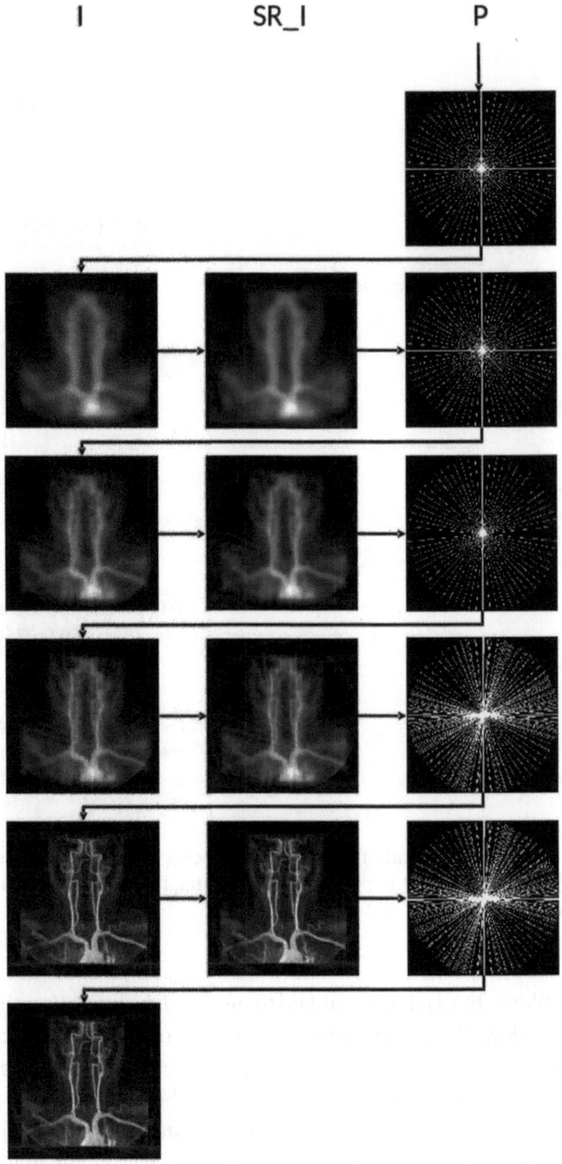

Fig. 3.7 The progression of GRADE. Image reconstruction (I, left column) and the corresponding super-resolved image (SR_I, middle column) are obtained by a projection dataset (P, right column). The starting set P is composed by 32 regularly sampled projections (upper right corner). The final I is in the lower left corner. At each step, reconstruction is obtained by different datasets (32-64-128-256-512). The example reports an angiography image (MRA)

3.3.5 Noise Threshold *T*

Each of the two channels representing the real and the imaginary components of the MR signal is affected by a Gaussian random noise of the type $N(0, \sigma^2)$. When we calculate the power spectrum of the signal, we construct the new variable $Z = \sqrt{X^2 + Y^2}$ where X and Y are the real and imaginary components of the signal, respectively. The density distribution of Z is of the type (Rayleigh):

$$f(z) = \frac{z}{\sigma^2} e^{\frac{-z^2}{2\sigma^2}} \tag{3.16}$$

If we want to calculate the probability p of the occurrence of noise, we have to find in Z the value h such as:

$$\int_0^h f(z)dz = p \tag{3.17}$$

that is

$$\int_0^h \frac{z}{\sigma^2} e^{\frac{-z^2}{2\sigma^2}} dz = p \tag{3.18}$$

that we can calculate as:

$$-\int_0^h \frac{z}{\sigma^2} e^{\frac{-z^2}{2\sigma^2}} dz = e^{\frac{-z^2}{2\sigma^2}} |_h^0 = 1 - e^{\frac{-h^2}{2\sigma^2}} = p \tag{3.19}$$

to obtain

$$e^{\frac{-h^2}{2\sigma^2}} = 1 - p \tag{3.20}$$

and, finally;

$$h = \sigma\sqrt{2ln(1-p)} \tag{3.21}$$

Having selected p, the level of probability that we want to consider for noise (given σ the standard deviation of noise in each of the real and/or imaginary channels), we can calculate the corresponding value of h as a function of σ. The value of h corresponds to the level of z above which we consider it as a useful information ($1 - p$ of uncertainty) and below which we consider it as noise with a probability equal to p. We have used $p = 0.9$, corresponding to $h \approx 2.146\sigma$ (that is $T = h$), to mediate between noise conservation (low T), corresponding to the measurement of a high number of projections and complete noise elimination (high T), corresponding to the measurement of a very low number of projections with the risk of leaving out useful information. The noise level σ is estimated by $s(t)$ as described above.

3.4 Results and Discussion

In order to test its effectiveness, GRADE has been tested on images of known quality whose data were collected by using different imaging sequences, equipment and sampling patterns (cartesian, radial, spiral, etc.): in this way we avoided favorable sampling patterns for different images. The images, downloaded by a freely accessible database (www.radiopedia.org), were all in 512×512 to avoid changes in the proposed framework. To perform our tests, radial acquisitions were calculated by Radon transforming the completely sampled images.

Following the scheme in [34], we used GRADE for images of different types (T1 and T2-weighted, proton density, etc.) and from different body districts (brain, articulations, thorax, angiography, etc.), which are sparse in different domains and have different SNR. Though GRADE is capable to support any resolution amplification, we performed a x4 amplification at each step of the algorithm, starting from 32×32, to simplify the comparison. The original images were all not negative (each image was in the modulus form) and, hence, represented in ideal conditions. To reproduce rough experimental conditions, we applied random zero and first-order phase errors on the Fourier Transform of each of the resulting projections calculated by Radon transforming the 512×512 images (this allows to eliminate symmetry from raw data). An angularly oversampled dataset of 512 regular projections, each of 512 samples, was obtained by each of the treated images. The resulting dataset consisted of projections composed by real and imaginary components simulating a radial acquisition process. The complete dataset of projections was used to reconstruct the complete image used as ground truth, in order to make the effects of the reconstruction negligible with respect to those due to undersampling. Regarding the measurement of the quality of reconstruction, we should have used different metrics, since a metric that allows to evaluate all the characteristics of a reconstruction does not exist [71]. However, we just used the mean squared error (MSE) [72] and structural similarity index metric (SSIM) [73]. Results, obtained for 20 images, are summarized in Table 3.1. For each image, the number of relevant wavelet coefficients used in JPEG compression, the number of projections selected by GRADE, the corresponding MSE and SSIM calculated with respect to the image reconstructed by using the complete dataset of 512 projections, are also reported.

As can be noticed, the number of selected projections increased with the number of relevant coefficients, thus demonstrating that GRADE: a) allows to select relevant information; b) is sensitive to the increasing of "data relevance"; c) allows to define an acquisition termination criterium, thus eliminating the problem of "blindness" that, being unknown the sparsity of the underlying image, requires "oversampling" above sparsity to ensure high image quality. The last point is particularly relevant: in fact, data collected by GRADE (roughly obtained by multiplying the data per projection by the number of collected projections) was well below those necessary for "blind" CS, though it was always above the number of relevant coefficients for each image. That demonstrates, from one side, that GRADE is capable to reduce the acquisition time with respect to classical CS and, from the other, that GRADE

Table 3.1 Evaluation of 20 images collected from different anatomical districts with different imaging sequences. For each image, a rough estimate of the sparsity value (the number of wavelet coefficients above noise), the number of projections collected by the proposed framework, MSE and SSIM, with respect to the image obtained with the complete dataset, are reported. To avoid dispersion between different images, MSE is normalized to the value of the image obtained with 32 projections. Regarding the imaging sequences [55], T1-w and T2-w correspond to T1-weighted and T2-weighted sequences, respectively, PD stands for Proton Density, SSFP stands for Steady-State Free Precession, and T1-w fat sat. stands for T1-weighted with fat saturation

District	Contrast	Wav. Coeff.	N. proj.	MSE	SSIM
Brain	T1-w	71835	156	0.015	0.82
	T1-w	73198	161	0.045	0.78
	T2-w	68747	143	0.034	0.83
	T2-w	69521	147	0.051	0.69
Chest	T1-w	72615	152	0.041	0.79
	T2-w	71645	148	0.053	0.81
Joints	PD	73521	155	0.019	0.76
	T1-w	80154	172	0.034	0.81
	T2-w	69166	146	0.025	0.74
	T2-w	74356	157	0.041	0.88
Angio		25148	98	0.036	0.64
		17132	77	0.051	0.78
		31457	103	0.064	0.82
		20453	91	0.043	0.73
		33125	107	0.072	0.81
Heart	SSFP	28562	89	0.058	0.79
	T1-w	14531	61	0.074	0.61
Abdom.	T2-w	83121	167	0.061	0.82
	T1-w	78143	151	0.056	0.79
	T1-w fat sat.	31457	164	0.076	0.82

has a "conservative" behavior (data redundancy is also present) to avoid that relevant information are left out. From data in Table 3.1, it can also be noticed that the number of relevant coefficients is greatly dependent on the examined region and on the acquisition sequence, and that can greatly oscillate. In fact, by imaging the same anatomical region with different acquisition sequences, a huge variation of contrast could result which implies a different number of relevant coefficients. Since GRADE follows those variations (to an increment of the relevant coefficients corresponds an increment of the data collected by GRADE and vice-versa), it could obtain a relevant advantage compared to "blind" CS regarding the number of data to be collected, that is to the acquisition time reduction. Another important aspect is that wavelet CS reconstruction [49, 50] can be applied on GRADE data to obtain a very effective reconstruction. To better highlight the effects of GRADE, some of the treated images have been also reported in Figs. 3.8-3.10 where, besides the

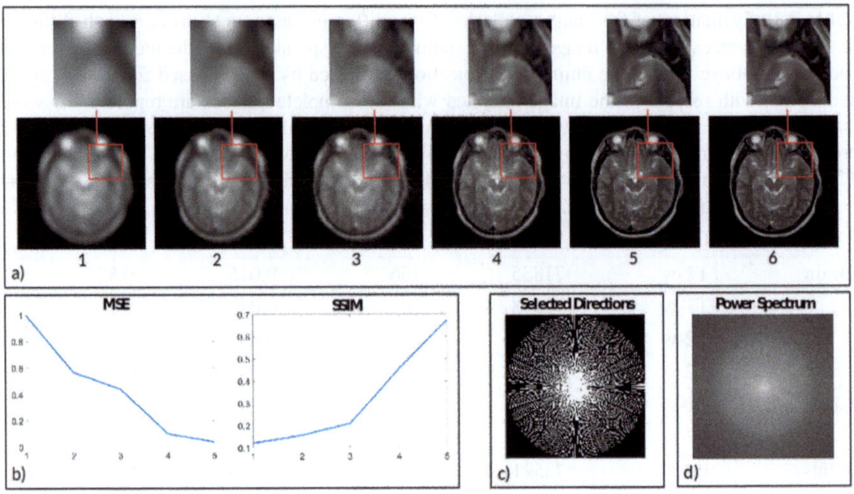

Fig. 3.8 MRI of the brain: projections collected by GRADE (**a**). Steps 1–5 (**a**) shows the image at 32×32, 64×64, 128×128, 256×256 and 512×512, respectively. In a.6 the image obtained by using the whole theoretical dataset P is shown. For each image, an inset is also shown in the highest part. For each step 1–5, also MSE and SSIM, calculated with respect to the complete image, are reported (**b**). MSE is normalized to the value of the 32×32 image. The selected directions to obtain the image a.5 and the power spectrum of the complete image, in logarithm form, are reported in **c** and **d**, respectively

progressive reconstructions, also the power spectrum of the complete image and its coverage by the collected projections are shown. The obtained results show that GRADE defines a subset of projections which approximately maximize the power spectrum coverage of the unknown images without having any a-priori knowledge of its distribution.

Moreover, it also allowed to estimate the number of relevant information to be collected for obtaining an image that greatly resembles the complete one (to a careful observation, a trained expert cannot find any relevant difference between the image obtained by undersampled projections and the corresponding complete one). Finally, it also demonstrates that a simple reconstruction algorithm, FR, could be effectively used for image reconstruction because a complete dataset is always ensured by calculating the missing projections directly by the previously reconstructed and SR image. By analyzing the images of Figs. 3.8-3.10 it can also be argued that the quality of the image improves monotonically (as confirmed both by MSE and SSIM) and greatly improves when the number of projections converges to the "GRADE number".

A confirmation was obtained by adding more directions above the number of GRADE: starting from the GRADE number, MSE reached a plateau and the improvement in SSIM did not correspond to visually appreciable improvements, as can be also noticed by the fact that the images in Figs. 3.8, 3.9 and 3.10.a.5 greatly resembled the corresponding complete images used for comparison (Figs. 3.8, 3.9 and 3.10.a.6).

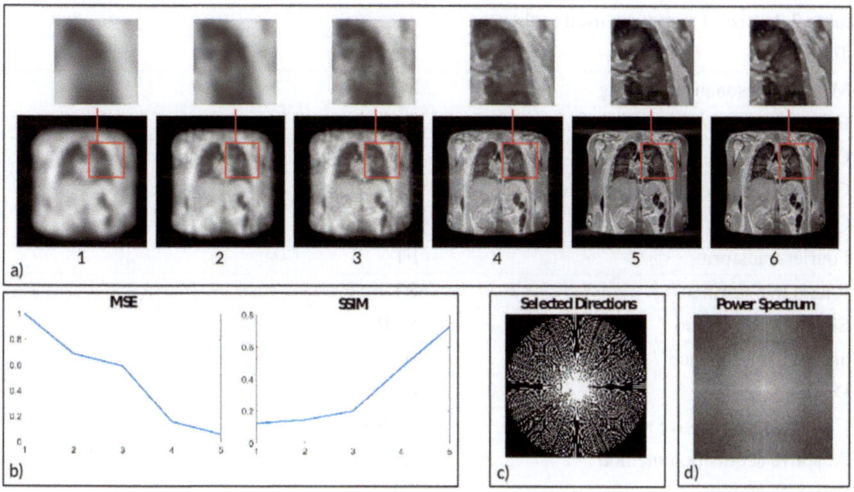

Fig. 3.9 MRI of the chest. Figure parameters and significance are the same as in Fig. 3.8

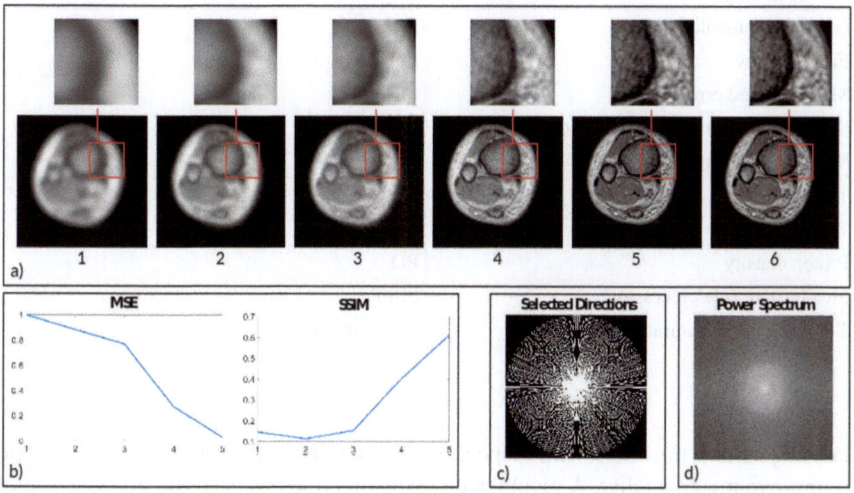

Fig. 3.10 MRI of a leg. Figure parameters and significance are the same as in Fig. 3.8

3.5 Conclusion

We have shown how a data driven strategy can be used with success in MRI to improve image quality and temporal resolution, to reduce redundancy and to construct an effective, sample specific, stopping criteria for the adaptive acquisition. To this aim, we have presented GRADE, a framework for MRI from radial projections that, using a successive acquisition/super-resolution/reprojection method, is capable to reduce

Table 3.2 List of acronyms used in the text

Term	Acronym
Magnetic resonance imaging	MRI
Functional MRI	fMRI
Compressed sensing	CS
GReedy adaptive data-driven environment	GRADE
Golden angle	GA
Fourier transform	FT
Radon transform	RT
Signal to noise ratio	SNR
artificial intelligence	AI
Distilled sensing	DS
Compressive adaptive sense and search	CASS
Adaptive acquisition method	AAM
Super-resolution	SR
High-resolution	HR
Low-resolution	LR
Fourier reconstruction	FR
Field of view	FOV
Mean squared error	MSE
Structural similarity index metric	SSIM
Magnetic resonance angiography	MRA
T1-weighted	T1-w
T2-weighted	T2-w
Proton density	PD
Steady-state free precession	SSFP
T1-weighted fat saturation	T1-w fat sat.

data acquisition time also with respect to CS, by selecting most powerful data, and to improve image quality. A pivotal role in the pipeline has been the introduction of the AI-based super-resolution strategy which allows to predict the future resolution of the image, a fundamental step to predict the positions of the future directions to be acquired. Further, GRADE uses also very fast reconstruction methods, as FR, to produce aliasing free reconstructions during the acquisition process, thus avoiding waste of time and without requiring any assumption on random distribution of the data (as required by non linear optimization). In fact, complete sampling is ensured at each step by using both the projections selected by GRADE or those estimated by the SR version of the reconstructed image. Wavelet sparsity of the underlying image is used when the reconstructed image is super-resolved: this is translated into the SR image by which a decision about the selection of some projections is assumed and, at the same time, other projections, those not selected by GRADE, are calculated. In this sense, GRADE can be considered as a tool to join the space of signal acquisition (Fourier space) with that where the image is sparsely represented (Wavelet space) but in a different way with respect to non linear optimization.

Finally, the proposed GRADE framework has allowed to estimate the sparsity of an image and to improve the image quality monotonically. In fact, results demonstrated that the trend of the number of relevant coefficients of each image was followed also by the number of selected data obtained by GRADE (to an increment/decrease of the first has always corresponded an increment/decrease of the second).

In the next future, we can imagine that AI-based strategies could play an ever more central role in the MRI radial sparse sampling/reconstruction. In fact, AI-based techniques have been recently applied with success in medical imaging in general [74–76] and in MRI in particular [45, 77–85]. Indeed, in the last years MRI image reconstruction has been rapidly changed thanks to the successful demonstration of of the deep learning-based MR reconstruction technologies [45, 77–82, 84, 85] thanks to the significant improvement of the image quality. When originally presented, these techniques were regarded as totally different technology having nothing to do with sparse sampling. However, recent theoretical results [83] showed that the deep convolutional neural network is closely related to sparse sampling and reconstruction. Therefore, we can argue that, besides super-resolution, radial sparse sampling MRI pipeline could benefit of deep learning also for image reconstruction to improve image quality while further reducing the number of radial projections, that is to increase temporal resolution, a major milestone for functional imaging Table 3.2.

Acknowledgements The Authors wish to thank the anonymous Reviewers for the constructive comments.

References

1. Lauterbur, P.C.: Image formation by induced local interactions: examples employing nuclear magnetic resonance. Nature **242**, 190–191 (1973)
2. Hingorani, D.V., Bernstein, A.S., Pagel, M.D.: A review of responsive mri contrast agents: 2005–2014. Contrast Media Mol. Imag. **10**, 245–265 (2015)
3. Glover, G.H.: Overview of functional magnetic resonance imaging. Neurosurg. Clin. North Am. **22**, 133–139 (2011)
4. Lufkin, R., Teresi, L., Chiu, L., Hanafee, W.: A technique for mr-guided needle placement. Am. J. Roentgenol. **151**, 193–196 (1988)
5. Adam, G., Neuerburg, J., Bücker, A., Glowinski, A., Vorwerk, D., Stargardt, A., Vaals, J.J.V., Günther, R.W.: Interventional magnetic resonance: initial clinical experience with a 1.5-tesla magnetic resonance system combined with c-arm fluoroscopy. Invest. Radiol. **32**, 191–197 (1997)
6. Matsumoto, R., Selig, A.M., Colucci, V.M., Jolesz, F.A.: Mr monitoring during cryotherapy in the liver: predictability of histologic outcome. J. Magn. Reson. Imag. **3**, 770–776 (1993)
7. Dumoulin, C., Souza, S., Darrow, R.: Real-time positioning of invasive devices using magnetic resonance. Magn. Reson. Med. **29**, 411–415 (1993)

8. Glowinski, A., Adam, G., Bücker, A., Neuerburg, J., Vaals, J.J.V., Günther, R.W.: Catheter visualization using locally induced, actively controlled field inhomogeneities. Magn. Reson. Medi. **38**, 253–258 (1997)
9. Kerr, A.B., Pauly, J.M., Hu, B.S., Li, K.C., Hardy, C.J., Meyer, C.H., Macovski, A., Nishimura, D.G.: Real-time interactive mri on a conventional scanner. Magn. Reson. Med. **38**, 355–367 (1997)
10. Rasche, V., Holz, D., Proksa, R.: Mr fluoroscopy using projection reconstruction multi-gradient-echo (prmge) MRI. Magn. Reson. Med. **42**, 324–334 (1999)
11. Block, K.T., Uecker, M., Frahm, J.: Undersampled radial mri with multiple coils. iterative image reconstruction using a total variation constraint. Magn. Reson. Med. **57**, 1086–1098 (2007)
12. Glover, G.H., Pauly, J.M.: Projection reconstruction techniques for reduction of motion effects in mri. Magn. Reson. Med. **28**, 275–289 (1992)
13. Gai, N., Axel, L.: Correction of motion artifacts in linogram and projection reconstruction mri using geometry and consistency constraints. Med. Phys. **23**, 251–262 (1996)
14. Sodickson, D.K., Manning, W.J.: "Simultaneous acquisition of spatial harmonics (smash): Fast imaging with radiofrequency coil arrays. Magn. Reson. Med. **38**, 591–603 (1997)
15. Pruessmann, K.P., Weiger, M., Scheidegger, M.B., Boesiger, P.: Sense: Sensitivity encoding for fast mri. Magn. Reson. Med. **42**, 952–962 (1999)
16. Griswold, M.A., Jakob, P.M., Heidemann, R.M., Nittka, M., Jellus, V., Wang, J., Kiefer, B., Haase, A.: Generalized autocalibrating partially parallel acquisitions (grappa). Magn. Reson. Med. **47**, 1202–1210 (2002)
17. Xu, D., King, K.F., Liang, Z.P.: Improving k-t sense by adaptive regularization. Magn. Reson. Med. **57**, 918–930 (2007)
18. Alecci, M., Brivati, J.A., Placidi, G., Testa, L., Lurie, D.J., Sotgiu, A.: A submicrosecond resonator and receiver system for pulsed magnetic resonance with large samples. J. Magn. Reson. Imag. **132**, 162–166 (1998)
19. Giuseppe, S.D., Placidi, G., Sotgiu, A.: New experimental apparatus for multimodal resonance imaging: Initial epri and nmri experimental results. Phys. Med. Biol. **46**, 1003–1016 (2001)
20. Eldar, Y.C.: Sampling theory: beyond bandlimited systems. In: Sampling Theory: Beyond Bandlimited Systems, pp. 1–800 (2014)
21. Tsao, J., Boesiger, P., Pruessmann, K.P.: k-t blast and k-t sense: Dynamic mri with high frame rate exploiting spatiotemporal correlations. Magn. Reson. Med. **50**, 1031–1042 (2003)
22. Huang, F., Akao, J., Vijayakumar, S., Duensing, G.R., Limkeman, M.: K-t grappa: a k-space implementation for dynamic mri with high reduction factor. Magn. Reson. Med. **54**, 1172–1184 (2005)
23. Vaals, J.J.V., Brummer, M.E., Dixon, W.T., Tuithof, H.H., Engels, H., Nelson, R.C., Gerety, B.M., Chezmar, J.L., Boer, J.A.D.: keyhole method for accelerating imaging of contrast agent uptake. J. Magn. Reson. Imag. **3**, 671–675 (1993)
24. Jones, R.A., Haraldseth, O., Müller, T.B., Rinck, P.A., Øksendal, A.N.: K-space substitution: a novel dynamic imaging technique. Magn. Reson. Med. **29**, 830–834 (1993)
25. Kim, D., Dyvorne, H.A., Otazo, R., Feng, L., Sodickson, D.K., Lee, V.S.: Accelerated phase-contrast cine mri using k-t sparse-sense. Magn. Reson. Med. **67**, 1054–1064 (2012)
26. Feng, L., Srichai, M.B., Lim, R.P., Harrison, A., King, W., Adluru, G., Dibella, E.V., Sodickson, D.K., Otazo, R., Kim, D.: Highly accelerated real-time cardiac cine mri using k-t sparse-sense. Magn. Reson. Med. **70**, 64–74 (2013)
27. Feng, L., Grimm, R., Block, K.T., Chandarana, H., Kim, S., Xu, J., Axel, L., Sodickson, D.K., Otazo, R.: Golden-angle radial sparse parallel mri: Combination of compressed sensing, parallel imaging, and golden-angle radial sampling for fast and flexible dynamic volumetric mri. Magn. Reson. Med. **72**, 707–717 (2014)
28. Baldassarre, L., Li, Y.H., Scarlett, J., Gozcu, B., Bogunovic, I., Cevher, V.: Learning-based compressive subsampling. IEEE J. Sel. Top. Sign. Process. **10**, 809–822 (2016)
29. Placidi, G., Alecci, M., Sotgiu, A.: Theory of adaptive acquisition method for image reconstruction from projections and application to epr imaging. J. Magn. Reson. Imag. Ser. B **108**, 50–57 (1995)

30. Placidi, G., Alecci, M., Sotgiu, A.: ω-space adaptive acquisition technique for magnetic resonance imaging from projections. J. Magn. Reson. Imag. **143**, 197–207 (2000)
31. Placidi, G., Alecci, M., Sotgiu, A.: Angular space-domain interpolation for filtered back projection applied to regular and adaptively measured projections. J. Magn. Reson. Imag. Ser. B **110**, 75–79 (1996)
32. Placidi, G.: Adaptive compression algorithm from projections: application on medical greyscale images. Comput. Biol. Med. **39**, 993–999 (2009)
33. Placidi, G., Cinque, L., Petracca, A., Polsinelli, M., Spezialetti, M.: Iterative adaptive sparse sampling method for magnetic resonance imaging. In: ICPRAM 2017—Proceedings of the 6th International Conference on Pattern Recognition Applications and Methods, vol. 2017, pp. 510–518 (2017)
34. Placidi, G., Cinque, L., Mignosi, F., Polsinelli, M., Spezialetti, M.: Sparse sampling for magnetic resonance imaging. In: Proceedings on 15th International Symposium on Computer Methods in Biomechanics and Biomedical Engineering (2018)
35. Ravishankar, S., Bresler, Y.: Mr image reconstruction from highly undersampled k-space data by dictionary learning. IEEE Trans. Med. Imag. **30**, 1028–1041 (2011)
36. Qu, X., Hou, Y., Lam, F., Guo, D., Zhong, J., Chen, Z.: Magnetic resonance image reconstruction from undersampled measurements using a patch-based nonlocal operator. Med. Imag Anal. **18**, 843–856 (2014)
37. Mairal, J., Bach, F., Ponce, J.: Sparse modeling for image and vision processing. Found. Trends Comput. Graph. Vision **8**, 85–283 (2014)
38. Timofte, R., De, V., Gool, L.V.: Anchored neighborhood regression for fast example-based super-resolution. In: Proceedings of the IEEE International Conference on Computer Vision, pp. 1920–1927 (2013)
39. Song, P., Weizman, L., Mota, J.F., Eldar, Y.C., Rodrigues, M.R.: Coupled dictionary learning for multi-contrast mri reconstruction. In: Proceedings—International Conference on Image Processing, ICIP, pp. 2880–2884 (2018)
40. Yang, G., Yu, S., Dong, H., Slabaugh, G., Dragotti, P.L., Ye, X., Liu, F., Arridge, S., Keegan, J., Guo, Y., Firmin, D.: Dagan: deep de-aliasing generative adversarial networks for fast compressed sensing mri reconstruction. IEEE Trans. Med. Imag. **37**, 1310–1321 (2018)
41. Ikram, S., Shah, J.A., Zubair, S., Qureshi, I.M., Bilal, M.: Improved reconstruction of mr scanned images by using a dictionary learning scheme. Sensors (Switzerland) **19** (2019)
42. Trzasko, J., Manduca, A.: Highly undersampled magnetic resonance image reconstruction via homotopic l0-minimization. IEEE Trans. Med. Imag. **28**, 106–121 (2009)
43. Dwork, N., Baron, C.A., Johnson, E.M., O'Connor, D., Pauly, J.M., Larson, P.E.: Fast variable density poisson-disc sample generation with directional variation for compressed sensing in MRI. Magn. Reson. Imag. **77**, 186–193 (2021)
44. Gözcü, B., Mahabadi, R.K., Li, Y.H., Ilicak, E., Çukur, T., Scarlett, J., Cevher, V.: Learning-based compressive MRI. IEEE Trans. Med. Imag. **37**, 1394–1406 (2018)
45. Bahadir, C.D., Wang, A.Q., Dalca, A.V., Sabuncu, M.R.: Deep-learning-based optimization of the under-sampling pattern in MRI. IEEE Trans. Comput. Imag. **6**, 1139–1152 (2020)
46. Candes, E.J., Tao, T.: Near-optimal signal recovery from random projections: Universal encoding strategies?," *IEEE Transactions on Information Theory*, vol. 52, pp. 5406–5425, 12 2006
47. Donoho, D.L.: Compressed sensing. IEEE Trans. Inf. Theory **52**, 1289–1306 (2006)
48. Haupt, J., Castro, R., Nowak, R.: Distilled sensing: Selective sampling for sparse signal recovery. J. Mach. Learn. Res. **5**, 216–223 (2009)
49. Lustig, M., Donoho, D., Pauly, J.M.: Sparse MRI: the application of compressed sensing for rapid mr imaging. Magn. Reson. Med. **58**, 1182–1195 (2007)
50. Lustig, M., Donoho, D.L., Santos, J.M., Pauly, J.M.: Compressed sensing mri: A look at how cs can improve on current imaging techniques. IEEE Signal Processing Magazine **25**, 72–82 (2008)
51. Foucart, S., Rauhut, H.: A mathematical introduction to compressive sensing. Appl. Numer. Harmonic Anal. 1–615 (2013)

52. Candès, E.J., Romberg, J., Tao, T.: Robust uncertainty principles: exact signal reconstruction from highly incomplete frequency information. IEEE Trans. Inf. Theory **52**, 489–509 (2006)
53. Rao, N., Nowak, R.: Adaptive sensing with structured sparsity. In: Proceedings on IEEE Conference on Acoustics, Speech, and Signal Processing (2013)
54. Haupt, J.D., Baraniuk, R.G., Castro, R.M., Nowak, R.D.: Compressive distilled sensing: sparse recovery using adaptivity in compressive measurements. In: Conference Record—Asilomar Conference on Signals, Systems and Computers, pp. 1551–1555 (2009)
55. Placidi, G.: MRI: Essentials for innovative technologies. In: MRI: Essentials for Innovative Technologies, pp. 1–195 (2012)
56. Arias-Castro, E., Candes, E.J., Davenport, M.A.: On the fundamental limits of adaptive sensing. IEEE Trans. Inf. Theory **59**, 472–481 (2013)
57. Placidi, G., Alecci, M., Colacicchi, S., Sotgiu, A.: Fourier reconstruction as a valid alternative to filtered back projection in iterative applications: Implementation of fourier spectral spatial epr imaging. J. Magn. Reson. Imag. **134**, 280–286 (1998)
58. Sung, K., Hargreaves, B.A.: High-frequency subband compressed sensing mri using quadruplet sampling. Magn. Reson. Med. **70**, 1306–1318 (2013)
59. Malloy, M.L., Nowak, R.D.: Near-optimal adaptive compressed sensing. IEEE Trans. Inf. Theory **60**, 4001–4012 (2014)
60. Ma, Y., Garnett, R., Schneider, J.: Active search for sparse signals with region sensing. In: 31st AAAI Conference on Artificial Intelligence, AAAI 2017, pp. 2315–2321 (2017)
61. Castro, R.M.: Adaptive sensing performance lower bounds for sparse signal detection and support estimation. Bernoulli **20**, 2217–2246 (2014)
62. Ciancarella, L., Avola, D., Placidi, G.: Adaptive sampling and reconstruction for sparse magnetic resonance imaging. Lect. Notes Comput. Vision Biomech. **15**, 115–130 (2014)
63. Lai, M.-J., Wang, Y.: Sparse solutions of underdetermined linear systems and their applications. Soc. Indus. Appl. Math, Philadelphia (2021)
64. Natterer, F.: The mathematics of computerized tomography. SIAM (2001)
65. Gottlieb, D.: On the direct fourier method for computer tomography. IEEE Trans. Med. Imaging **19**, 223–232 (2000)
66. Penczek, P.A., Renka, R., Schomberg, H.: Gridding-based direct fourier inversion of the three-dimensional ray transform. J. Opt. Soc. Am. A **21**, 499 (2004)
67. Averbuch, A., Coifman, R.R., Donoho, D.L., Elad, M., Israeli, M.: Fast and accurate polar fourier transform. Appl. Comput. Harmonic Anal. **21**, 145–167 (2006)
68. Placidi, G., Alecci, M., Sotgiu, A.: Post-processing noise removal algorithm for magnetic resonance imaging based on edge detection and wavelet analysis. Phys. Med. Biol. **48**, 1987–1995 (2003)
69. Anbarjafari, G., Demirel, H.: Image super resolution based on interpolation of wavelet domain high frequency subbands and the spatial domain input image. ETRI J. **32**, 390–394 (2010)
70. Guo, T., Mousavi, H.S., Vu, T.H., Monga, V.: Deep wavelet prediction for image super-resolution. In: IEEE Computer Society Conference on Computer Vision and Pattern Recognition Workshops, vol. 2017-July, pp. 1100–1109 (2017)
71. Placidi, G., Cinque, L., Mignosi, F., Polsinelli, M.: Multiple sclerosis lesions identification/segmentation in magnetic resonance imaging using ensemble cnn and uncertainty classification. *arXiv*, vol. https://arxiv.org/abs/2108.11791(2021)
72. Gonzalez, R., Woods, R.: Digital image processing. In: MRI: Essentials for Innovative Technologies (2008)
73. Wang, Z., Bovik, A.C., Sheikh, H.R., Simoncelli, E.P.: Image quality assessment: from error visibility to structural similarity. IEEE Trans. Image Process. **13**, 600–612 (2004)
74. Hosny, A., Parmar, C., Quackenbush, J., Schwartz, L.H., Aerts, H.J.: Artificial intelligence in radiology. Nat. Rev. Cancer **18**, 500–510 (2018)
75. A. Barragán-Montero, U. Javaid, G. Valdés, D. Nguyen, P. Desbordes, B. Macq, S. Willems, L. Vandewinckele, M. Holmström, F. Löfman, S. Michiels, K. Souris, E. Sterpin, and J. A. Lee, "Artificial intelligence and machine learning for medical imaging: A technology review," *Physica Medica*, vol. 83, pp. 242–256, 3 2021

76. D. in Eun, R. Jang, W. S. Ha, H. Lee, S. C. Jung, and N. Kim, "Deep-learning-based image quality enhancement of compressed sensing magnetic resonance imaging of vessel wall: comparison of self-supervised and unsupervised approaches," *Scientific Reports*, vol. 10, 12 2020
77. K. Hammernik, T. Klatzer, E. Kobler, M. P. Recht, D. K. Sodickson, T. Pock, and F. Knoll, "Learning a variational network for reconstruction of accelerated mri data," *Magn. Reson. Med.*, vol. 79, pp. 3055–3071, 6 2018
78. Y. Han, J. Yoo, H. H. Kim, H. J. Shin, K. Sung, and J. C. Ye, "Deep learning with domain adaptation for accelerated projection-reconstruction mr," *Magn. Reson. Med.*, vol. 80, pp. 1189–1205, 9 2018
79. B. Zhu, J. Z. Liu, S. F. Cauley, B. R. Rosen, and M. S. Rosen, "Image reconstruction by domain-transform manifold learning," *Nature*, vol. 555, pp. 487–492, 3 2018
80. J. Schlemper, J. Caballero, J. V. Hajnal, A. N. Price, and D. Rueckert, "A deep cascade of convolutional neural networks for dynamic mr image reconstruction," *IEEE Transactions on Medical Imaging*, vol. 37, pp. 491–503, 2 2018
81. S. Wang, Z. Su, L. Ying, X. Peng, S. Zhu, F. Liang, D. Feng, and D. Liang, "Accelerating magnetic resonance imaging via deep learning," *Proceedings - International Symposium on Biomedical Imaging*, vol. 2016-June, pp. 514–517, 6 2016
82. K. Kwon, D. Kim, and H. Park, "A parallel mr imaging method using multilayer perceptron:," *Med. Phys.*, vol. 44, pp. 6209–6224, 12 2017
83. Ye, J., Han, Y., Cha, E.: Deep convolutional framelets: A general deep learning framework for inverse problems. SIAM Journal on Imaging Sciences **11**(2), 991–1048 (2018)
84. Gassenmaier, S., Küstner, T., Nickel, D., Herrmann, J., Hoffmann, R., Almansour, H., Afat, S., Nikolaou, K., Othman, A.E.: Deep learning applications in magnetic resonance imaging: Has the future become present? Diagnostics **11**, 12 (2021)
85. Wang, S., Cao, G., Wang, Y., Liao, S., Wang, Q., Shi, J., Li, C., Shen, D.: Review and prospect: artificial intelligence in advanced medical imaging. Front. Radiol. 15 (2021)

Chapter 4
Unsupervised Domain Adaptation Approach for Liver Tumor Detection in Multi-phase CT Images

Rahul Kumar Jain, Takahiro Sato, Taro Watasue, Tomohiro Nakagawa, Yutaro Iwamoto, Xianhua Han, Lanfen Lin, Hongjie Hu, Xiang Ruan, and Yen-Wei Chen

Abstract For computer-aided diagnosis, automatic and accurate liver tumor detection in multi-phase CT images is essential. Nowadays, deep learning has been widely used in various medical applications. Deep learning-based AI systems require a large amount of training data for model learning. However, acquiring sufficient training data with high-quality annotation is a major challenge in Healthcare. As a result, deep learning-based models face a lack of annotated training data problem. While

---

R. K. Jain · Y. Iwamoto · Y.-W. Chen (✉)
College of Information Science and Engineering, Ritsumeikan University, Shiga, Japan
e-mail: chen@is.ritsumei.ac.jp

R. K. Jain
e-mail: rahulkumarjain16@gmail.com

Y. Iwamoto
e-mail: yiwamoto@fc.ritsumei.ac.jp

T. Sato · T. Watasue · T. Nakagawa · X. Ruan
tiwaki Co. Ltd., Shiga, Japan
e-mail: sato@tiwaki.com

T. Watasue
e-mail: watasue@tiwaki.com

T. Nakagawa
e-mail: nakagawa@tiwaki.com

X. Ruan
e-mail: ruanxiang@tiwaki.com

X. Han
Artificial Intelligence Research Center, Yamaguchi University, Yamaguchi, Japan
e-mail: hanxhua@yamaguchi-u.ac.jp

L. Lin
College of Computer Science and Technology, Zhejiang University, Hangzhou, China
e-mail: llf@zju.edu.cn

H. Hu
Department of Radiology, Sir Run Run Shaw Zhejiang University, Hangzhou, China
e-mail: hongjiehu@zju.edu.cn

© The Author(s), under exclusive license to Springer Nature Switzerland AG 2023
C.-P. Lim et al. (eds.), *Artificial Intelligence and Machine Learning for Healthcare*, Intelligent Systems Reference Library 228,
https://doi.org/10.1007/978-3-031-11154-9_4

the generalization of a label-rich training domain (source) to a new test domain (target) causes a domain shift problem in deep learning-based models. To solve the lack of training data and domain shift problem, domain adaptation-based methods have recently been developed as a technique to bridge the domain gap across datasets with different feature characteristics and data distributions. In this chapter, we have proposed domain adaptation-based technique for liver tumor detection in multi-phase CT images. We discuss the domain-shift problem in different phases of multiphase liver CT images and introduce our domain adaptation technique for multi-phase CT images. We have used PV phase images to learn a model and applied the learnt model to ART and NC phase images (i.e. different domains) by adapting the domain knowledge. To address the domain gap between the different phases of CT images, we employ adversarial learning scheme using an anchor-free object detector. Further, we propose to use the maximum square loss for mid-level output feature maps to improve the performance. Our method does not require separate object-level annotations for each phase of Multiphase CT image while training. The results of the experiments show that models trained using our proposed domain adaptation technique perform much better than those trained in normal setting.

Keywords Liver tumor detection · Multi-phase ct image · Anchor-free object detectors · Domain adaptation · Adversarial learning · Maximum square loss

Table of Acronyms

ART	Arterial phase
AUC	Area under the curve
CT	Imaging and computed tomography imaging
DA	Domain adaptation
DL	Deep learning
DLA	Deep layer aggregation network
FNH	Focal nodular hyperplasia
GT	Ground truth
HCC	Hepatocellular carcinoma
HEM	Epithelioid Hemangioendothelioma
IoU	Intersection over union
mAP	Mean average precision
METs	Metastatic tumors
MRI	Imaging and magnetic resonance imaging
NC	Non-contract enhanced phase
PV	Portal venous phase
ReLU	Rectified linear unit
tSNE	t-Distributed stochastic neighbor embedding

4.1 Introduction

Tumor detection is an important function for medical applications. The identification of malignant tumors from high-resolution multi-phase computed tomography (CT) images is a critical task in computer-aided diagnosis of various diseases. The malignant liver tumor is one of the most life-threatening diseases. The use of CT scan images in the early recognition of malignant liver tumors has become very common. This chapter focuses on the advancement of deep learning in healthcare by describing the domain-shift problem and novel deep learning-based domain adaption approaches for liver tumor recognition in multi-phase liver CT images.

4.1.1 Domain-Shift Problem

Nowadays, deep learning-based techniques are widely used for various tasks in medical images such as tumor classification, tumor detection and tumor segmentation [1–4]. Deep learning is a data-driven task-specific approach that automatically learns high-level feature representations from the given input training images. Most of the existing deep learning-based methods for CT images follow a supervised learning approach and need a large amount of object-level annotated images for model training. Whereas object-level annotations (segmentation mask and bounding box annotations) are a laborious, time-consuming and costly task. The task of recognizing malignancies in multi-phase CT images (slice by slice) for annotation increases the workload of radiologists/experts correspondingly. It is difficult to recruit experts to annotate large amount of medical data collected from different domains/medical-centers (multi-center data) for various diseases. Moreover, it is a tedious task for any expert to annotate every single tiny tumor for training deep learning-based models. As a result, deep learning-based models face a lack of training data problem. The transfer of knowledge (model generalization) from a label-rich source domain (in terms of quality and samples) to a target domain (without labels) can be used to address the lack of training data problem. In particular medical images requires high quality annotated data. But knowledge transfer from a label-rich source domain to a unlabeled target domain can cause domain-shift problems for various tasks [5–8]. In practice, domain-shift from the source domain (training data) to the target domain (testing data) limits the performance of deep learning-based detection and segmentation models during inference time.

In medical images, domain shift is also a major problem for model learning. Different medical image datasets may have different data distributions and feature information due to variation in acquisition devices/equipment, parameters configurations and medical-center [6, 9]. The distribution of data in different phases of multi-phase CT and MRI images may also differ substantially. Multi-phase CT imaging, also known as contrast-enhanced dynamic CT, is widely used to diagnose a variety of malignant tumors. The difference between the multiphase CT images a causes domain shift problem, which is one of the major challenges in liver tumor detection [4]. A multi-phase CT scan mainly consists of three phases (i.e. different domains). The first phase is the non-contrast enhanced (NC) phase, in which an examination is performed before contrast enhancement injection. After the contrast injection, further examinations are obtained in several phases. One is arterial (ART) phase, that is obtained in 30-40 seconds after the contract injection. Another is portal venous (PV) phase, which obtains in 70-80 seconds after the contract injection. The CT images of different phases might also be affected due to various factors such as patient's body position, movement, respiration, and heartbeat. Texture and spatial information of liver and tumors might also vary significantly in these different phases (i.e. different domains) due to various technical factors. Fig.1 shows images of corresponding liver tumors slices in different phases. The texture and spatial information of liver tumors varies significantly in these different phases due to duration of time the contrast enhancement agent is administered, as seen in the figure. As a result, deep learning models that are trained on one phase of multiphase CT image perform inadequately when evaluated on other CT phase images (Fig. 4.1).

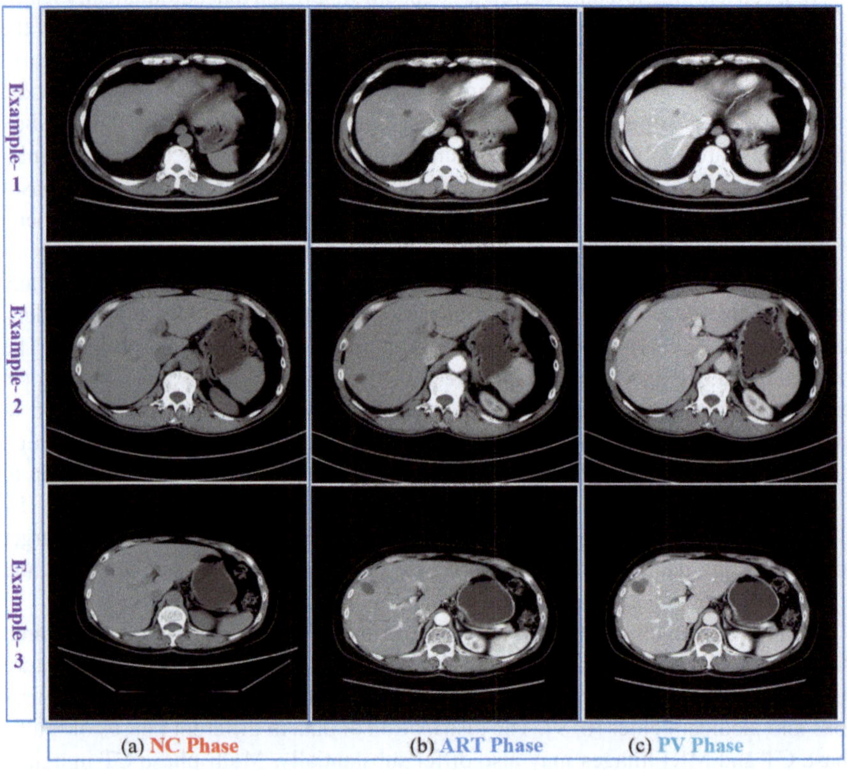

Fig. 4.1 Examples of corresponding slices from different phases of CT images

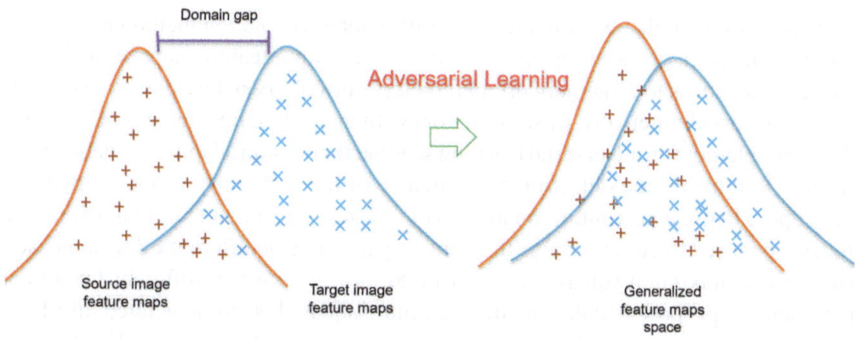

Fig. 4.2 Domain adaptation using adversarial learning

4.1.2 Domain Adaptation

In medical applications, tumor detection in different CT phase images is highly valuable, as the identification of each tiny tumor is crucial for decision-making. Different CT phase images may have some underlying correlated complementary information that might be useful for accurate detection of liver tumors. If CT scan data from distinct CT phases (NC, ART, and PV) is not considered by decision-making systems, this information can be lost. But the independent annotation process for each phase takes enormous efforts and resources. To overcome the domain-shift problem and minimize the performance degradation, recently domain adaptation-based techniques have been introduced as a way to bridge the domain gap between images with varying data styles, characteristics, features, and distributions. By adapting object detectors to bridge the domain gap between two different domains (distinct CT phases), domain adaptation techniques provide an appealing solution. Domain adaptation-based techniques use adversarial learning [5–8] scheme to align the feature space between source (training) and target (test) datasets. Fig. 4.2 depicts the generalization process of different domains to reduce the domain gap.

Recently, domain adaptation techniques have also been used to address the problem of domain shift in medical images [6, 9]. To address the data annotation and domain shift problems, in this chapter, we present domain adaptation frameworks for liver tumor detection that are capable of aligning domain gaps between different CT phase images. For model training we need annotations only for a single phase, so this technique reduces the dependency on annotations for other phases. Our method reduces the dependency on separate annotation for each CT phase images by adopting knowledge from unlabeled images. In our experiments, we use PV phase CT images as the source domain images for model training (with bounding box annotations) whereas CT images of ART and NC phases are used as target (test) domain images (i.e. different domains). Note that we use these target domain images (ART and NC Phase) without annotations. The proposed framework improves the performance and offers more accurate detection of liver tumors.

Among some of the existing methods, our domain adaptation method is based on our previous work [8], we propose to use mid-level output feature maps of the feature extractor networks to align network parameters between two domains. We combine a domain classifier network (discriminator) with an anchor-free detector, CenterNet [10], to implement an adversarial learning scheme for domain adaptive detection task. Further, to improve the detection performance of the previously proposed method, we propose to use a maximum square loss of mid-level feature maps of target domain images to more effectively bridge the domain gap between different CT scan phases. The idea of maximum square loss is inspired by [7]. However different from their approach, we propose to calculate the maximum square loss for generated mid-level feature maps instead of calculating for predicted segmentation maps. For the first time, we suggest using the adversarial domain classification loss with maximum square loss to improve detection performance in a domain adaptation scenario in our novel proposed method. The network parameters are effectively aligned between two domains using a combination of maximum square loss and adversarial learning loss for training. The preliminary study of our research has been reported in [11, 12]. As an extension of our previous studies, in this chapter, we have evaluated and analyzed the performance of domain adaptation for liver tumor detection and further investigated the feature distribution using our proposed methods.

4.2 Domain Adaptation Using Adversarial Learning

The framework for our domain adaptive detector using adversarial learning is described in this section. Adversarial learning is one of the successful ideas to bridge the domain gaps. For liver tumor detection, we employ domain adaptive approach using an adversarial learning scheme with an anchor-free object detector—CenterNet [10].

4.2.1 Anchor-free Detector

We use CenterNet as the detection network (detection-head), which is an anchor-free detector introduced in [10]. CenterNet recognizes objects by their bounding box's center point and generates a shape-vector to estimate the height and width of objects. CenterNet detection head includes three sub-heads: the heatmap head, size head and offset head. The heatmap head generates class-wise heatmaps. The size head generates shape vectors to determine the size of an object, while the offset head handles the discretization error caused by the down sampling during locating the position of an object. The pixel activation intensity value score is used to recognize the objects. The class-wise heatmaps are used to define the category of recognized objects. Based on these different functions, the training objective loss function of CenterNet can be given as:

$$L_{det} = L_k + \lambda_{size} L_s + \lambda_{off} L_{off} \tag{4.1}$$

where L_k is the focal loss classification function [13] for heatmaps, L_s and L_{off} are $L1$ loss functions for size and offset, λ_{size} and λ_{off} are loss weights. To perform feature extraction, we use deep layer aggregation (DLA-34) [14] CNNs network as the backbone of the CenterNet detection head. The design of of DLA-34 backbone network is similar to [10] and the detailed design structure is available in the author's paper [14].

4.2.1.1 Discriminator Network

We employ an adversarial learning scheme by combining a domain discriminator network with the anchor-free detection framework. The discriminator network has 5 convolutional layers with a kernel size of 4 × 4 and a stride of 2. The number of channels in each layer is [64, 128, 256, 512, 1]. After the first four convolutional layers, a Leaky-ReLU activation is applied. A fixed negative slope of 0.2 is used for the Leaky-ReLU activation layer. Finally, a pixel-wise classification loss has been calculated using the final output of the network. The detailed structure and operations of the discriminator network are given in Table 4.1.

4.2.2 Proposed Multi-phase Domain Adaptation Framework Using Adversarial Domain Classification Loss

We intend to address model learning towards the distribution of the target domain images by aligning the output feature maps of the source and target domains as close to each other to improve the generalization of the model. We use an adversarial learning scheme to align the model between two domains by including a domain discriminator network in the training phase of the detection framework. The overall structure of the detection framework with an adversarial learning scheme is depicted in Fig. 4.3. In our previous work [8], we proposed to align the domain gap for the logo detection task using a mid-level feature maps with anchor-free detector. We

Table 4.1 Design of domain classifier network

Layer	Output dimension	Operation, kernel size, output channels, stride
Layer-1	128 × 128	Conv, 4 × 4, 64, 2
Layer-2	64 × 64	Conv, 4 × 4, 128, 2
Layer-3	32 × 32	Conv, 4 × 4, 256, 2
Layer-4	16 × 16	Conv, 4 × 4, 512, 2
Layer-5	4 × 4	Conv, 4 × 4, 1, 2

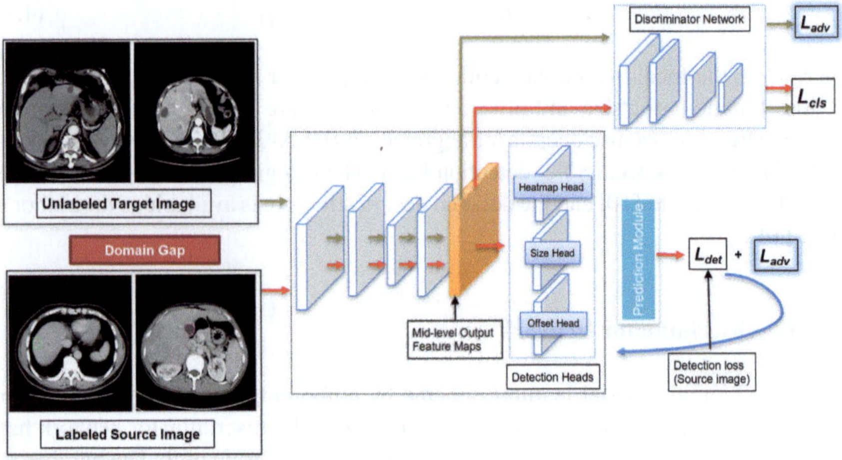

Fig. 4.3 Our proposed domain adaptation based training strategy using mid-level output feature maps

observed that using the most appropriate output feature maps is essential to align the domain gap since anchor-free detectors train the network to recognize objects in terms of some keypoints. As a result, we propose to use the mid-level output of the feature extraction network for domain adaptation. The main advantage of using mid-level output is that it contains important domain-specific semantic and spatial information, making adversarial learning more successful.

CenterNet generates mid-level output feature maps for images from both the source and target domains. Only mid-level output feature maps of source images are provided to different detection heads (heatmap-head, offset-head, size-head) to compute their respective objective losses to train the framework for tumor detection task (i.e. Equation.4.1). For the source images, object-level annotations are required. An adversarial domain classification loss is calculated using the mid-level output feature maps of the target images to match the data distribution of the source and target domains. Therefore, object-level annotations are not required for the target images. During training, we provide the generated mid-level output feature maps of the source domain and target domain images as inputs to the discriminator network. These input mid-level feature maps are classified as either source or target domains to optimize the discriminator network classification capability. While an adversarial domain classification loss (i.e. adversarial learning scheme) is computed to train the detector network in order to mock the discriminator network. The adversarial classification loss can be computed by assigning an inverted domain label to the target images (i.e. the domain label of the source images). To minimize the gap between the source and target domains, the adversarial loss is beneficial for aligning network parameters in a common shared space.

In our experiments, we use labeled source images (PV phase) and unlabeled target images (NC or ART phase) for model training. We assign domain label '0' to source images (source-domain) and domain label '1' to target images (target-domain). During training, at first, mid-level output feature maps of the target image (Mid_X_T) are provided to the discriminator network to calculate the adversarial domain classification loss. We provide the inverted domain label (*i.e.* '0' instead of '1') to obtain the adversarial loss. The adversarial binary classification loss L_{adv} can be defined as:

$$L_{adv} = \frac{1}{|X_T|}\sum_{i=1}^{|X_T|} L_{cls}(Mid\_X_T^i, 0) \tag{4.2}$$

where $Mid\_X_T^i$ is the mid-level features of the ith target domain image. $|X_T|$ are the number of images form target domain. Adversarial loss is combined with detection loss of source images to update the gradients of detection framework. Now using Eq. 4.1, the objective optimization loss for the detection framework can be given as:

$$L_{det} = L_k + \lambda_{size} L_s + \lambda_{off} L_{off} + \lambda_{adv} L_{adv} \tag{4.3}$$

λ_{adv} is loss weight. We use a value of 0.001 in our experiments.

At the same time, a domain classification loss (training objective of the discriminator network) is also calculated to build the ability of the discriminator network to distinguish the inputs into the relevant domains. The binary cross entropy classification loss L_{cls} can be defined as:

$$L_{cls} = \frac{1}{|X_S|}\sum_{i=1}^{|X_s|} L_{cls}(Mid\_X_S^i, 0) + \frac{1}{|X_T|}\sum_{i=1}^{|X_T|} L_{cls}(Mid\_X_T^i, 1) \tag{4.4}$$

where $Mid\_X_s^i$ and $Mid\_X_T^i$ are the mid-level features of the ith source domain and target domain image, respectively. $|X_s|$ and $|X_T|$ are the number of images from source domain and target domain. The detection and discriminator networks are jointly trained in an end-to-end manner. During inference, we drop the discriminator network and the normal detection pipeline is used for liver tumor detection.

4.3 Proposed Multi-phase Domain Adaptation Framework Using Adversarial Learning with Maximum Square Loss

To enhance the performance of the proposed method, we introduce maximum square loss for mid-level output feature maps and combine it with adversarial domain classification loss for domain adaptive training. To effectively reduce the gap between the source and target domains, we use both maximum square loss and adversarial domain classification loss to train network parameters in a common shared space. The maximum square loss for predicted segmentation masks of target domain images was proposed by the author in [7]. However, different from their proposed method, in this study, we propose to compute maximum square loss for mid-level feature maps. In comparison to using the maximum square loss to align domains at heatmaps, our proposed approach significantly increases performance.

4.3.1 Maximum Square Loss

To calculate the maximum square loss for an input feature space of the target domain image x_t, we first apply a linear transformation of the feature map using 1×1 convolutional operation followed by softmax normalization across the channel dimension. The resulting feature maps $x_t'(x, y, c) = softmax\{x_t(x, y, c)\}$ has newly synthesized scalar values ensuring the sum of all predictions is equal to one along the dimension c, where x and y are coordinates and c is the number of channels. Finally, a maximum square loss for this output can be calculated using the following equation.

$$L_{msl\_t} = -\frac{1}{2N}\sum_{n=1}^{N}\sum_{c=1}^{C}(p_t^{n,c})^2 \tag{4.5}$$

where p_t is a scalar value, n is pixel position and c is the number of channels in feature maps $x_t'(x, y, c)$.

4.3.2 Overall Framework with Adversarial Domain Classification and Maximum Square Loss

The overall structure of our network is shown in Fig. 4.4. During training, we calculate a maximum square loss for the mid-level feature of target domain images using Eq. 4.5. Maximum square loss and adversarial loss are combined with detection loss of source images to update the gradients of the network. Now the objective optimization function can be given as using Eq. 4.3:

$$L_{det} = L_k + \lambda_{size} L_s + \lambda_{off} L_{off} + L_{msl\_t} + \lambda_{adv} L_{adv} \tag{4.6}$$

The adversarial domain classification (Eq. 4.2) and binary domain classification loss for the discriminator network (Eq. 4.4) is calculated using the procedure described in Sect. 4.2.2.

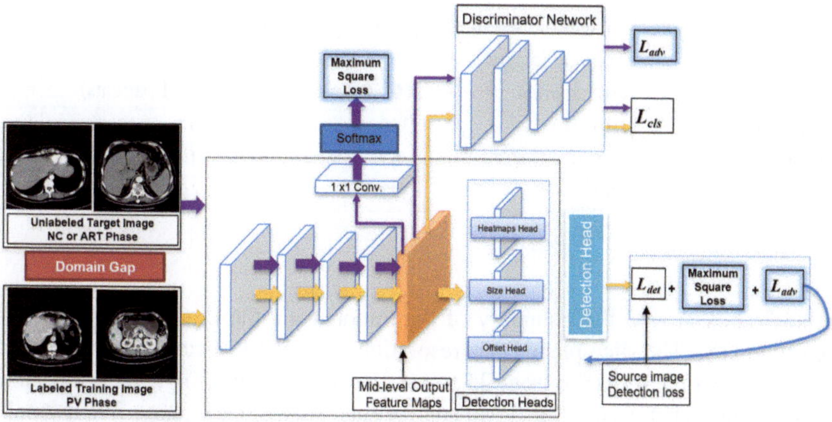

Fig. 4.4 Our proposed domain adaptation based training strategy using adversarial learning with maximum square loss

4.4 Experiments

4.4.1 Implementation Details

We train our network for 140 epochs using a batch size of 8. We use Adam optimizer with an initial learning rate of 0.000125. The learning rate is multiplied by 0.1 at epochs 90 and 120. Input image slices with a size of 512×512 resolution are used. The network is pre-trained on the MS COCO dataset. We trained the discriminator network from scratch with Adam optimizer and a learning rate of 0.0001. The learning rate of the discriminator is dropped by 0.1 at epochs 90 and 120. The same batch-sized images from source and target domains are fed to the model during training. The proposed method is implemented using the publicly available framework Pytorch and CenterNet projects [10]. Following CenterNet, the flip test is used for the final prediction. In the flip test, outputs from the network are flipped and averaged before decoding bounding boxes.

4.4.2 Dataset

In this study, we have used an in-house MPCT-FLLs (Multi-Phase CT dataset of Focal Liver Lesions) database retrospectively collected by Sir Run Run Shaw Hospital, Zhejiang University. It has been used in some previous works [4, 15–17]. The MPCT-FLLs dataset has 121 sets of multi-phase abdominal CT images. The annotations of liver and lesions are manually performed by experienced radiologists. The segmentation masks for liver and tumors are provided by the experts. We draw a

Table 4.2 The details of images (slices) in each phase

Phase	Training images (80 patients)	Test images (41 patients)	Total (121 patients)
PV phase	630	360	990
NC phase	635	367	1002
ART phase	632	377	1009

rectangle box around the boundary of the tumor using the Canny edge detection algorithm [18]. The slice-plane has a resolution of 512×512 pixels. The number of slices for each phase varies from 25 to 99. For image processing, we select pixel intensity values between -70 to +180 HU for each slice of each phase. We use only tumor images of each phase for model training and testing. This dataset contains five different types of liver tumors (Cyst, FNH, HCC, HEM, METs). We use multi-phase information of PV, ART and NC phases for our experiments. In order to validate the effectiveness of our proposed domain adaptation method we use the PV phase as the source domain for model training while ART and NC phase as the target domain. A total of 121 patients are randomly divided into 80 and 41 for training and testing, respectively. The details of training and test slices for each phase are given in the Table 4.2.

4.4.3 Evaluation

There are five different types of tumors in the MPCT-FLLs dataset (Cyst, FNH, HCC, HEM, METs). The performance of the detection frameworks is evaluated considering all tumor classes as a single tumor class. We measure the detection accuracy in terms of Average Precision (AP) accuracy score for tumor class (i.e. localisation and classification of tumors). Average precision (AP) accuracy score based on True Positive and False Positive samples is a popular evaluation technique for the object detection tasks. We can calculate Precision and Recall using IoU value for a given threshold. A predicted candidate region is considered True Positive if the Intersection over Union (IoU) of the predicted candidate region and the ground truth (GT) bounding box overlap by more than a certain value. For our experiments, we considered a correct object region true for IoU 50% (IoU-0.5) and 30% (IoU-0.3) overlapping. The Intersection over Union value (IoU) can be defined as:

$$IoU = \frac{Area\ of\ Overlap\ between\ Predicted\ and\ GT\ Bounding\ Box}{Area\ of\ Union\ between\ Predicted\ and\ GT\ Bounding\ Box} \tag{4.7}$$

The Precision value for any given category is the percentage of correct predictions. i.e.,

Table 4.3 Results of liver tumor detection on different CT phase images using Deep Layer Aggregation (DLA34) as feature extractor (**Case:** No domain shift)

Network	Phase	AP IoU-0.5	AP IoU-0.3
CenterNet-DLA34	NC to NC phase	57.2	63.8
CenterNet-DLA34	ART to ART phase	65.3	72.2
CenterNet-DLA34	PV to PV phase	64.6	72.3

$$Precision = \frac{True\ Positive}{True\ Positive + False\ Positive} \tag{4.8}$$

Whereas Recall measures the proportion of true positive that can be determined as:

$$Recall = \frac{True\ Positive}{True\ Positive + False\ Negative} \tag{4.9}$$

In general, the Average Precision (AP) for any given category is the area under the Precision-Recall curve (AUC - area under the curve). Average Precision (AP) is the weighted sum of Precision values where the weight is the increase in Recall.

4.4.4 Results

4.4.4.1 Case-I: No Domain Shift

For each CT-image phase, we train the network using the images from the same phase to obtain the oracle accuracy rate. The training has been done in a target-to-target manner (No Domain-Shift) when images from the same domain are used for training. Table.4.3 shows accuracies for the NC, ART and PV phases using the DLA34 network as the backbone. For NC phase, the network achieves an of accuracy 57.2% AP (IoU-0.5) and 63.8% AP (IoU-0.3). The experiments results show a relatively higher accuracy rate for the ART and PV Phase in comparison to the NC phase. The reason is that the ART and PV phase are obtained after the contract enhancement. During the ART phase, the network achieves an accuracy of 65.3% AP (IoU-0.5) and 72.2% AP (IoU-0.3) for model training utilizing images from the same domain (target-to-target). Whereas for PV phase it achieves 64.6% AP (IoU-0.5) and 72.3% AP (IoU-0.3) accuracy.

Table 4.4 Results of liver tumor detection on ART phase images (**Case:** Domain shift from PV to ART Phase)

Network	Phase	Max. Square Loss	Adversarial Loss	AP IoU-0.5	AP IoU-0.3
CenterNet-DLA34 [9] Baseline	PV to ART			61.7	67.4
Advent [5] (Entorpy Minimization)	PV to ART			62.9	67.7
MSL [7] (Max. Sqaure Loss)	PV to ART			62.4	67.3
Proposed Method-I	PV to ART		✓	63.9	68.6
Proposed Method-II	PV to ART	✓	✓	64.4	70.2

4.4.4.2 Case-II: Domain Shift PV to ART Phase

In this section, we show the results of the experiments for domain shift from the PV phase to the ART phase. During the training, we use PV phase images as the source domain. While only training images of the ART phase are used as the target domain. We use these target domain images of the ART phase without the bounding box annotations. The evaluation (testing) is conducted on the unseen ART phase images. The results for normal training, entropy minimization-based domain adaptation [5], maximum sqaure loss using heatmaps [7], adversarial learning-based domain adaptation (proposed method-I) and adversarial learning with maximum square loss (proposed method-II) using the DLA34 backbone are shown in Table 4.4. For normal training, in case of a domain shift from PV to ART phase (source-to-target), the network achieves 61.7% AP (IoU-0.5) and 67.4% AP (IoU-0.3) accuracy. In comparison to training on same phase images (ART-to-ART), the performance degradation occurs due to the domain shift as we used PV phase images for training whereas ART phase images for testing. Entropy minimization-based domain adaptation at heatmaps-level achieves 62.9% AP (IoU-0.5) and 67.7% AP (IoU-0.3). We also implement domain adaptation using the maximum square loss method at the heatmaps-level, proposed in [7], with the detection framework. This method achieves 62.4% AP (IoU-0.5) and 67.3% AP (IoU-0.3) accuracy. Our domain adaptation method, adversarial loss using mid-level output feature maps (proposed method-I), shows significant improvement in performance while achieving 63.9% AP (IoU-0.5) and 68.6% AP (IoU-0.3) accuracy. Our proposed method-II, which utilizes adversarial domain classification loss and maximum square loss for domain adaptation, achieves 64.4% AP (IoU-0.5) and 70.2% AP (IoU-0.3) accuracy obtaining significant performance increases.

Figure 4.5 shows the detection results for some images from the ART phase. The proposed domain-adaptation approaches improve tumor detection performance, as shown in the figure. The proposed method-II, which is an improved version of the proposed method-I, is more effective at detecting tumors. Figure 4.6 depicts the t-SNE [19] feature distribution of ART and PV liver images for normal training and proposed

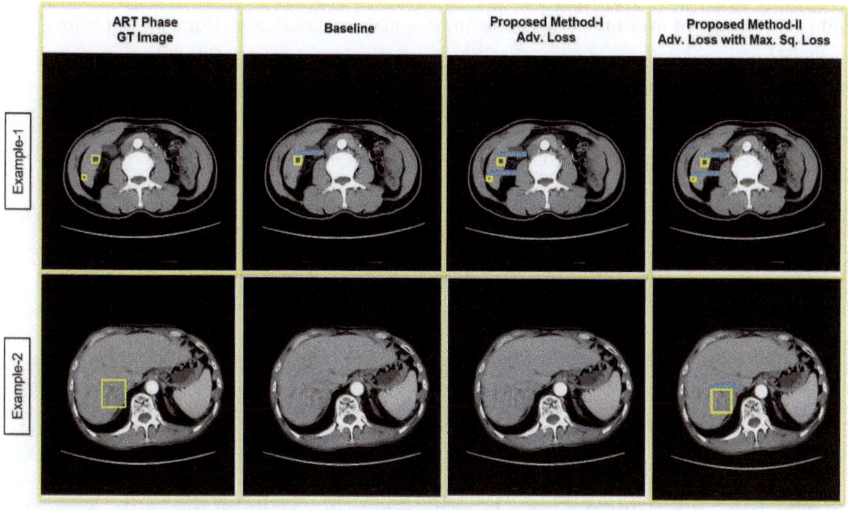

Fig. 4.5 Examples of liver tumor detection on ART phase images

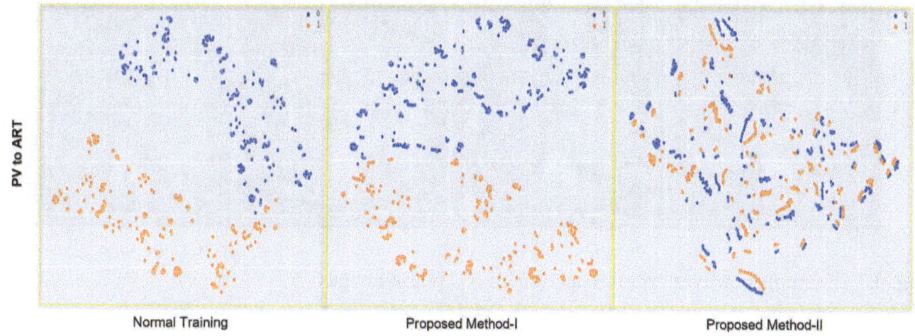

Fig. 4.6 Visualization of the t-SNE feature distributions of **ART** and **PV** liver tumor images. Feature maps distribution in normal training (Left), Proposed Method-I (middle) and Proposed Method-II (Right)

methods. Normal training scheme for ART and PV images has substantially distinct feature distributions. On the other hand, the Proposed Method-I (adversarial learning) brings the domain closer. Whereas Proposed Method-II (maximum square loss with adversarial learning) is more effective at bringing the domain closer together.

4.4.4.3 Case-III: Domain Shift PV to NC Phase

In this section, we show the results for domain shift from the PV phase to the NC phase. This time we use PV phase images as the source domain (labeled) and NC

Table 4.5 Results of liver tumor detection on NC phase images (**Case:** Domain shift from PV to NC Phase)

Network	Phase	Max. Square loss	Adversarial Loss	AP IoU-0.5	AP IoU-0.3
CenterNet-DLA34 [9]	PV to NC			47.7	52.8
Baseline					
Proposed method-I	PV to NC		✓	51.7	57.3
Proposed method-II	PV to NC	✓	✓	53.4	59.5

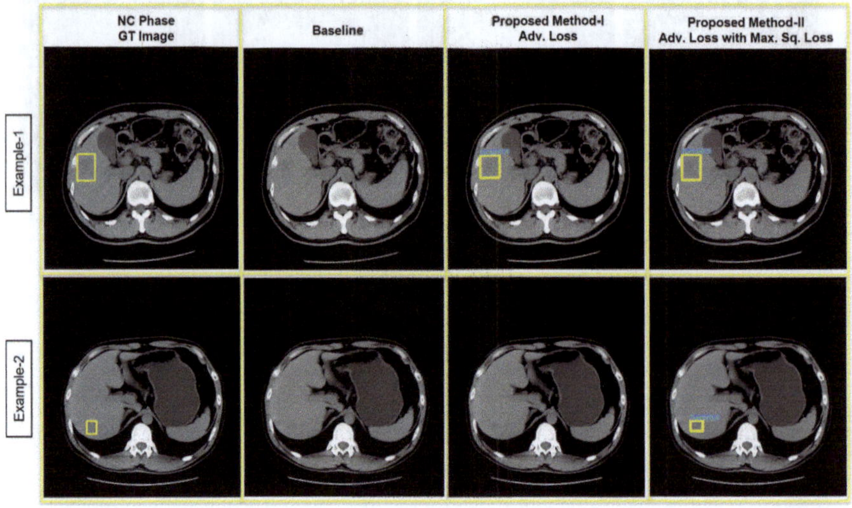

Fig. 4.7 Examples of liver tumor detection on NC phase images

phase images as the target domain (unlabeled). Table.4.5 shows the results using DLA34 backbone.

In the case of target-to-target training (NC-to-NC Phase) network obtains 57.2% (IoU-0.5) and 63.8% (IoU-0.3) accuracy. In direct transfer (model is trained in normal setting) from PV to NC phase, the network achieves 47.7% AP (IoU-0.5) and 52.8% AP (IoU-0.3) accuracy. Again, in comparison to training on the same phase images (NC-to-NC), the performance degradation occurs due to the domain shift as we used PV phase images for training whereas NC phase images for testing. Our domain adaptation method using adversarial learning (proposed method-I) shows an improvement and achieves 51.7% AP (IoU-0.5) and 57.3% AP (IoU-0.3) accuracy. Our domain adaptation-based approach using adversarial learning and maximum square loss (proposed method-II) shows a significant improvement and achieves 53.4% AP (IoU-0.5) and 59.5% AP (IoU-0.3) accuracy.

Figure 4.7 shows the detection results for some images from the NC phase. The proposed domain-adaptation approaches improve tumor detection performance in the NC phase as well. The t-SNE feature distribution of NC and PV liver images is shown

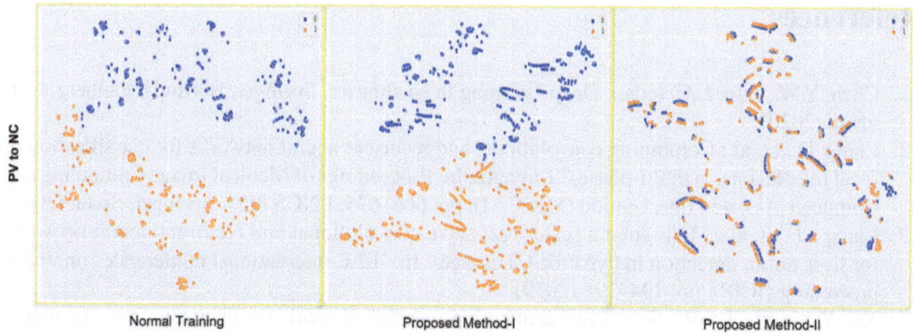

Fig. 4.8 Visualization of the t-SNE feature distributions of **NC** and **PV** liver tumor images. Feature maps distribution in normal training (Left), Proposed Method-I (middle) and Proposed Method-II (Right)

in Fig. 4.8 for normal training and proposed approaches. The feature distributions for NC and PV images are noticeably different in the normal training scheme. On the other hand, the proposed method-I (adversarial learning) brings the domain closer. Proposed method-II (maximum square loss and adversarial learning) is more effective at bringing the domain closer.

4.5 Conclusions

This chapter discusses maximum square loss and adversarial learning-based domain adaptation methods using an anchor-free object detector to address the domain-shift problem in multi-phase CT scan. To address data annotation and domain shift problems, in this chapter, we introduce a novel domain adaptation-based technique to align the domain gap between different CT phase images for liver tumor detection. We evaluate the proposed method on different phases of CT scan images. Our experimentation shows that the method can significantly improve model generalization towards new domains. Our methods significantly improve tumor detection accuracy in CT scans without using annotation of target domain images, according to the feature distribution analysis. Our approach reduces the labor-intensive annotations tasks for different CT scan phases. In future, we will investigate and develop more domain adaptation-based methods to mitigate the domain-shift problem.

Acknowledgements This work is supported in part by Grant-in Aid for Scientific Research from the Japanese Ministry for Education, Science, Culture and Sports (MEXT) under Grant No. 20KK0234, 21H03470 and 20K21821, in part by the Natural Science Foundation of Zhejiang Province under Grant No. LZ22F020012, in part by Major Scientific Research Project of Zhejiang Lab under Grant No. 2020ND8AD01

References

1. Chen, Y.W., Jain, L.C. (eds.): Deep Learning in Healthcare. Springer, Berlin/Heidelberg, Germany (2020)
2. Liang, D., et. al.: Combining convolutional and recurrent neural networks for classification of focal liver lesions in multi-phase CT images. In: Proceedings of Medical Image Computing and Computer Assisted Intervention (MICCAI), pp. 666–675. LNCS7951, Springer, Spain (2018)
3. Liang, D., et. al.: Multi-stream scale-insensitive convolutional and recurrent neural networks for liver tumor detection in dynamic CT images. In: IEEE international conferences on image processing (ICIP), pp. 794–798 (2019)
4. Xu, Y., et. al.: PA-ResSeg: a phase attention residual network for liver tumor segmentation from multi-phase CT images. Med. Phys. (**48**)(7), 3752-3766 (2021)
5. Vu, T.H., Jain, H., Bucher, M., Cord, M., Perez, P.: ADVENT: adversarial entropy minimization for domain adaptation in semantic segmentation. In: IEEE International Conferences on Computer Vision and Pattern Recognition, pp. 2512–2521. U.S. (2019)
6. Rongbo, S., Jianhua, Y., Yan, K., Tan, K., Jiang, C., Zhou, K.: Unsupervised domain adaptation with adversarial learning for mass detection in mammogram. Neurocomputing **393**, 27–37 (2020)
7. Chen, M., Xue, H., Cai, D.: Domain adaptation for semantic segmentation with maximum squares loss. In IEEE International Conferences on Computer Vision, pp. 2090–2099, Seoul, S. Korea (2019)
8. Jain, R.K., Watasue, T., Nakagawa, T., Sato, T., Iwamoto, Y., Ruan, X., Chen, Y.-W.: LogoNet: A robust layer-aggregated dual-attention ancho free logo detection framework with an adversarial domain adaptation approach. Appl. Sci. (**11**)(20), 9622 (2021)
9. Panfilov, E., Tiulpin, A., Klein, S., Nieminen, M.T., Saarakkala, S.: Improving robustness of deep learning based knee MRI segmentation Mixup and adversarial domain adaptation. In: IEEE International Conferences on Computer Vision Workshops (ICCVW), pp. 450–459. Seoul, S. Korea (2019)
10. Zhou, X., Wang, D., Kráhenbühl P.: Objects as Points. arXiv, arXiv:1904.07850 (2019)
11. Jain R.K., Sato T., Watasue T., Nakagawa T., Iwamoto Y., Han X., Lin L., Hu H., Ruan X., Chen Y.W.: Unsupervised domain adaptation with adversarial learning for liver tumors detection in multi-phase CT images. In: 10th International KES-InMed 2022 Conference (2022). (accepted)
12. Jain R.K., Sato T., Watasue T., Nakagawa T., Iwamoto Y., Han X., Lin L., Hu H., Ruan X., Chen Y.W.: Unsupervised domain adaptation using adversarial learning and maximum square loss for liver tumors detection in multi-phase CT images. In: 44th Annual International Conference of the IEEE Engineering in Medicine and Biology Society (EMBC) (2022). (accepted)
13. Lin, T.Y., Goyal, P., Girshick, R., He, K., Dollar, P.: Focal loss for dense object detection. In: IEEE International Conferences on Computer Vision, pp. 2999–3007. Venice, Italy (2017)
14. Yu, F., Wang, D., Shelhamer, E., Darrell, T.: Deep layer aggregation. In IEEE International Conference on Computer Vision and Pattern Recognition, pp. 2403–2412. Utah, U.S. (2018)
15. Xu, Y., et al.: Texture-Specific bag of visual words model and spatial cone matching based method for the retrieval of focal liver lesions using multiphase contrast-enhanced CT images. Int. J. Comput. Assisted Radiol. Surgery **13**, 151–164 (2018)
16. Wang, J., et al.: Tensor-based sparse representations of multi-phase medical images for classification of focal liver lesions. Pattern Recogn. Lett. **130**, 207–215 (2020)
17. Hasegawa, R., et al.: Automatic detection and segmentation of liver tumors in multi-phase CT images by phase attention mask R-CNN. In: IEEE International Conference on Consumer Electronics (ICCE), pp. 1–5. U.S. (2021)
18. Canny, J.: A Computational approach to edge detection. IEEE Trans. Pattern Anal. Mach. Intell. (**PAMI-8**)(6), 679-698 (1986)
19. Maaten, L.V.D., Hinton, G.: Visualizing data using t-SNE. J. Mach. Learn. Res. (**9**)(86), 2579–2605 (2008)

Chapter 5
Multi-stage Synthetic Image Generation for the Semantic Segmentation of Medical Images

Paolo Andreini, Simone Bonechi, Giorgio Ciano, Caterina Graziani, Veronica Lachi, Natalia Nikoloulopoulou, Monica Bianchini, and Franco Scarselli

Abstract Recently, deep learning methods have had a tremendous impact on computer vision applications, from image classification and semantic segmentation to object detection and face recognition. Nevertheless, the training of state-of-the-art neural network models is usually based on the availability of large sets of supervised data. Indeed, deep neural networks have a huge number of parameters which, to be properly trained, require a fairly large dataset of supervised examples. This problem is particularly relevant in the medical field due to privacy issues and the high cost of image tagging by medical experts. In this chapter, we present a new approach that allows to reduce this limitation by generating synthetic images with their corresponding supervision. In particular, this approach can be applied in semantic segmentation,

P. Andreini (✉) · G. Ciano · C. Graziani · V. Lachi · M. Bianchini · F. Scarselli
Department of Information Engineering and Mathematics, University of Siena, Siena, Italy
e-mail: paolo.andreini@unisi.it

G. Ciano
e-mail: giorgio.ciano@unifi.it

C. Graziani
e-mail: caterina.graziani@student.unisi.it

V. Lachi
e-mail: veronica.lachi@student.unisi.it

M. Bianchini
e-mail: monica@diism.unisi.it

F. Scarselli
e-mail: franco@diism.unisi.it

S. Bonechi
Department of Social, Political and Cognitive Sciences, University of Siena, Siena, Italy
e-mail: simone.bonechi@unisi.it

N. Nikoloulopoulou
Computer Engineering and Informatics, University of Patras, Patras, Greece
e-mail: nikoloul@ceid.upatras.gr

G. Ciano
Department of Information Engineering, University of Florence, Florence, Italy

© The Author(s), under exclusive license to Springer Nature Switzerland AG 2023

C.-P. Lim et al. (eds.), *Artificial Intelligence and Machine Learning for Healthcare*, Intelligent Systems Reference Library 228,
https://doi.org/10.1007/978-3-031-11154-9_5

where the generated images (and label-maps) can be used to augment real datasets during network training. The main characteristic of our method, differently from other existing techniques, lies in the generation procedure carried out in multiple steps, based on the intuition that, by splitting the procedure in multiple phases, the overall generation task is simplified. The effectiveness of the proposed multi-stage approach has been evaluated on two different domains, retinal fundus and chest X-ray images. In both domains, the multi-stage approach has been compared with the single-stage generation procedure. The results suggest that generating images in multiple steps is more effective and computationally cheaper, yet allowing high resolution, realistic images to be used for training deep networks.

5.1 Introduction

Deep Neural Networks (DNNs) have become the standard approach in semantic segmentation [1–3] and in many other computer vision tasks [4–7]. DNN training, however, requires large sets of accurately labeled data, making the availability of annotated images increasingly critical. Many real world applications exist for which collecting a huge amount of labeled data is hard and, to overcome this issue, some approaches were proposed to exploit weaker bounding-box annotations [8, 9]. From a different perspective, architectures with a reduced number of parameters, like U-net [10], were employed. In particular, in the medical field, the presence of privacy concerns and the high cost of image labeling makes it almost impossible to collect amounts of data comparable to ImageNet [11] or Coco [12].

Nevertheless, in recent years, the number of collaborations between machine learning experts and clinicians have grown exponentially, particularly for the automatic analysis of medical images. Many applications have been developed based on DNNs, ranging from the prediction of the risk of pneumonia [13], to the analysis of cerebral Nuclear Magnetic Resonance (NMR) for the diagnosis of neurodegenerative disorders [14], to the prognostic classification of skin lesions [15–17] up to segmentation of the 3D NMR images of the aorta for aneurysm and dissection prognosis [18]. Collecting a huge amount of data for these applications is critical because, in addition to privacy issues (meaning that the patients must give their consent), there is the difficulty in providing an appropriate supervision. In semantic segmentation, for example, a ground truth label-map is needed, where a class is assigned to each pixel in the image. Therefore, to obtain such a label-map, a doctor or an expert has to manually examine the image pixel by pixel—a very expensive task both in terms of time (in some cases could take hours for a single image) and resources. For this reason, generating synthetic labeled data is of great interest in this field, even if synthesizing high-resolution realistic medical images remains an open challenge.

Several techniques have been used to generate synthetic data over time. In addition to classical data augmentation approaches, Deep Learning (DL) methods can be applied to implicitly acquire a specific domain model from real data, which can be used to generate new data. A popular DL approach for this purpose is the Generative Adversarial Network (GAN) [19]. In this chapter, we propose new methods, based on GANs, to generate both realistic images and the corresponding label-maps. Their main feature is that, unlike other methods described in the literature, they are multi-stage, that is, they are composed of several phases. By splitting the generation procedure in steps, in fact, we simplify the generation task so that simpler models can be used and, more importantly, a smaller number of examples are required for their training. The experiments have confirmed that, with a multi-stage generation procedure, we were able to produce images with a higher quality, which can be used to enrich semantic segmentation datasets. In particular, the proposed methods were employed on two medical image tasks with different characteristics: retinal and Chest X-ray (CXR) image segmentation. The aim of the former task is to identify blood vessels in retinal images while, in the latter, the goal is to determine which pixels belong to lungs and heart.

From the medical point of view, retinal vessels are very important because the ocular fundus is the only part of human circulation that can be directly and non-invasively visualized in vivo [20]. Hence, it can be easily acquired and analyzed by automatic tools, allowing the diagnosis of diseases that go well beyond the eye pathologies, but extend to all major circulatory and metabolic disorders [21, 22]. In all these applications an important processing step is the correct segmentation of the retinal vessels, which can be used to extract various quantitative vessels' parameters, helping more objective and accurate medical diagnoses, treatments, and monitoring of diseases such as diabetic retinopathy, hypertension, and arteriosclerosis [23, 24]. Moreover, retinal fundus images have a multitude of applications, including biometric identification and computer-assisted laser surgery. We propose a generative approach, that can be used as a data augmentation tool for the automatic segmentation of retinal images, which consists of two distinct phases. In the first stage, the typical distribution of blood vessels is learned from data by a GAN, thus defining the semantic label-map. In the second phase, an image-to-image translation algorithm is trained to transform the label-map into a synthetic image.

As for chest radiography (CXR), it is one of the most used techniques in the world for the diagnosis of various diseases, such as pneumonia, tuberculosis, infiltration, heart failure and lung cancer. Chest radiographs have enormous advantages: they are inexpensive, radiographic equipment is available even in the poorest areas of the world, and, in addition, the interpretation/reporting of radiographs is less operator dependent than the results of other more advanced techniques, such as computed tomography (CT) and magnetic resonance imaging (MRI). Furthermore, undergoing this exam is very fast and minimally invasive [25]. Recently, CXR images have gained even greater importance due to COVID-19, which mainly causes lung infection and, after healing, often leaves widespread signs of pulmonary fibrosis: the respiratory tissue affected by the infection loses its characteristics and its normal structure. Consequently, CXR images are often used for the diagnosis of COVID-19 and for the treatment of the after-effects of SARS-CoV-2 [26–28]. For the segmentation of chest X-ray images, which involves the identification of multiple classes, a three-stage approach is employed, which adds a further step at the beginning of the generative procedure. In particular, in the first stage, the position of each anatomical part is generated and represented by a "dot" within the image; in the second stage, semantic labels are obtained from the dots; finally, the CXR image is generated. It is worth noting that, while in the procedure described in this chapter the positions of the dots are automatically generated, the dots may be manually positioned within the image in order to have a tool that can generate objects at predefined positions.

The chapter is organized as follows. In Sect. 5.2, an overview of the literature related to this work is given. In Sect. 5.3, we describe the proposed generation models and the segmentation network used. In Sect. 5.4, we present some images generated for the two tasks and the respective results obtained in the segmentation phase. Finally, some conclusions and possible future developments are reported in Sect. 5.5.

5.2 Related Works

This chapter is focused mainly on image generation and segmentation. In this section we will present a review of the literature on these topics. Moreover, we will see how the latest synthetic image generation and segmentation techniques have been used in the two applications considered in this work.

5.2.1 Synthetic Image Generation

Methods for generating images can be classified into two main categories: model-based and learning-based approaches. The standard procedure is to formulate a model of the observed data and to render the images using a dedicated engine. For example, this approach has been used to extend the available datasets of driving scenes in urban environments [29, 30] or for object detection [31]. One of the fields that has mostly employed the generation of synthetic images is that of medical image analysis. For instance, realistic digital brain-phantom has been synthesized in [32], while, more recently, synthetic agar plate images have been generated for image segmentation [33–35]. A deep understanding of the specific domain and an accurate model of the scene are required for designing specialized engines for data generation. For this reason, in recent years, the learning-based approach has attracted increasing research resources. Through machine learning techniques, the probability distribution underlying the set of real images can be learned. The information obtained is exploited to generate synthetic images that can be used to extend existing datasets for training machine learning models. One of the most successful machine learning model for data generation is represented by Generative Adversarial Networks (GANs) [19] that are normally used to create images that resemble real data. An extension of the GAN architecture is the Progressive Growing of GAN (PGGAN) [36] that allows a more stable training and is capable of producing High Definition (HD) images. Two further upgrades of PGGANs were made in [37, 38]. GANs have been used in [39] to augment data for a patch-based approach to OCT chorio-retinal boundary segmentation. In [40], synthetic CXR images are generated by developing an Auxiliary Classifier Generative Adversarial Network (ACGAN) model, called CovidGAN. Synthetic images produced by CovidGAN were used to improve the performance of a standard CNN for detecting COVID-19. In [41], Wasserstein GANs (WGANs) and InfoGANs have been combined to classify histopathological images, whereas in [42] WGAN and CatGAN generated images were used to improve the classification of dermoscopic images. In [43], synthetic abnormal MR images containing brain tumors were generated. An image-to-image translation algorithm was employed to construct semantic label-maps of real MR brain images, with distortions introduced on the generated segmentation (i.e., tumors are shrunk or enlarged, or their position is changed), and then the segmentation is translated back to images. Indeed, the manual introduction of distortions on the generated label-maps is not trivial because they can alter the semantics of the image. We solve this problem directly by learning the semantic label-map distribution with a GAN.

5.2.2 *Image-to-Image Translation*

Recently, beside image generation, adversarial learning has also been extended to image-to-image translation, which is aimed at converting an input image from one domain to another. In general, both unsupervised [44–47] and supervised approaches [36, 48, 49] can be used. For the proposed applications, the unsupervised category is not relevant. Supervised training uses a set of pairs of corresponding images $\{(s_i, t_i)\}$, where s_i is an image of the source domain and t_i is the corresponding image in the target domain. Usually, Conditional GANs (CGANs), a particular type of GAN which constrain the generation based on some auxiliary information, are used for translation. For an example, Pix2Pix [49] is a CGAN that operates with supervision, and Pix2PixHD [50] employs a coarse-to-fine generator and discriminator, along with a feature-matching loss function, to translate images with higher resolution and quality.

5.2.3 *Retinal Image Synthesis and Segmentation*

One of the first applications of retinal image synthesis has been described in the seminal work [51], in which an anatomic model of the eye and of the surrounding face has been implemented for surgical simulations. Thereafter, several approaches has been used for retinal image synthesis. In particular, many models rely on a pre-existing vessel network. In [52], for example, an image-to-image translation model has been employed to transform existing vessel networks into realistic retinal images. Vessel networks used for learning have been obtained using a suitable segmentation technique applied to a set of real retinal images. However, the quality of the generated images heavily depends on the segmentation module performance. Instead, in order to avoid the dependence of the model on the availability of pre-existent vessel maps, in [53], an adversarial auto-encoder for retinal vessel synthesis has been adopted. Nevertheless, this approach is able to generate only low resolution images, and the performance for vessel segmentation using synthesized data is far below the state-of-the-art. Higher resolution retinal images, along with their segmentation label-maps, have been generated in [54], using Progressively Growing GANs (PGGANs) [36], though without evaluating their quality. Differently, in this chapter, generated images are indirectly evaluated by measuring their effectiveness as a data augmentation tools. Retinal vessel segmentation is a challenging task because of the retina complex structure. Nonetheless, it plays a fundamental role in automatic disease diagnosis. During the last decades, several approaches for retinal vessel segmentation have been proposed. Among them, deep learning methods are those providing better results. For instance, in [55], a fully convolutional network [2] was described, with an AlexNet [7] encoder. Fully convolutional networks have also been used in [56, 57] and [58], where a stationary wavelet transform pre-processing step is introduced to improve the network performance. Finally, in [59], a CNN was pre-trained on image patches and then fine-tuned at the image level. Also other neural network architectures have been used for the segmentation of retinal images. A modified U-Net [10] was used in [60] to exploit a combination between a segment-level loss and a pixel-level loss to deal with the unbalanced ratio between thick and thin vessels in fundus images. Moreover, a deep supervision was incorporated in some intermediate layers of a VGG network [61] in [62, 63].

5.2.4 Chest X-ray Image Synthesis and Segmentation

X-rays are inexpensive, non-invasive and fast examinations; for this reason, they are one of the most widely used techniques in medical diagnostics. However, due to overlapping organs, low resolution and subtle anatomical shape and size variations, interpreting CXRs accurately remains challenging and requires highly qualified and trained personnel. Therefore, it is of great clinical and scientific interest to develop computer-based systems that support the analysis of CXRs. In particular, the segmentation of CXR images is important in medical applications as it allows for the extraction of anatomical structures in view of the diagnosis of related diseases. Because of the lack of publicly available datasets of chest radiographs, an image generation process is needed in order to succeed in the segmentation task. In the related literature, several methods has been used for CXR image generation. Only in a few cases have GANs been used to generate chest X-ray images, as in [64], where images for cardiac abnormality classification were obtained with a semi-supervised architecture, or in [65], where GANs were used to generate low resolution (64×64) CXRs to diagnose pneumonia.

Detecting and segmenting the lung region out of the chest X-ray images is fundamental for computer-aided diagnosis of lung diseases. A method for lung field segmentation, based on joint shape and appearance sparse learning, was proposed in [66], while a technique for landmark detection was presented in [67]. *Inverted-Net*, an architecture able to segment the heart, clavicles and lungs, was introduced in [68]. This network employs a loss function based on the Dice Coefficient, Exponential Linear Unit (ELU) activation functions, and a model architecture that aims at containing the number of parameters. Moreover, the U-Net [10] architecture has been widely used for lung segmentation, as in [69–71]. In the Structure Correcting Adversarial Network (SCAN) [72], a segmentation network and a critic network were jointly trained with an adversarial mechanism for organ segmentation in chest X-rays.

5.3 Multi-stage Image Synthesis

The main objective of this chapter is to present the proposed multi-stage generation approach. The rationale behind this method is that by dividing the generation problem into several simpler stages, the quality of the synthetic images should improve while also reducing the computational burden required to generate them. Each step of the proposed multi-stage generation approach is implemented by a GAN. More precisely, we adopt Progressively Growing GANs (PGGANs) [36], an extension of GANs that allows the generation of high resolution images, and Pix2PixHD [50] for the translation step. In Sect. 5.3.1 the single-stage approach, used as baseline, the two-stage and the three-stage generation approaches were presented. It should be noted that, in principle, the number of steps that can be used to generate an image depends on the semantics of the image to be synthesized. In this work, we have compared the two and three-step approaches; however, the proposed procedure could be extended using more steps if needed for a specific domain.

5.3.1 Image Generation

In the following, the three different image generation approaches, based on a different number of steps, are briefly sketched.

Single-Stage Generation

With the single-stage method (see Fig. 5.1) the label-map and the image are generated simultaneously, stacked in two different channels of the generation network output. This means that a single GAN architecture is used and optimized to learn the distribution of both the semantic label-maps and the corresponding images. The GAN architecture that was used for the single-stage generation is the PGGAN. In this model, the generation procedure starts at a low resolution, which is then progressively increased by adding new layers to the networks. Indeed, the generator and the discriminator are symmetric and grow in sync (see Fig. 5.2). The transition from the generation of low to high resolution images allows to increase the quality and the stability of the procedure. In our setup, the training starts with both the generator and

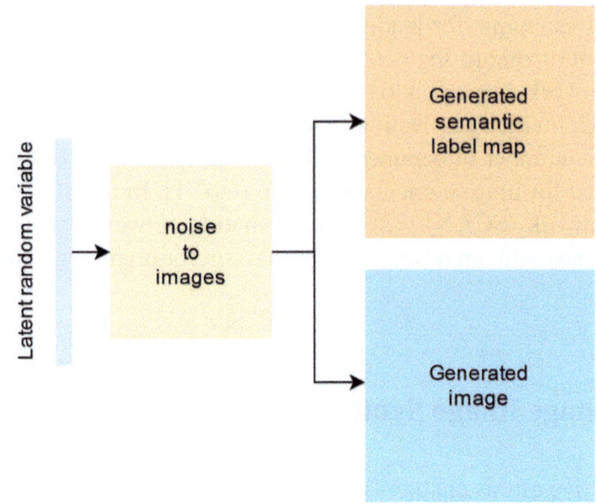

Fig. 5.1 Single-stage image generation scheme

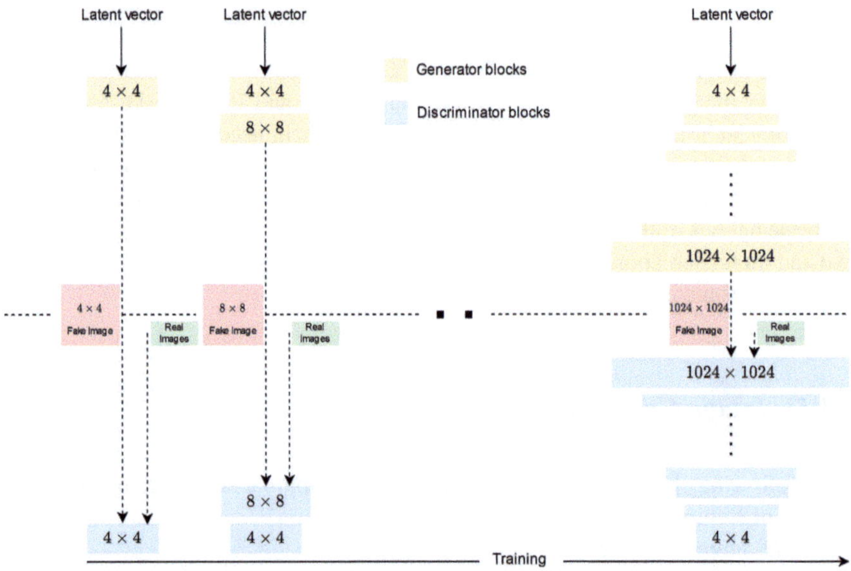

Fig. 5.2 PGGAN training scheme. The resolution of the generator (G) and the discriminator (D) was progressively increased until the final desired resolution is reached

the discriminator having a spatial resolution of 4×4 pixels, progressively increasing until the final resolution is reached. The Wasserstein loss, with a gradient penalty [73], was used as the loss function for the discriminator.

Images and label-maps are generated simultaneously by the network; the generator output is a four channel image where the three color channels are concatenated with

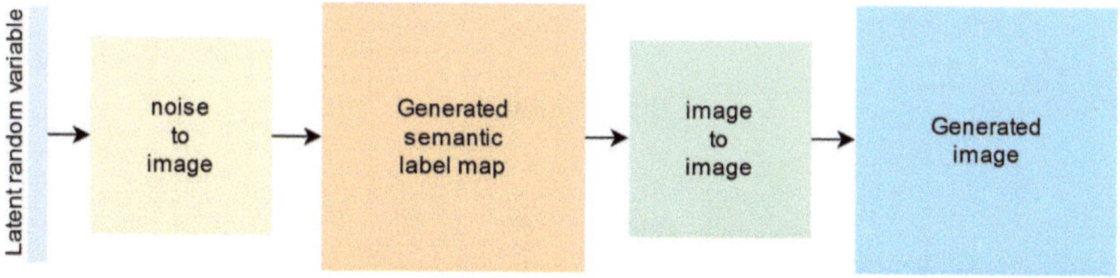

Fig. 5.3 The proposed two-step image generation method

the label-map. PGGANs have also been employed, in different ways, in the first phase of both the multi-stage approaches presented below. In particular, they will be used to generate the label-maps in the two-stage approach and to generate the points, which represent the position of the objects, in the three-stage approach.

Two-Stage Generation

The proposed generation procedure is composed of two steps (see Fig. 5.3): the first one involves the generation of semantic label-maps while, in the second, the synthesis of realistic images, based on the label-maps, is carried out.
In particular, the first stage is based on a PGGAN, like in the single-stage approach, but trained to produce only semantic label-maps. The semantic label-maps encapsulate the semantic structure of the scene by indicating the type of object that would be generated in each pixel of the image. Once the semantic label-maps are obtained, they are translated in the output image by using an image-to-image translation approach. The translation is based on Pix2PixHD [50], a supervised image-to-image translation framework derived from Pix2Pix [49]. In Pix2Pix, a conditional GAN learns to generate the output conditioned on the corresponding input image. The generator has an encoder-decoder structure: it takes in input images belonging to a certain domain A, and generates images in a different domain B. The discriminator observes pairs of images, and the image of A is provided as input along with the corresponding image of B (real or generated). The discriminator aims to distinguish between real and fake (generated) pairs. Pix2PixHD improves upon Pix2Pix by introducing a coarse to fine generator consisting of two subnets operating at different resolutions. A multiscale discriminator was also employed, with an adversarial loss that incorporates a feature-matching loss for training stabilization. In our setup, the semantic label-maps, previously generated, were fed into the generator, which is trained to generate the final images. An overview of the proposed setup is given in Fig. 5.4.

Three-Stage Generation In this approach, a further, preliminary step is added which allows to generate the position and type of objects, that will be generated later, regardless of their shape or appearance. In particular, label-maps containing "dots"—that can be considered as "seeds"—with a specific value for each object, are created. The position of the "dot" center is given by the centroid of each labeled object. This map was generated in low resolution (64×64), as a high level of detail is not needed, since at this stage we are only interested in the position of the object regardless of its shape. It should be observed that this also allows a significant reduction in the

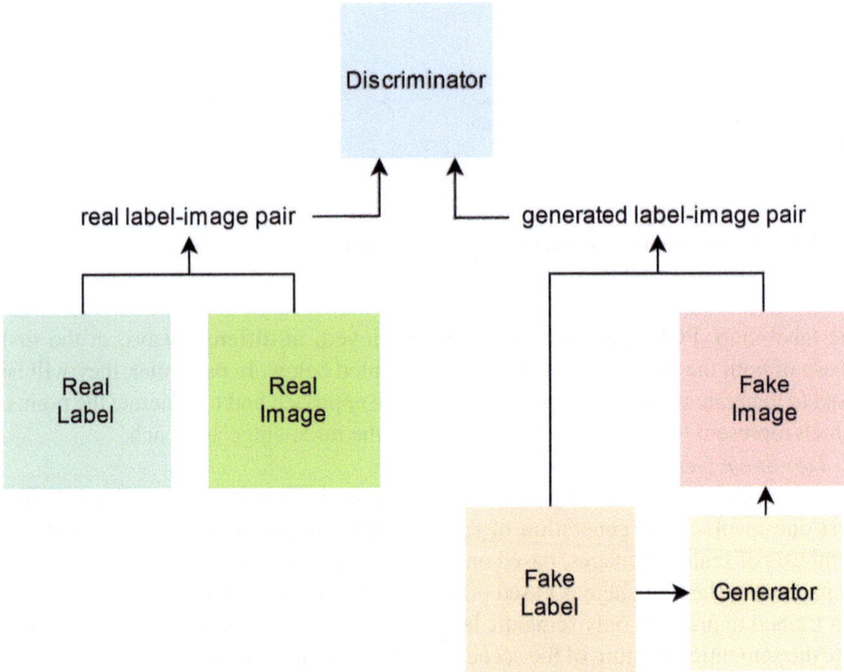

Fig. 5.4 Scheme of the Pix2PixHD training framework employed to translate label-maps into images

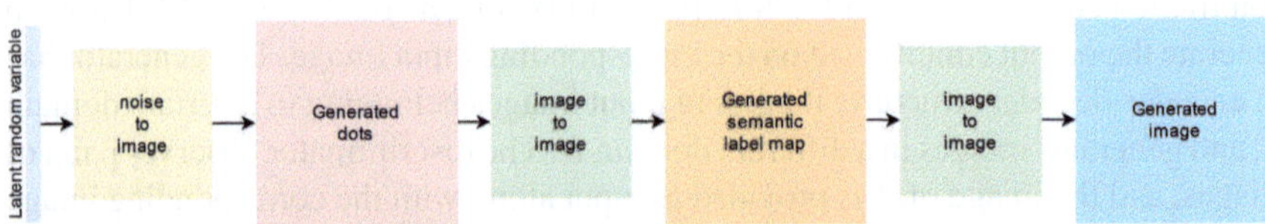

Fig. 5.5 The proposed three-stage image generation method

computational burden of this stage and speeds up the computation. The generated object map must be subsequently resized to the original image resolution, using a nearest neighbour interpolation approach, to maintain the original code of each object. The maps should have the same resolution of the original images before their translation into labels and then into images, using Pix2PixHD (see Fig. 5.5).

5.4 Evaluation of Multi-stage Methods

In this section the experiments that were carried out to evaluate the quality of the different generation methods are described. In particular, in Sect. 5.4.1 we introduce the datasets used to generate the syntetic images and to train the segmentation network. The neural network employed for semantic segmentation is briefly illustrated in Sect. 5.4.2 and the experimental setup is described in Sect. 5.4.3. Finally, Sect. 5.4.4 and Sect. 5.4.5 show the results obtained with the two and the three-stage generation methods on retinal images and chest radiographic images, respectively.

5.4.1 Datasets

The experiments were conducted in two different domains, blood vessel segmentation in retinal images and organ segmentation in chest X-rays. The datasets used for the experiments in both domains are described below.

5.4.1.1 Retinal Image Datasets

Two publicly available datasets, both containing a very small number of examples, were employed for retinal image analysis.

- DRIVE dataset—The DRIVE dataset [74] includes 40 retinal fundus images of size $584 \times 565 \times 3$ (20 images for training and 20 for test). The images were collected by a screening program for diabetic retinopathy in the Netherlands. Among the 40 photos, 33 showed no diabetic retinopathy, while 7 showed mild early diabetic retinopathy. The segmentation ground-truth was provided both for the training and the test sets.
- CHASE_DB1 dataset—The CHASE_DB1 dataset [75] is composed by 28 fundus images of size $960 \times 999 \times 3$, corresponding to the left and right eyes of 14 children. Each image is annotated by two independent human experts. An officially defined split between training and test is not provided for this dataset. In our experiments, we adopted the same strategy as [60, 76], selecting the first 20 images for training and the remaining 8 for testing the network.

5.4.1.2 Chest X-ray Dataset

The experiments in this domain were carried out using the JSRT [77] dataset collected by the Japanese Society of Radiological Technology (JSRT). The dataset consists of 247 CXRs. The image size is 2048×2048 pixels, with a spatial resolution of 0.175 mm/pixel and 12 bit gray levels. Furthermore, segmentation supervisions for the JSRT database are available in the Segmentation in the Chest Radiographs (SCR) dataset [78]. More precisely, this dataset provides chest X-ray supervisions which correspond with the pixel-level positions of the different anatomical parts. Such supervisions were produced by two observers who annotated five classes in each image: the two lungs, the heart and the two clavicles. The first observer was a medical student and his segmentation was used as the gold standard, while the second observer was a computer science student, specialized in medical imaging, and his segmentation was considered that of a human expert. The SCR dataset comes with an official splitting, which is employed in our experiments and consists of 124 images for learning and 123 for testing.

5.4.2 Segmentation Network

All the experiments in this work were carried out with the Segmentation Multiscale Attention Network (SMANet), originally proposed for scene text segmentation [79]. The SMANET comprises three main components: a ResNet encoder, a multi-scale attention module, and a convolutional decoder. The architecture is based on the PSPNet [3], a deep fully convolutional neural network with a ResNet [80] encoder followed by a pooling pyramid to gather context information. In the encoder, dilated convolutions (i.e., atrous convolutions [81]) were used in place of standard convolutions. In addition, in the SMANet, a multi-scale attention mechanism is employed to focus on the relevant objects present in the image, while a two-level convolutional decoder is added to the architecture to better handle the presence of thin objects.

5.4.3 Experimental Setup

To evaluate the different generation methods presented in Sect. 5.3, a fixed number of images with the corresponding label-maps have been generated, by employing the single-stage, the two-stage and the three-stage approaches. The generated data have been used to train a segmentation network which has been tested on a common test set. The rationale behind this approach is that higher quality images, that better capture the underlying distribution of real data, should produce better results when used to train the segmentation network. In particular, the following experimental configurations were used:

- SYNTH (S)—the segmentation network was trained using only the generated synthetic images;
- REAL (R)—only real data were used to train the semantic segmentation network;
- SYNTH + REAL (SR)—synthetic data were used to pre-train the semantic segmentation network and real data were employed for fine-tuning.

This experimental setup was used to evaluate the different multi-stage generation procedures on two distinct domains. Specifically, retinal images were used to assess improvement in the effectiveness of a two-stage generation approach compared to a single-stage generation. An effective generation method can be particularly useful in this domain since, when synthetic images are used for data augmentation, they compensate for the lack of large annotated datasets. The number of generation steps that is worth employing depends on the domain; for instance, if multiple objects are present in the image, an additional generation stage can be useful to model the position of the objects. Retinal images cannot be used with this aim, having only a single entity to be segmented (the blood vessels). For this reason, chest X-ray images, that contain multiple organs in different positions, have been employed to evaluate the three-stage procedure.

5.4.4 Two-Stage Method Evaluation

To demonstrate that a two-stage generation is capable of producing higher quality images than a single-stage approach, we decided to compare these two strategies. In particular, following the method described in Sect. 5.3.1, we generated synthetic images using both the single and the two-stage approach and evaluated them both qualitatively and quantitatively. Some qualitative results of the generated images, with the single and the two-stage approach, compared with real images of the DRIVE and CHASE_DB1 datasets are given in Figs. 5.6 and 5.7.

Moreover, in Fig. 5.8, a zoom on a random patch of a high resolution generated image shows that the image-to-image translation allows us to effectively translate the generated vessel structures in retinal images by maintaining the semantic information provided by the semantic label-map.

It is worth noting that, although most of the generated samples closely resemble real retinal fundus images, few examples are clearly sub-optimal (see Fig. 5.9, which shows disconnected vessels and an unrealistic optical disc).

To further validate the quality of the two-stage generation process, a sub-sample of 100 synthetically generated retinal images were examined by an expert ophthalmologist. The evaluation showed that 35% of the images are of medium-high quality. The remaining 65% is visually appealing but contains small details that reveal an unnatural anatomy, such as an optical disc with feathered edges—which actually occur only in the case of specific diseases—or blood vessels that pass too close to the macula—while usually, except in the case of malformations, the macular region is avascular or at least paucivascular.

The proposed method was also compared with other learning-based approaches for retinal image generation that can be found in literature [52–54, 82] and we observed that our system is capable of synthesizing higher resolution images, with fewer training samples. Unfortunately, a direct quantitative comparison with them was not possible because they did not evaluate the use of synthetic images for semantic segmentation. Instead, in this work, to further demonstrate the effectiveness of synthetic images, we evaluated the effect of their inclusion during network training, which indirectly guarantees the high quality of the generated data. This approach, similar to [83], is based on the assumption that the performance of a deep learning architecture on real images can be directly related with the quality and vari-

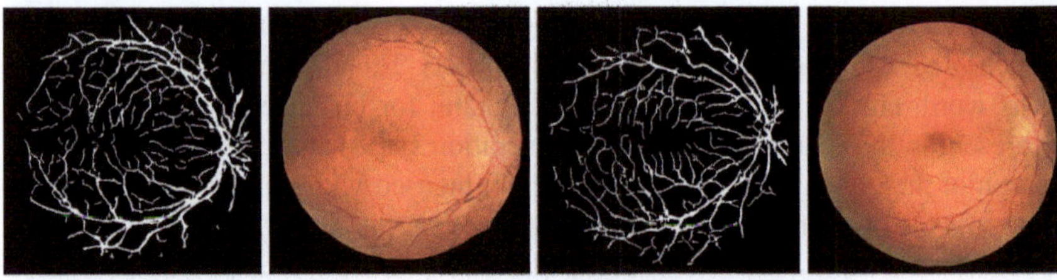

(a) Generated DRIVE images with the two–step method.

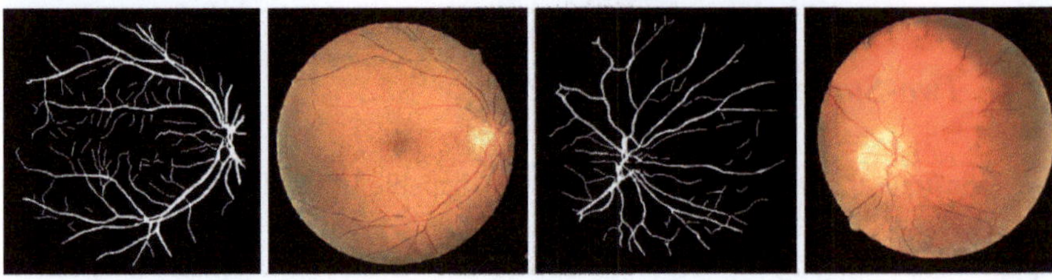

(b) Generated DRIVE images with the single–step method.

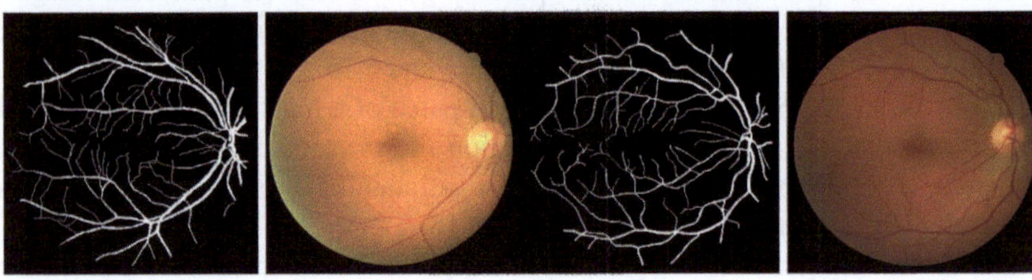

(c) Real DRIVE images.

Fig. 5.6 Examples of real and generated DRIVE images along with their label-maps

ety of GAN-generated images. The experimental setup described in Sect. 5.4.3 was employed to compare the quality of the generated images, with the single and two-stage methods, for both the DRIVE and the CHASE_DB1 datasets. The results obtained for the vessel segmentation are shown in Table 5.1. The Jaccard Index J, also called Intersection Over Union (IOU), the Area Under the Roc Curve (AUC) and the Accuracy were employed to measure the quality of the produced segmentation. The Jaccard Index is a standard measure to evaluate segmentation and it measures the similarity between two finite sample sets—the predicted segmentation and the target mask in this case—and is defined as the size of their intersection divided by the size of their union. We choose also to employed AUC to evaluate the quality of the segmentation network because it was widely used in the other retinal images segmentation approaches found in literature.

It can be observed that better results are obtained in all the configurations when using the two-stage generation approach. In particular, if we consider the SYNTH setup, we can notice that the AUC increases respectively by 5.01% and 31.68% in

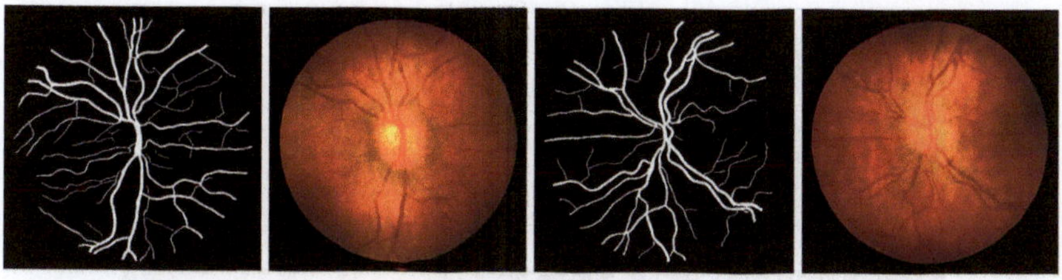

(a) Generated CHASE_DB1 images with the two–step method.

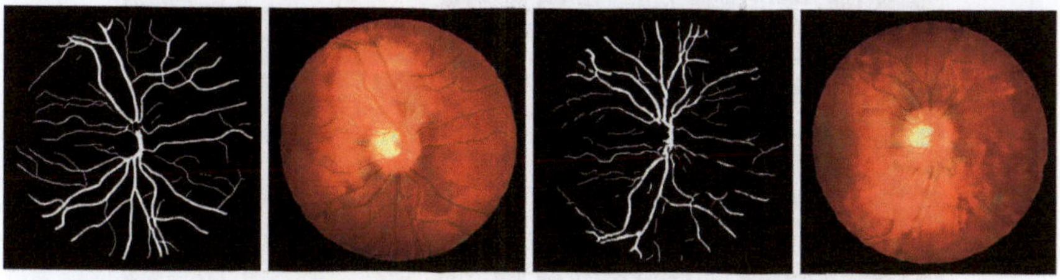

(b) Generated CHASE_DB1 images with the single–step method.

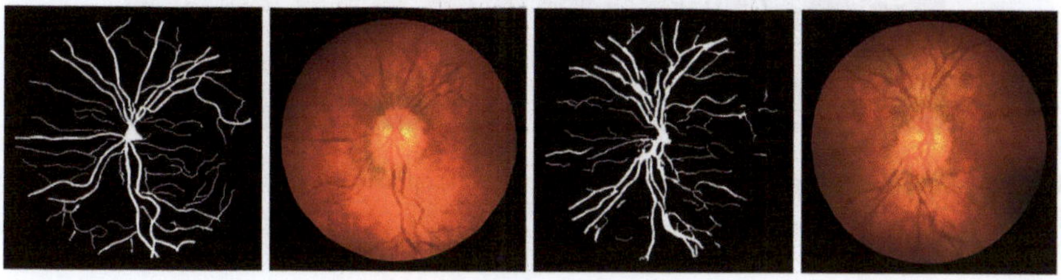

(c) Real CHASE_DB1 images.

Fig. 5.7 Examples of real and generated CHASE_DB1 images along with their label-maps

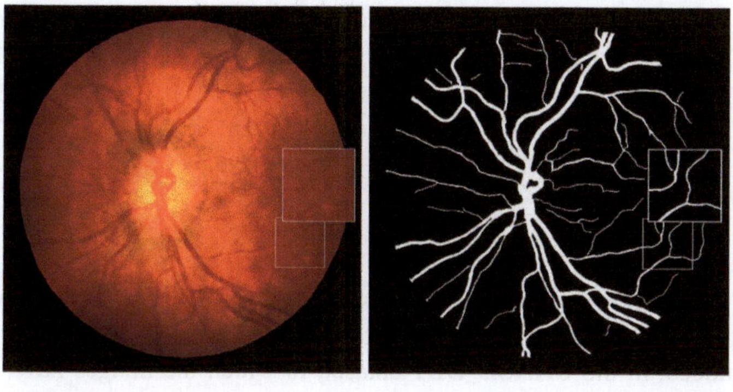

Fig. 5.8 Example of a generated image (resolution 1024 × 1024) with the corresponding label-map from the CHASE_DB1 dataset

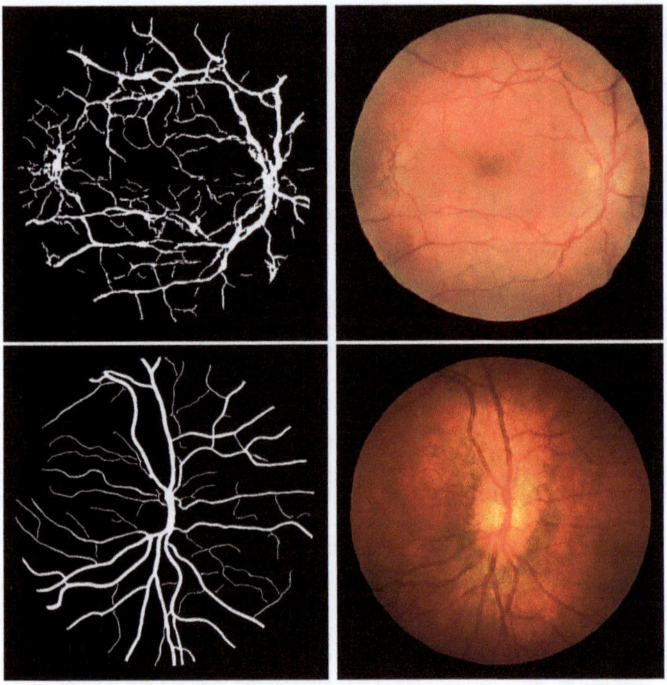

Fig. 5.9 Examples of generated images with an unrealistic optical disc and vasculature from DRIVE (**top**) and CHASE _DB1 (**bottom**)

Table 5.1 Segmentation performance on DRIVE and CHASE_DB1 datasets

Dataset	Metric	Real (%)	Single-stage		Two-stage	
			S (%)	**SR** (%)	**S** (%)	**SR** (%)
DRIVE	AUC	98.48	93.49	98.57	98.50	98.65
	Accuracy	96.87	91.01	96.88	96.88	96.90
	J	82.51	63.53	82.82	82.67	82.60
CHASE_DB1	AUC	98.82	66.96	98.87	98.64	99.16
	Accuracy	97.50	92.62	97.65	97.49	97.72
	J	81.31	46.76	82.95	82.36	83.63

the DRIVE and CHASE_DB1 datasets, respectively, when the two-stage approach is used instead of the single-stage. As expected, the gap increases for higher resolution images; indeed, in the CHASE_DB1 dataset, in which the images have twice the resolution of the DRIVE dataset, the single-step generated images alone are not enough to properly train a deep network. Furthermore, the semantic segmentation network, trained on the synthetic data generated in two steps, produces results very similar to those obtained by training only on real data. This demonstrates that the two-stage generation procedure effectively captures the real distribution of the data,

Table 5.2 A comparison with the state-of-the-art vessel segmentation methods on the DRIVE and CHASE_DB1 datasets

	DRIVE		CHASE_DB1	
Methods	AUC (%)	Acc (%)	AUC (%)	Acc (%)
[55]	96.80	95.93	95.80	95.91
[76]	97.38	95.27	97.16	95.81
[56]	97.44	95.33	–	–
[60]	97.52	95.42	97.81	96.10
[63]	97.82	95.21	98.12	95.99
[84]	97.90	95.35	98.45	95.77
[57]	97.92	95.60	–	–
[58]	98.21	95.76	98.55	96.53
[59]	**98.74**	**96.90**	98.78	97.37
Our	98.65	**96.90**	**99.16**	**97.72**

so that the produced images can be used to adequately train a deep neural network. If fine-tuning with real data is applied, after pre-training with synthetic data only, the results further improve with respect to the use of real data only. This fact indicates that the generated data can be effectively used to enlarge small training sets, such as DRIVE and CHASE_DB1.

Finally, Table 5.2 compares the segmentation results obtained with our best model (network trained with the two-stage synthetic images and fine-tuning on real images) with other state-of-the-art techniques.

The results show that our approach achieves state-of-the-art on the DRIVE dataset, where it is only surpassed by [59] based on the AUC, and outperforms all other methods on CHASE_DB1. It is worth pointing out that the experimental setups adopted by the previous approaches are various and that a perfect comparison was impossible. For example, CHASE_DB1 does not provide an explicit training/test split and, in [60, 76], the same split as in this paper was employed, while in [58, 59, 63] a four fold cross-validation strategy was applied. Moreover, in [84], only patches that were fully inside the field of view were considered. However, even with such inevitable experimental limits, the results of Table 5.2 suggest that the proposed method is promising and is at least as good as the best state-of-the-art techniques.

5.4.5 Three-Stage Method Evaluation

To evaluate the three-stage generation approach, images containing multiple objects were needed. For this reason we have chosen chest X-rays, where we have to generate different types of objects (organs) within the image. The results of the three-stage generation approach were compared with those obtained with only one and two steps. A

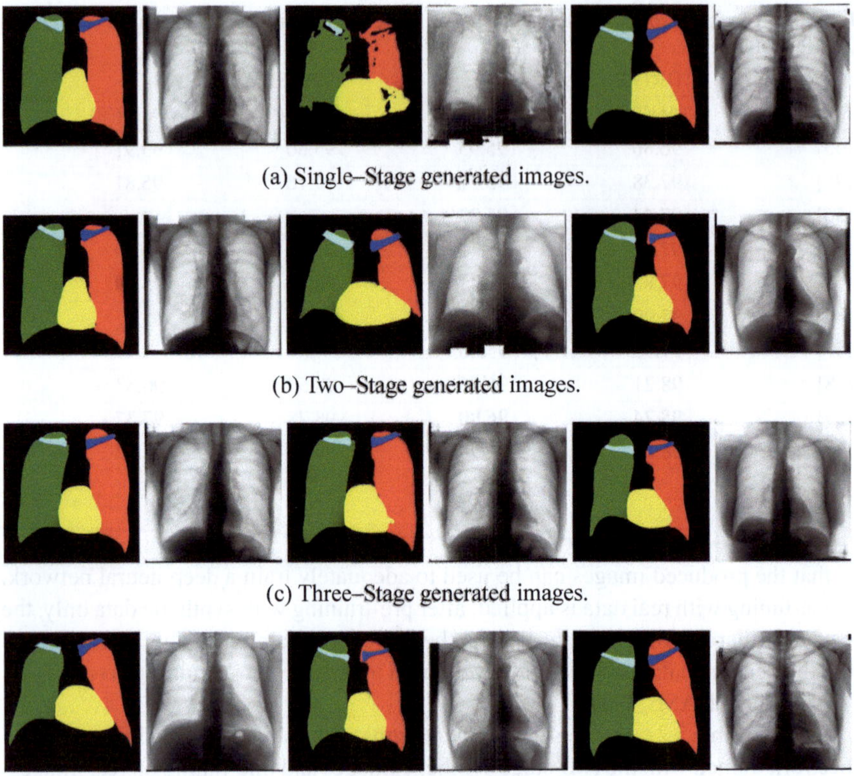

(a) Single–Stage generated images.

(b) Two–Stage generated images.

(c) Three–Stage generated images.

(d) Real images.

Fig. 5.10 Examples of generated images, with their label-maps, based on the SCR dataset

generation procedure is normally used when few images are available. In the present study, to simulate this situation, we employed only 10% of the SCR dataset and we generated synthetic images, with single, two and three-stage, following the procedure described in Sect. 5.3.1. Synthetic images generated with different strategies were evaluated both qualitatively and quantitatively. Some qualitative results are given in Fig. 5.10, where generated images are compared with real images extracted from the SCR dataset.

We can observe that, with the single and two-stage methods, the images tend to be more similar to those belonging to the training set. For example, in most of the generated images there are white rectangles, which resemble those present in the training images, used to cover the names of both the patient and the hospital. Instead, the three-stage method does not produce such artifacts, suggesting that it is less prone to overfitting. To quantitatively asses the quality of the generated images we employed the experimental setup described in Sect. 5.4.3 to compare the three strategies based on the SCR dataset. A good performance of the segmentation network indicates

Table 5.3 Segmentation performance on the SCR datasets

Metric	Organ	Real	Single-stage		Two-stage		Three-stage	
			S (%)	SR (%)	S (%)	SR (%)	S (%)	SR (%)
J	Left lung	93.70	55.59	74.11	94.91	94.4	94.96	95.29
	Heart	85.50	0.07	37.47	86.98	85.21	87.27	87.47
	Right lung	93.70	52.78	79.99	95.90	95.44	95.90	95.92
	Average	90.97	36.15	63.86	92.60	91.68	92.71	92.89
DSC	Left lung	96.75	71.46	85.13	97.39	97.12	97.42	97.59
	Heart	92.18	0.13	54.51	93.04	92.02	93.20	93.32
	Right lung	96.74	69.09	88.89	97.91	97.66	97.90	97.92
	Average	95.22	46.89	76.18	96.11	95.60	96.17	96.28

that the generated data successfully capture the true distribution of real samples. The Jaccard Index J and the Dice Score, a *quotient of similarity between sets* that ranges between 0 and 1, were used to evaluate the segmentation. Table 5.3 reports the segmentation results for the SCR dataset.

As we can notice the three-stage method outperforms both the two-stage and the single-stage procedures, even when both the other two approaches were followed by a fine-tuning on real data. The training with the three-stage generation process allowed to obtain better performance on the segmentation of all the organs. These results confirm our claim that splitting the generation procedure may provide a better performance when multiple objects should be generated within the same image. Finally, it is worth noting that fine-tuning improves the performance of the three-stage method but not of the two-stage one. This behaviour may be explained by some complementary information that is captured from real images only with the three-stage method. Actually, we may argue that, in different phases of a multi-stage approach, different types of information can be collected: such a diversification seems to provide an advantage to the three-stage method, which develops some capability to model the data domain with more orthogonal information.

Moreover, in order to evaluate the three-stage method, we assessed the quality of the segmentation results based on three human experts, who were asked to check 20 chest X-ray synthetic images, along with the corresponding synthetic label-maps and the segmentation obtained by the SMANet. Such images were chosen among those that can be considered difficult, at least based on the high error obtained by the segmentation algorithm. The three physicians were asked to choose the best organ segmentation and to motivate their choice. The three doctors shared the common opinion that, on average, the images generated are of good quality and that both the network segmentation and the label-map provided by the three-step method are fairly accurate. Surprisingly, they often tended to prefer the generated image because of a more precise organ segmentation.

Table 5.4 Comparison of segmentation results among different methods on the SCR dataset (CV stands for cross-validation). The values in parentheses in the evaluation scheme of the SCAN method correspond to the split between the training and test sets

Method	Image size	Augmentation	Evaluation scheme	Lungs		Heart	
				DSC	J	DSC	J
Human [78]	2048 × 2048	No	–	–	94.6	–	87.8
U-Net [71]	256 × 256	No	5–fold CV	–	95.9	–	89.9
InvertedNet [68]	256 × 256	No	3-fold CV	97.4	95	93.7	88.2
SegNet [69]	256 × 256	No	5-fold CV	97.9	95.5	94.4	89.6
FCN [69]	256 × 256	No	5-fold CV	97.4	95	94.2	89.2
SCAN [68]	400 × 400	No	(209/38)	97.3	94.7	92.7	86.6
Our	512 × 512	Yes	official split	98.2	96.5	95.36	91.1

Finally, Table 5.4 shows our best results and the segmentation performance published by all recent methods, of which we are aware, on the SCR dataset. According to the results in the table, the network trained with synthetic images, generated with the three-stage method, obtained the best performance score both for the lungs and the heart.

However, it is worth mentioning that Table 5.4 gives only a rough idea of the state-of-the-art, since a direct comparison between the proposed method and other approaches is not feasible. In fact, the previous methods used different partitions of the SCR dataset to obtain the training and the test set, such as two-fold, three-fold, five-fold cross-validation or ad hoc splittings, which are often not publicly available, while, in our experiments, we preferred to use the original partition, provided with the SCR dataset.

5.5 Conclusions

In this chapter, we investigated the use of GAN-based deep learning techniques for synthetic image generation, along with the corresponding label-maps, for segmentation purposes. In the proposed procedure, the generation is split into several steps. The main idea supporting the proposal is that, if the difficulty of the problem increases, the generation can benefit from this division into simpler problems. Thus, compared to other generation methods, we can generate the label-maps and images with a simpler network and a smaller number of examples. The generated images can be used to augment the training set of semantic segmentation networks. To demonstrate the effectiveness of the multi-stage method, we applied the method on two important applications in medical image analysis. In the first case, we used a two-stage approach for the generation of retinal images that can be used to train a segmentation network which has to decide whether a pixel belongs to a retinal vessel or to the background. The second application is a multi-class task, aimed at creating CXR images, which is more complex and which is faced based on a three-stage generation procedure. The approach proposed is general and can be applied to different tasks, not only to the medical field. Indeed, it is future matter of research the experimentation of the multi-stage methods on different application fields. In fact, both the two-stage and three-stage methods can be applied to other domains, where the latter approach is probably more suitable for more complex tasks. Another advantage of the three-stage method is its use of "seeds", which can be employed to generate objects in given positions in any type of image. For example, regarding the generation of CXR images, we can generate cancer nodules, in addition to the anatomical parts. The images generated in this way can be used to expand the dataset and to train a segmentation network, the aim of which is to work out whether there is a nodule in a chest X-ray image or not and, possibly, localizing the nodule. Moreover, since dots can be posed in any position inside the image, CXRs with nodules in rare locations can be generated.

Finally, given the generality of the method and the possibility of dividing the generative process into an even greater number of steps, we are confident that techniques similar to the one proposed here can also be used for the generation of natural images. In the latter case, possibly starting from a single image, we will be able to capture the internal distribution of patches within the image and to generate high quality, diverse samples that carry the same visual content as the image, possibly reorganizing them to create new "synthesized" environments.

References

1. Chen, L.C., Papandreou, G., Kokkinos, I., Murphy, K., Yuille, A.L.: DeepLab: semantic image segmentation with deep convolutional nets, atrous convolution, and fully connected CRFs. IEEE Trans. Pattern Anal. Mach. Intell. **40**(4), 834–848 (2017)
2. Long, J., Shelhamer, E., Darrell, T.: Fully convolutional networks for semantic segmentation. In: Proceedings of the IEEE Conference on Computer Vision and Pattern Recognition, pp. 3431–3440 (2015)
3. Zhao, H., Shi, J., Qi, X., Wang, X., Jia, J.: Pyramid scene parsing network. In: Proceedings of the IEEE Conference on Computer Vision and Pattern Recognition, pp. 2881–2890 (2017)
4. Chéron, G., Laptev, I., Schmid, C.: P–CNN: Pose–based CNN features for action recognition. In: Proceedings of the IEEE International Conference on Computer Vision, pp. 3218–3226 (2015)
5. He, K., Gkioxari, G., Dollár, P., Girshick, R.: Mask R–CNN. In: Proceedings of the IEEE International Conference on Computer Vision, pp. 2961–2969 (2017)
6. Huynh, T.C.: Vision-based autonomous bolt-looseness detection method for splice connections: design, lab-scale evaluation, and field application. Autom. Constr. **124**, 103591 (2021)
7. Krizhevsky, A., Sutskever, I., Hinton, G.E.: ImageNet classification with deep convolutional neural networks. Adv. Neural Inf. Process. Syst. **25**, 1097–1105 (2012)
8. Bonechi, S., Andreini, P., Bianchini, M., Scarselli, F.: Generating bounding box supervision for semantic segmentation with deep learning. In: IAPR Workshop on Artificial Neural Networks in Pattern Recognition, pp. 190–200. Springer (2018)

9. Bonechi, S., Andreini, P., Bianchini, M., Scarselli, F.: COCO_TS dataset: pixel–level annotations based on weak supervision for scene text segmentation. In: International Conference on Artificial Neural Networks, pp. 238–250. Springer (2019)
10. Ronneberger, O., Fischer, P., Brox, T.: U–net: Convolutional networks for biomedical image segmentation. In: International Conference on Medical Image Computing and Computer–Assisted Intervention, pp. 234–241. Springer (2015)
11. Deng, J., Dong, W., Socher, R., Li, L.J., Li, K., Fei-Fei, L.: ImageNet: A large–scale hierarchical image database. In: 2009 IEEE Conference on Computer Vision and Pattern Recognition, pp. 248–255 (2009). https://doi.org/10.1109/CVPR.2009.5206848
12. Lin, T.Y., Maire, M., Belongie, S., Hays, J., Perona, P., Ramanan, D., Dollár, P., Zitnick, C.L.: Microsoft COCO: common objects in context. In: European Conference on Computer Vision, pp. 740–755. Springer (2014)
13. Caruana, R., Lou, Y., Gehrke, J., Koch, P., Sturm, M., Elhadad, N.: Intelligible models for healthcare: predicting pneumonia risk and hospital 30–day readmission. In: Proceedings of the 21th ACM SIGKDD International Conference on Knowledge Discovery and Data Mining, pp. 1721–1730 (2015)
14. Rossi, A., Vannuccini, G., Andreini, P., Bonechi, S., Giacomini, G., Scarselli, F., Bianchini, M.: Analysis of brain NMR images for age estimation with deep learning. Procedia Comput. Sci. **159**, 981–989 (2019)
15. Bonechi, S., Bianchini, M., Bongini, P., Ciano, G., Giacomini, G., Rosai, R., Tognetti, L., Rossi, A., Andreini, P.: Fusion of visual and anamnestic data for the classification of skin lesions with deep learning. In: International Conference on Image Analysis and Processing, pp. 211–219. Springer (2019)
16. Esteva, A., Kuprel, B., Novoa, R.A., Ko, J., Swetter, S.M., Blau, H.M., Thrun, S.: Dermatologist-level classification of skin cancer with deep neural networks. Nature **542**(7639), 115–118 (2017)
17. Tognetti, L., Bonechi, S., Andreini, P., Bianchini, M., Scarselli, F., Cevenini, G., Moscarella, E., Farnetani, F., Longo, C., Lallas, A., et al.: A new deep learning approach integrated with clinical data for the dermoscopic differentiation of early melanomas from atypical nevi. J. Dermatol. Sci. **101**(2), 115–122 (2021)
18. Bonechi, S., Andreini, P., Mecocci, A., Giannelli, N., Scarselli, F., Neri, E., Bianchini, M., Dimitri, G.M.: Segmentation of aorta 3D CT images based on 2D convolutional neural networks. Electronics **10**(20), 2559 (2021)
19. Goodfellow, I., Pouget-Abadie, J., Mirza, M., Xu, B., Warde-Farley, D., Ozair, S., Courville, A., Bengio, Y.: Generative adversarial nets. Adv. Neural Inf. Process. Syst. **27** (2014)
20. Patton, N., Aslam, T.M., MacGillivray, T., Deary, I.J., Dhillon, B., Eikelboom, R.H., Yogesan, K., Constable, I.J.: Retinal image analysis: concepts, applications and potential. Prog. Retinal Eye Res. **25**(1), 99–127 (2006)
21. Fraz, M.M., Remagnino, P., Hoppe, A., Uyyanonvara, B., Rudnicka, A.R., Owen, C.G., Barman, S.A.: Blood vessel segmentation methodologies in retinal images–a survey. Comput. Methods Prog. Biomed. **108**(1), 407–433 (2012)
22. Patil, D.D., Manza, R.R.: Design new algorithm for early detection of primary open angle glaucoma using retinal optic cup to disc ratio. In: 2016 International Conference on Electrical, Electronics, and Optimization Techniques (ICEEOT), pp. 148–151 (2016). 10.1109/ICEEOT.2016.7754905
23. Abràmoff, M.D., Garvin, M.K., Sonka, M.: Retinal imaging and image analysis. IEEE Rev. Biomed. Eng. **3**, 169–208 (2010)
24. Kanski, J.J., Bowling, B.: Kanski's clinical ophthalmology e–book: a systematic approach. Elsevier Health Sciences (2015)
25. Mettler, F.A., Jr., Huda, W., Yoshizumi, T.T., Mahesh, M.: Effective doses in radiology and diagnostic nuclear medicine: a catalog. Radiology **248**(1), 254–263 (2008)
26. Hussain, E., Hasan, M., Rahman, M.A., Lee, I., Tamanna, T., Parvez, M.Z.: CoroDet: a deep learning based classification for COVID-19 detection using chest X-ray images. Chaos, Solitons Fractals **142**, 110495 (2021)

27. Ismael, A.M., Şengür, A.: Deep learning approaches for COVID-19 detection based on chest X-ray images. Expert Syst. Appl. **164**, 114054 (2021)
28. Nayak, S.R., Nayak, D.R., Sinha, U., Arora, V., Pachori, R.B.: Application of deep learning techniques for detection of COVID-19 cases using chest X-ray images: a comprehensive study. Biomed. Sign. Process. Control **64**, 102365 (2021)
29. Richter, S.R., Vineet, V., Roth, S., Koltun, V.: Playing for data: ground truth from computer games. In: European Conference on Computer Vision, pp. 102–118. Springer (2016)
30. Ros, G., Sellart, L., Materzynska, J., Vazquez, D., Lopez, A.M.: The Synthia dataset: a large collection of synthetic images for semantic segmentation of urban scenes. In: Proceedings of the IEEE Conference on Computer Vision and Pattern Recognition, pp. 3234–3243 (2016)
31. Hodaň, T., Vineet, V., Gal, R., Shalev, E., Hanzelka, J., Connell, T., Urbina, P., Sinha, S.N., Guenter, B.: Photorealistic image synthesis for object instance detection. In: 2019 IEEE International Conference on Image Processing (ICIP), pp. 66–70. IEEE (2019)
32. Collins, D., Zijdenbos, A., Kollokian, V., Sled, J., Kabani, N., Holmes, C., Evans, A.: Design and construction of a realistic digital brain phantom. IEEE Trans. Med. Imag. **17**(3), 463–468 (1998). https://doi.org/10.1109/42.712135
33. Andreini, P., Bonechi, S., Bianchini, M., Mecocci, A., Scarselli, F.: A deep learning approach to bacterial colony segmentation. In: International Conference on Artificial Neural Networks, pp. 522–533. Springer (2018)
34. Andreini, P., Bonechi, S., Bianchini, M., Mecocci, A., Scarselli, F.: Image generation by GAN and style transfer for agar plate image segmentation. Comput. Methods Prog. Biomed. **184**, 105268 (2020)
35. Bonechi, S., Bianchini, M., Mecocci, A., Scarselli, F., Andreini, P.: Segmentation of Petri plate images for automatic reporting of urine culture tests. In: Handbook of Artificial Intelligence in Healthcare, pp. 127–151. Springer (2022)
36. Karras, T., Aila, T., Laine, S., Lehtinen, J.: Progressive growing of GANs for improved quality, stability, and variation. arXiv preprint arXiv:1710.10196 (2017)
37. Karras, T., Laine, S., Aila, T.: A style–based generator architecture for generative adversarial networks. In: Proceedings of the IEEE/CVF Conference on Computer Vision and Pattern Recognition, pp. 4401–4410 (2019)
38. Karras, T., Laine, S., Aittala, M., Hellsten, J., Lehtinen, J., Aila, T.: Analyzing and improving the image quality of StyleGAN. In: Proceedings of the IEEE/CVF Conference on Computer Vision and Pattern Recognition, pp. 8110–8119 (2020)
39. Kugelman, J., Alonso-Caneiro, D., Read, S.A., Vincent, S.J., Chen, F.K., Collins, M.J.: Data augmentation for patch–based OCT chorio–retinal segmentation using generative adversarial networks. Neural Comput. Appl. 1–16 (2021)
40. Waheed, A., Goyal, M., Gupta, D., Khanna, A., Al-Turjman, F., Pinheiro, P.R.: CovidGAN: data augmentation using auxiliary classifier GAN for improved COVID-19 detection. IEEE Access **8**, 91916–91923 (2020)
41. Hu, B., Tang, Y., Eric, I., Chang, C., Fan, Y., Lai, M., Xu, Y.: Unsupervised learning for cell-level visual representation in histopathology images with generative adversarial networks. IEEE J. Biomed. Health Inf. **23**(3), 1316–1328 (2018)
42. Yi, X., Walia, E., Babyn, P.: Unsupervised and semi–supervised learning with categorical generative adversarial networks assisted by Wasserstein distance for dermoscopy image classification. arXiv preprint. arXiv:1804.03700 (2018)
43. Shin, H.C., Tenenholtz, N.A., Rogers, J.K., Schwarz, C.G., Senjem, M.L., Gunter, J.L., Andriole, K.P., Michalski, M.: Medical image synthesis for data augmentation and anonymization using generative adversarial networks. In: International Workshop on Simulation and Synthesis in Medical Imaging, pp. 1–11. Springer (2018)
44. Liu, M.Y., Breuel, T., Kautz, J.: Unsupervised image–to–image translation networks. In: Advances in Neural Information Processing Systems, pp. 700–708 (2017)
45. Liu, M.Y., Tuzel, O.: Coupled generative adversarial networks. Adv. Neural Inf. Process. Syst. **29**, 469–477 (2016)

46. Yi, Z., Zhang, H., Tan, P., Gong, M.: Dualgan: unsupervised dual learning for image-to-image translation. In: Proceedings of the IEEE International Conference on Computer Vision, pp. 2849–2857 (2017)
47. Zhu, J.Y., Park, T., Isola, P., Efros, A.A.: Unpaired image–to–image translation using cycle–consistent adversarial networks. In: Proceedings of the IEEE International Conference on Computer Vision, pp. 2223–2232 (2017)
48. Chen, Q., Koltun, V.: Photographic image synthesis with cascaded refinement networks. In: Proceedings of the IEEE International Conference on Computer Vision, pp. 1511–1520 (2017)
49. Isola, P., Zhu, J.Y., Zhou, T., Efros, A.A.: Image–to–image translation with conditional adversarial networks. In: Proceedings of the IEEE Conference on Computer Vision and Pattern Recognition, pp. 1125–1134 (2017)
50. Wang, T.C., Liu, M.Y., Zhu, J.Y., Tao, A., Kautz, J., Catanzaro, B.: High–resolution image synthesis and semantic manipulation with conditional GANs. In: Proceedings of the IEEE Conference on Computer Vision and Pattern Recognition, pp. 8798–8807 (2018)
51. Sagar, M.A., Bullivant, D., Mallinson, G.D., Hunter, P.J.: A virtual environment and model of the eye for surgical simulation. In: Proceedings of the 21st Annual Conference on Computer Graphics and Interactive Techniques, pp. 205–212 (1994)
52. Costa, P., Galdran, A., Meyer, M.I., Abramoff, M.D., Niemeijer, M., Mendonça, A.M., Campilho, A.: Towards adversarial retinal image synthesis. arXiv preprint arXiv:1701.08974 (2017)
53. Costa, P., Galdran, A., Meyer, M.I., Niemeijer, M., Abràmoff, M., Mendonça, A.M., Campilho, A.: End-to-end adversarial retinal image synthesis. IEEE Trans. Med. Imag. **37**(3), 781–791 (2017)
54. Beers, A., Brown, J., Chang, K., Campbell, J.P., Ostmo, S., Chiang, M.F., Kalpathy-Cramer, J.: High–resolution medical image synthesis using progressively grown generative adversarial networks. arXiv preprint arXiv:1805.03144 (2018)
55. Jiang, Z., Zhang, H., Wang, Y., Ko, S.B.: Retinal blood vessel segmentation using fully convolutional network with transfer learning. Comput. Med. Imag. Graph. **68**, 1–15 (2018)
56. Dasgupta, A., Singh, S.: A fully convolutional neural network based structured prediction approach towards the retinal vessel segmentation. In: 2017 IEEE 14th International Symposium on Biomedical Imaging (ISBI 2017), pp. 248–251 (2017). 10.1109/ISBI.2017.7950512
57. Feng, Z., Yang, J., Yao, L.: Patch–based fully convolutional neural network with skip connections for retinal blood vessel segmentation. In: 2017 IEEE International Conference on Image Processing (ICIP), pp. 1742–1746 (2017). 10.1109/ICIP.2017.8296580
58. Oliveira, A., Pereira, S., Silva, C.A.: Retinal vessel segmentation based on fully convolutional neural networks. Expert Syst. Appl. **112**, 229–242 (2018)
59. Sekou, T.B., Hidane, M., Olivier, J., Cardot, H.: From patch to image segmentation using fully convolutional networks—application to retinal images. arXiv preprint arXiv:1904.03892 (2019)
60. Yan, Z., Yang, X., Cheng, K.T.: Joint segment-level and pixel-wise losses for deep learning based retinal vessel segmentation. IEEE Trans. Biomed. Eng. **65**(9), 1912–1923 (2018). https://doi.org/10.1109/TBME.2018.2828137
61. Liu, S., Deng, W.: Very deep convolutional neural network based image classification using small training sample size. In: 2015 3rd IAPR Asian Conference on Pattern Recognition (ACPR), pp. 730–734 (2015). 10.1109/ACPR.2015.7486599
62. Maninis, K.K., Pont-Tuset, J., Arbeláez, P., Van Gool, L.: Deep retinal image understanding. In: Ourselin, S., Joskowicz, L., Sabuncu, M.R., Unal, G., Wells, W. (eds.) Medical Image Computing and Computer-Assisted Intervention–MICCAI 2016, pp. 140–148. Springer International Publishing, Cham (2016)
63. Mo, J., Zhang, L.: Multi-level deep supervised networks for retinal vessel segmentation. Int. J. Comput. Assist. Radiol. Surg. **12**(12), 2181–2193 (2017)
64. Madani, A., Moradi, M., Karargyris, A., Syeda-Mahmood, T.: Semi–supervised learning with generative adversarial networks for chest X–ray classification with ability of data domain adaptation. In: 2018 IEEE 15th International Symposium on Biomedical Imaging (ISBI 2018), pp. 1038–1042. IEEE (2018)

65. Srivastav, D., Bajpai, A., Srivastava, P.: Improved classification for pneumonia detection using transfer learning with GAN based synthetic image augmentation. In: 2021 11th International Conference on Cloud Computing, Data Science and Engineering (Confluence), pp. 433–437. IEEE (2021)
66. Shao, Y., Gao, Y., Guo, Y., Shi, Y., Yang, X., Shen, D.: Hierarchical lung field segmentation with joint shape and appearance sparse learning. IEEE Trans. Med. Imag. **33**(9), 1761–1780 (2014)
67. Ibragimov, B., Likar, B., Pernuš, F., Vrtovec, T.: Accurate landmark–based segmentation by incorporating landmark misdetections. In: 2016 IEEE 13th International Symposium on Biomedical Imaging (ISBI), pp. 1072–1075 (2016). 10.1109/ISBI.2016.7493451
68. Novikov, A.A., Lenis, D., Major, D., Hlalduvka, J., Wimmer, M., Bühler, K.: Fully convolutional architectures for multiclass segmentation in chest radiographs. IEEE Trans. Med. Imag. **37**(8), 1865–1876 (2018)
69. Islam, J., Zhang, Y.: Towards robust lung segmentation in chest radiographs with deep learning. arXiv preprint arXiv:1811.12638 (2018)
70. Oliveira, H., dos Santos, J.: Deep transfer learning for segmentation of anatomical structures in chest radiographs. In: 2018 31st SIBGRAPI Conference on Graphics, Patterns and Images (SIBGRAPI), pp. 204–211. IEEE (2018)
71. Wang, C.: Segmentation of multiple structures in chest radiographs using multi–task fully convolutional networks. In: Scandinavian Conference on Image Analysis, pp. 282–289. Springer (2017)
72. Dai, W., Dong, N., Wang, Z., Liang, X., Zhang, H., Xing, E.P.: SCAN: Structure correcting adversarial network for organ segmentation in chest X–rays. In: Deep Learning in Medical Image Analysis and Multimodal Learning for Clinical Decision Support, pp. 263–273. Springer (2018)
73. Gulrajani, I., Ahmed, F., Arjovsky, M., Dumoulin, V., Courville, A.: Improved training of Wasserstein GANs. In: Proceedings of the 31st International Conference on Neural Information Processing Systems, NIPS'17, pp. 5769—5779. Curran Associates Inc., Red Hook, NY, USA (2017)
74. Staal, J., Abramoff, M., Niemeijer, M., Viergever, M., van Ginneken, B.: Ridge-based vessel segmentation in color images of the retina. IEEE Trans. Med. Imag. **23**(4), 501–509 (2004). https://doi.org/10.1109/TMI.2004.825627
75. Fraz, M.M., Remagnino, P., Hoppe, A., Uyyanonvara, B., Rudnicka, A.R., Owen, C.G., Barman, S.A.: An ensemble classification-based approach applied to retinal blood vessel segmentation. IEEE Trans. Biomed. Eng. **59**(9), 2538–2548 (2012)
76. Li, Q., Feng, B., Xie, L., Liang, P., Zhang, H., Wang, T.: A cross-modality learning approach for vessel segmentation in retinal images. IEEE Trans. Med. Imag. **35**(1), 109–118 (2016). https://doi.org/10.1109/TMI.2015.2457891
77. Shiraishi, J., Katsuragawa, S., Ikezoe, J., Matsumoto, T., Kobayashi, T., Komatsu, K.I., Matsui, M., Fujita, H., Kodera, Y., Doi, K.: Development of a digital image database for chest radiographs with and without a lung nodule: receiver operating characteristic analysis of radiologists' detection of pulmonary nodules. Am. J. Roentgenol. **174**(1), 71–74 (2000)
78. Van Ginneken, B., Stegmann, M.B., Loog, M.: Segmentation of anatomical structures in chest radiographs using supervised methods: a comparative study on a public database. Med. Imag. Anal. **10**(1), 19–40 (2006)
79. Bonechi, S., Bianchini, M., Scarselli, F., Andreini, P.: Weak supervision for generating pixel-level annotations in scene text segmentation. Pattern Recogn. Lett. **138**, 1–7 (2020)
80. He, K., Zhang, X., Ren, S., Sun, J.: Deep residual learning for image recognition. In: Proceedings of the IEEE Conference on Computer Vision and Pattern Recognition, pp. 770–778 (2016)
81. Papandreou, G., Kokkinos, I., Savalle, P.A.: Untangling local and global deformations in deep convolutional networks for image classification and sliding window detection. arXiv preprint arXiv:1412.0296 (2014)

82. Zhao, H., Li, H., Maurer-Stroh, S., Cheng, L.: Synthesizing retinal and neuronal images with generative adversarial nets. Med. Imag. Anal. **49**, 14–26 (2018)
83. Shmelkov, K., Schmid, C., Alahari, K.: How good is my GAN? In: Proceedings of the European Conference on Computer Vision (ECCV), pp. 213–229 (2018)
84. Liskowski, P., Krawiec, K.: Segmenting retinal blood vessels with deep neural networks. IEEE Trans. Med. Imag. **35**(11), 2369–2380 (2016)

Chapter 6
Classification of Arrhythmia Signals Using Hybrid Convolutional Neural Network (CNN) Model

Evelyn Siao Yung Ern and Dzati Athiar Ramli

Abstract Arrhythmia is a fatal cardiovascular disease that presents an excessively fast heartbeat, excessively slow heartbeat or an irregular heartbeat rhythm. Atrial fibrillation (AF) is a common type of arrhythmia that can be diagnosed using an electrocardiogram (ECG) pattern. Identification of arrhythmia through ECG can be very challenging because the process is highly dependent on experts and very time consuming. The use of deep learning in automatically assisting the detection of arrhythmia using one-dimensional (1-D) input is proposed in this study. Deep learning is preferred over standard neural networks because it facilitates training in an end-to-end manner and directly trains the classification system with raw signals. This study aims to investigate the performance of 1-D convolutional neural network (CNN) for arrhythmia classification and improve its performance by introducing a hybrid approach based on long short-term memory (LSTM) approach. Experimental data are obtained from PhysioNet CinC Challenge 2017 database. ECG signals are preprocessed via filtering, QRS detection, segmentation and median wave selection. One-dimensional CNN, hybrid CNN–long short-term memory (CNN–LSTM) and hybrid CNN–bidirectional LSTM (CNN–biLSTM) models are developed and evaluated in this study to classify ECG signals into (1) normal rhythm, (2) AF rhythm, (3) other rhythms and (4) noisy signal. Accuracies of the 1-D CNN, hybrid CNN–LSTM and 1-D hybrid CNN–biLSTM models were 91.67%, 82.33% and 94.67%, respectively. The experimental results showed that the proposed CNN models can aid in atrial fibrillation (AF) diagnosis for healthcare advancement.

Keywords Arrhythmia · Convolutional neural network · Long short-term memory · Deep learning · Electrocardiogram

E. S. Y. Ern · D. A. Ramli (✉)
School of Electrical and Electronic Engineering, Universiti Sains Malaysia, USM Engineering Campus, Nibong Tebal, 14300 Penang, Malaysia
e-mail: dzati@usm.my

© The Author(s), under exclusive license to Springer Nature Switzerland AG 2023

C.-P. Lim et al. (eds.), *Artificial Intelligence and Machine Learning for Healthcare*, Intelligent Systems Reference Library 228,
https://doi.org/10.1007/978-3-031-11154-9_6

Nomenclature

ANN	Artificial Neural Network
ECG	Electrocardiogram
COVID-19	Coronavirus Disease 2019
CNN	Convolutional Neural Network
LSTM	Long Short-term Memory
AF	Atrial Fibrillation
VF	Ventricular Fibrillation
1-D	One-dimensional
2-D	Two-dimensional
CVD	Cardiovascular diseases
KNN	K-nearest Neighbors
SVM	Support Vector Machine
MLP	Multi Layer Perceptron
PAF	Paroxysmal atrial fibrillation
CCR	Correct Classification Rate
STFT	Short-time Fourier Transform
LS-SVM	Least Square SVM
GUI	Graphical User Interface
WFDB	Waveform-database
FIR	Finite Impulse Response
ReLU	Rectified Linear Unit
RNN	Recurrent Neural Network
SGD	Stochastic Gradient Descent
PHEIC	Public Health Emergency of International Concern

6.1 Introduction

Cardiovascular diseases (CVDs) are a leading cause of mortality worldwide. Ischemic heart disease and all forms of stroke were attributed causes of death for an estimated 18.6 million people, which is a quarter of the total global population, in 2019 [1]. According to the WebMD Medical Team, the human heart is an amazing organ that beats a steady and even rhythm of approximately 60–100 times each minute that results in around 100,000 beats a day. Arrhythmia is a kind of cardiovascular disease with a problematic heartbeat rate or rhythm. The heart of a patient with arrhythmia can beat excessively fast, excessively slow or with an irregular rhythm. This irregular rhythm can cause cardiovascular diseases and become fatal.

Atrial fibrillation (also called AFib or AF) is a type of irregular heartbeat (arrhythmia) that can lead to blood clots, stroke, heart failure and other heart-related complications. A human heart normally contracts and relaxes to a regular beat. Upper chambers of the heart (atria) beat irregularly (quiver) instead of beating effectively

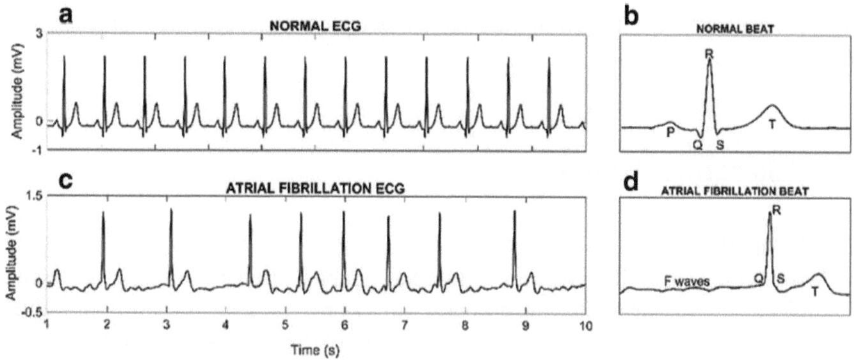

Fig. 6.1 ECG signal of (a, b) healthy person and (c, d) AF patient [4]

to move blood into ventricles in atrial fibrillation. If a clot breaks off, enters the bloodstream and lodges in an artery leading to the brain, then it will result in a stroke. Approximately 15–20% of people that suffer from strokes present this kind of heart arrhythmia [2]. Thus, diagnosing and detecting arrhythmia are very important. Dynamic electrocardiogram (ECG) monitoring is widely used in diagnosing and predicting cardiac arrhythmia and other heart diseases. AF can be detected by observing three main morphological features in the ECG, namely, P-wave absence, P-wave fluctuating waveforms (f-waves) and heart rate irregularity. Figure 6.1 shows the differences between the ECG of a normal person and an AF patient. ECG characteristics of AF are the absence of P waves, oscillating baseline f (fibrillation) waves, atrial rate of 350–600 bpm, irregular ventricular rhythm and ventricular rate of 100–180 bpm [3].

However, clinical experts must observe ECG recordings for a long period of time to detect arrhythmia. This process is time consuming, labour-intensive and susceptible to errors. This technique also requires a cardiologist expert with extensive domain knowledge. However, the limited number of specific experts may fail to meet the high demand. Automated ECG signal classification using machine learning approaches, including artificial (ANN) [5], backpropagation [6] and deep (DNN) neural networks [7, 8], have been proposed. Deep learning is a relatively better choice than ANN because it facilitates the training in an end-to-end manner and directly trains the classification system using raw signals without handcrafted features [9, 10]. Various methods, such as convolutional recurrent [7] and convolutional [8] neural networks, have been used in this category. Classification systems of convolutional neural network (CNN) arrhythmia are commonly developed in two dimensions although they require transformation of raw signals from time-series data into two-dimensional (2-D) data [10, 11]. The literature showed that the accuracy of developed one-dimensional (1-D) classification systems is unsatisfactory at less than 91% [7, 12, 13]. Hence, this study aims to investigate the performance of 1-D CNN for arrhythmia classification and improve its performance by introducing a hybrid approach on the basis of the long short-term memory (LSTM). The proposed hybrid model is expected to outperform the CNN model because it combines advantages of both CNN and LSTM.

6.2 Literature Review

Atrial Fibrillation.

Arrhythmia is a cardiovascular disease that can be caused by smoking, excessive alcohol or caffeine drinking, drug abuse, stress or even genetics. Normal values of resting heart rate of adults are between 60 and 90 bpm [14]. The normal sinus heart rate is between 60 and 100 bpm according to the American Heart Association [15]. Arrhythmias are classified into two types according to the speed of heart rate they cause (tachycardia) and from where arrhythmias originate (either from atria or ventricles, bradycardia) [16]. Tachycardia refers to a heartbeat faster than normal or a resting heart rate greater than 100 bpm. Bradycardia refers to a heart rate slower than normal or a resting heart rate of less than 60 bpm [17, 18].

The World Health Organisation declared that the outbreak of COVID-19 constitutes a Public Health Emergency of International Concern (PHEIC) in 2020. The COVID-19 outbreak can cause the death of countless lives even until 2021. Cardiovascular complications have been identified as common factors of mortality in patients with COVID-19 [19]. Amongst arrhythmias significantly associated with COVID-19 severity and mortality, AF is the most frequent arrhythmia type diagnosed [20] that increases the risk of stroke and heart disease. AF was mentioned in 175,326 death certificates and the underlying cause of death in 25,845 of those deaths in 2018 [21]. ECG is performed by placing several electrodes on the skin to record the heart's electrical activity in wavelengths and used to diagnose AF.

Artificial Neural Network

Machine learning is a branch of artificial intelligence that allows the system to learn from experience without explicit programming and improvement of data used [12]. Machine learning algorithms can build a model on the basis of training data to improve predictions and decisions in the future. These algorithms are often categorised as supervised and unsupervised learning. Other machine learning methods also include semisupervised and reinforcement learning.

ANNs are a type of technology based on studies of the brain and nervous system. These networks reproduce the function of a biological neural network but with a reduced set of concepts from the biological neural network [22]. ANN is composed of a layer of input nodes, followed by one or more layers of hidden nodes and lastly a layer of output nodes. Firing activation functions allows input layer nodes to pass information to hidden layer nodes. Weighting functions are then applied to hidden layers, and the value is passed to the output layer when the value of nodes h_n in the hidden layer achieves the particular threshold value [23]. For example, values in the input layer x_m are multiplied by the connection weight $W_{m,n}$ to obtain values in the hidden layer of an ANN model. Learning is emulated in ANNs through the

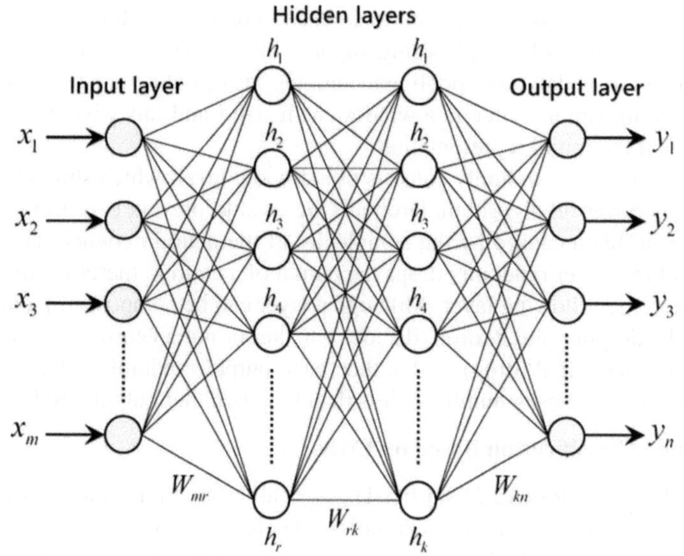

Fig. 6.2 Architecture of the ANN [25]

adjustment of the weightage. All values of hidden layers are then aggregated to a scalar function, such as summation (i.e. $y = \sum W_{mn}x_m$), averaging, input maximum or mode value, using a vector to produce a single input value. The hidden layer then uses a transfer function [24], such as sigmoid, hyperbolic tangent or other nonlinear functions, to produce its output when the input value is calculated. The process is repeated between layers of the hidden layer until a final output value y_n is produced by the neural network. Figure 6.2 shows the architecture of the artificial neural network.

Convolutional Neural Network

Fukushima [26] developed the convolutional neural network in the 1980s. CNN is the first deep learning approach in which hierarchical layers are trained robustly by means of stochastic gradient descent algorithm. This deep learning algorithm can used in an input image, assign importance (learnable weights and biases) to various aspects of the image and classify these aspects. The CNN has been widely used for feature extraction and signal classification problems in the literature. A Fourier transform was applied between convolutional and subsampling layers to switch EEG signals from the 1-D time domain to the 2-D frequency domain for detecting steady-state visually evoked potential [27]. P300 wave detection via arrhythmia signal classification and character recognition problems using a CNN with two convolutional layers and one subsampling layer was applied to solve two classification problems [28].

Although CNN is designed purposely in processing 2-D images, it can also perform properly when 1-D signals are used as input [29]. The operation of 1-D convolution starts by sliding a 1-D filter across the input one unit at a time, followed by calculating the dot product between 1-D filter and input kernels.

One-dimensional pooling is commonly used to reduce the dimensionality of the convolution output whilst emphasising important features [30] as well as overfitting. Max pooling is a widely used pooling technique. Max pooling can be performed by applying the maximum value in a window with size f and this window is slid over subregions of the initial representation.

The CNN model commonly consists of a dropout layer, which shows the importance of this powerful algorithm. Dropouts are used to prevent overfitting, which is a common problem caused by the complexity of the neural network. The working principle of this layer randomly drops the output of a neuron, thereby indicating the zero input to the following layer. Although a layer can be composed of a number of neurons, the dropout rate P (drop) decides whether or not a neuron drops the output [30]. For instance, if P (drop) = 0.6, then each output randomly selects a number from 0 to 1. If the chosen number is less than 0.6, then that output will be dropped.

Arrhythmia Classification Based on CNN

Xiong et al. [7] developed a 21-layer 1-D CNN called RhythmNet to classify normal heartbeat, AF, other arrhythmias and noisy signals. The dataset used was obtained from 12,186 single-lead ECG recordings, which are performed in waveform and recorded by patients from a self-diagnosis device called AliveCor Kardia [31]. The training set was subjected to fivefold cross validation and then each fold was used as the testing set at a particular point given that the testing set is not publicly accessible. The architecture of RhythmNet consisted of 16 convolution layers for direct feature extraction from the raw ECG signal. Three recurrent layers were applied after the convolution layer to process ECGs of different lengths and detect arrhythmia events in long recordings. Batch normalisation, rectified linear activation units and residual connections were utilised in RhythmNet to improve convergence during the training process. The ECG signal was inputted in 5 s windows, thereby indicating that the input length is 5 s. The signal is then passed through 16 repeated residual blocks containing convolutions of different depths. The output of these 16 residual blocks was then flattened into a 1-D vector and inputted in three recurrent layers to process windows sequentially whilst following the pace of 5 s at a time. Lastly, the output of the recurrent layer was mapped onto a fully connected layer with four nodes representing probabilities of the four classes for prediction. F1 score represents the average of individual F1 scores for the normal heartbeat (N), AF (A) and other arrhythmias (O) and was used as the evaluation metric in this study. Although the classification accuracy of noisy signals was excluded from this study, it impacted F1 scores of other classes when noisy signals were incorrectly predicted. This study obtained an F1 accuracy of 82% in the classification of sinus rhythm, AF and other arrhythmias after evaluating the algorithm on 3658 points of testing data.

Pourbabaee et al. [8] conducted two experiments to classify paroxysmal atrial fibrillation (PAF) and normal/healthy patients using the PAF prediction challenge database. The database was split into a training set containing 100 signals and a testing set with only 50 signals, of which 28 are from PAF patients. The 30 min-long ECG signal composed of 38,400 samples was separated into six 5 min duration signals to accelerate the training process. An end-to-end five-layer CNN network was developed in experiment 1 whilst only the first four layers of the CNN network was initially used to obtain feature vectors before utilising other conventional classifiers, including KNN, SVM and MLP, in experiment 2. The five-layer CNN network consisted of one input layer, one convolutional layer, one subsampling (pooling) layer, a fully connected layer and lastly the output layer. The results showed that the end-to-end CNN in experiment 1 obtained a correct classification rate (CCR) of 85.33% whilst the KNN classifier in experiment 2 exhibited a CCR of 91%. Thus, the KNN demonstrated higher accuracy in screening PAF patients compared with other methods.

Ullah et al. [27] classified the ECG signal into eight classes, namely, normal, premature ventricular contraction, paced, right-bundle branch block, left-bundle branch block, atrial premature contraction, ventricular flutter wave and ventricular escape beats, using the MIT-BIH Arrhythmia dataset. The ECG signal was initially preprocessed to remove noise and obtain a denoised ECG signal for further processing. The transformation of the one-dimensional ECG signal representing time series data into a 2-D image using short-time Fourier transform (STFT) to modify data as input for the designed CNN was the primary contribution of this study. Although 1-D CNN can be sufficiently used for the ECG signal, which was originally a time series signal, the 2-D CNN is more versatile because it uses 2-D kernels, which can supply more significant features for ECG signal data. A softmax layer with eight neurons was utilised as the output layer to provide the final classification. A fully connected layer representing features learned by the CNN model was used before the output layer. Accuracy, precision, sensitivity and specificity were utilised as the evaluation metrics. The results obtained in this study achieved an average sensitivity of 97.91%, specificity of 99.61%, average accuracy of 99.11% and positive predictive value (precision) of 98.59%. These results proved that the application of 2-D CNN, which used the 2-D ECG signal as the input, is reliable and can be applied to arrhythmia diagnosis.

Rajpurkar et al. [32] classified and segmented 12 arrhythmia types with a 34-layer CNN. A dataset 500 times larger than other widely used datasets, such as MIT-BIH Arrhythmia and PhysioNet Computing in Cardiology Challenge 2017 databases, was constructed by collecting datasets from patients who have used the Zio patch monitor [13]. Patients exhibiting abnormal rhythms were purposely selected to balance classes of the dataset. The high-level architecture composed of 33 convolution layers, followed by a fully connected layer and a softmax layer, was designed, with the network consisting of 16 residual blocks with two convolutional layers per block. Batch normalisation, rectified linear activation and dropout layer were applied. The model accuracy was measured using Sequence and Set F1 Level Accuracies. The average overlap between the prediction and the ground truth annotation for the Sequence F1 was measured whilst the set of unique arrhythmias presented in each 30 s record were considered the ground truth annotation for Set F1. The results for both Sequence and Set F1 values were then compared with the prediction to obtain the F1 score. The results of this study outperformed the average expert cardiologist performance in both Sequence and Set F1 scores. Accordingly, this model showed superiority over cardiologists with a precision of 80% and sensitivity of 83% whilst cardiologists presented a precision of 76% and sensitivity of 75%. However, this study also demonstrated some limitations. For example, many arrhythmia occurrences were erroneously identified as the sinus rhythm. This mistake was expected attributed to the ambiguous location of the accurate offset and onset of arrhythmia in the ECG signal.

Andreotti et al. [33] compared feature-based classifiers and convolutional neural networks to classify ECG signals into atrial fibrillation, normal rhythm, other rhythms and noisy recording. The training dataset denoted TRAIN-DB consists of 8528 10 s single-lead ECG segments whilst the test set was composed of a subset of 3,658 hidden records [11]. However, the second training dataset called AUG-BD was augmented by increasing the number of AF and noisy recordings to improve the training of classifiers. An additional 2000 AF rhythm databases were obtained from different PhysioNet databases [34] (INCART-DB, LTAFDB and AFDB). FECGSYN toolbox [35] was used to simulate 2000 additional noisy recordings and perform time reversal on 284 existing noisy segments to increase the number of noisy recordings in AUG-DB. QRS detections were applied to extract morphological features, such as P-wave power and QT interval. The 34-layer ResNet (33 layers of convolution and a fully connected layer) developed by Rajpurkar et al. [32] was used as the basic model. The network consisted of 16 residual blocks with two convolutional layers per block. Training and testing processes were carried out on both TRAIN-DB and AUG-DB using ResNet. As a result, the convolutional neural network scored 72.1% on the augmented database and 83% on the test set.

Mathunjwa et al. [36] applied a 2D CNN to group arrhythmia ECG signals into six classes, namely, noise, ventricular fibrillation (VF), atrial fibrillation (AF), normal, premature AF and premature VF. The first two classes were categorised in the first stage, and the remaining classes were labelled in the second stage. The database used in this study was from the MIT-BIH Arrhythmia, MIT-BIH Atrial Fibrillation and MIT-BIH Malignant Ventricular Ectopy Databases. The comparison amongst the CNN of 8, 16 and 19 layers was recorded. Maximum testing accuracies of 95.3% $\pm$ 1.27% and 98.41% $\pm$ 0.11% were achieved for arrhythmia detection in the first and second stages, respectively.

Billeci et al. [37] developed an algorithm to group ECG signals into four classes, namely, AF, normal, noisy and other arrhythmias, specifically for AF using MIT-BH AF and PhysioNet Computing in Cardiology Challenge 2017 Databases. This modified algorithm was a combination of RR, P-Wave and frequency spectrum analyses for detecting arrhythmia AF. Least square SVM (LS-SVM) classifier was used in this study. The results showed acceptable accuracy at 98% despite the limited classification.

Therefore, on the basis of methods used in [27, 36], a 2-D CNN that converts raw time-series ECG signals into 2-D input signals via Fourier transform is proposed. The remainder of the study applied 1-D CNN in which the raw ECG signal is used as input to the CNN although the accuracy of developed one-dimensional (1-D) classification systems is unsatisfactory at less than or equal to 91% [7, 12, 13]. The number of CNN layers is determined according to the researchers' design and number of signals inputted. Notably, a large number of convolutional layers is ideal because each convolutional layer reduces the number of input features to fully connected layers (output layer). Although the CNN proposed in [8] only contains five layers, it achieved an accuracy of 91% because it only needs to categorise two classes.

6.3 Methodology

Dataset

PhysioNet CinC Challenge 2017 Database [34] was used to create a dataset in this project. A total of 8528 short single-lead ECG recordings were collected using the AliveCor device in the training set. A subset of this database containing 300 records was designated as the validation set. ECG recordings with a length of 9–60 s were band pass filtered via the AliverCor device. Data were stored as 300 Hz 16-bit files with a bandwidth of 0.5–40 Hz and a dynamic range of $\pm$ 5 mV. The database presents corresponding labels (ground truth) that identify the type of rhythm present. Recordings were categorised into normal rhythm, atrial fibrillation, other rhythms and noisy recordings. These labels and annotations were assigned by expert cardiologists and used for supervised training.

All data are presented in MATLAB V4 WFDB-compliant format. Additional details of the training set are listed in Table 6.1. Figure 6.3 shows the examples of ECG waveforms for the four classes in this database.

Deep learning and CNN, with Keras and NumPy as primary libraries, are used in this project. The results requiring PANDAS and matplotlib libraries are displayed in graphical and table forms. A toolbox specifically designed for ECG signal processing called BioSPPy is installed. NumPy is a library for the Python programming language that adds support to large multi-dimensional arrays and matrices along with an extensive collection of high-level mathematical functions to operate on these arrays. Keras is an open-source software library that provides a Python interface for artificial neural networks. Keras acts as an interface for the TensorFlow library and supports multiple backends, including TensorFlow, Microsoft Cognitive Toolkit, Theano and PlaidML. PANDAS is a software library written for the Python programming language for data manipulation and analysis. Particularly, it offers data structures and operations for

Table 6.1 Data profile of the training set

Type	No of recording	Time length (seconds)				
		Mean	SD	Max	Median	Min
Normal	5154	31.9	10.0	61.0	30	9.0
AF	771	31.6	12.5	60.0	30.0	10.0
Other rhythms	2557	34.1	11.8	60.9	30.0	9.1
Noisy	46	27.1	9.0	60.0	30.0	10.2
Total	8528	32.5	10.9	61.0	30.0	9.0

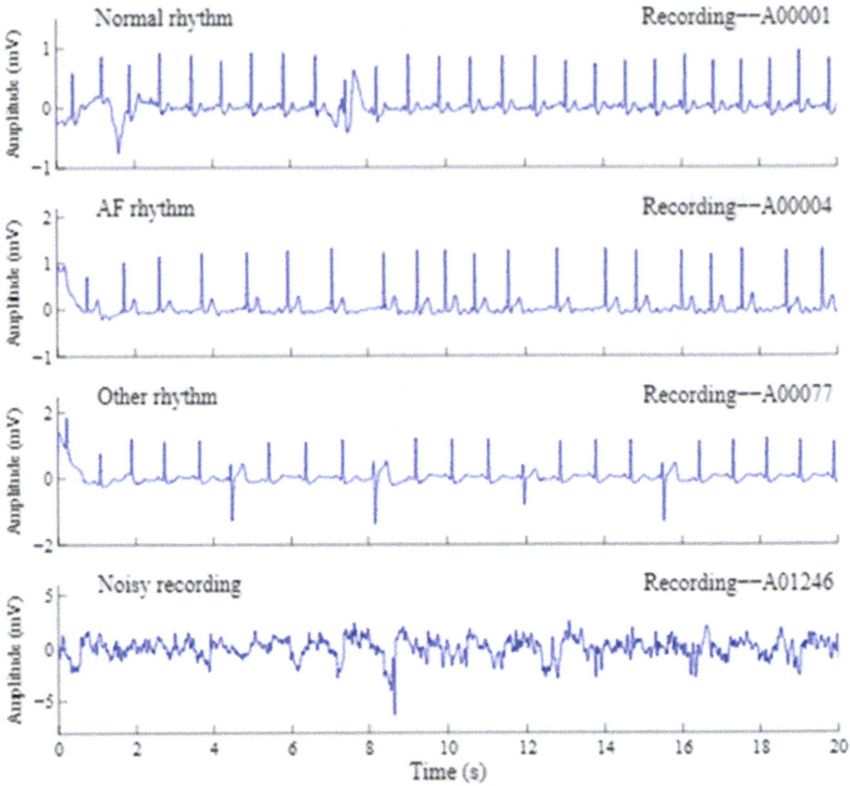

Fig. 6.3 Examples of ECG waveforms. ECG waveforms of normal rhythm, AF rhythm, other rhythms and noisy recordings are presented from top to bottom [34]

manipulating numerical tables and time series. Matplotlib is a plotting library for the Python programming language and its numerical mathematics extension NumPy that provides an object-oriented API for embedding plots into applications using general-purpose GUI toolkits, such as Tkinter, wxPython, Qt and GTK. BioSPPy is a toolbox for biosignal processing written in Python. The toolbox bundles together various signal processing and pattern recognition methods for the analysis of biosignals.

Preprocessing

Processes involved in the preprocessing stage were filtering, QRS complex detection, segmentation and median wave selection. A finite impulse response (FIR) filter within the frequency range of 3–45 Hz was applied to remove high—(50–60 Hz) and low—(0.5–0.6 Hz) frequency noises. Hamilton QRS complex detection algorithm [38] was used to locate R peaks of ECG signals after filtering. The waveform of a complete wave cycle can be obtained in this case. Segmentation was carried out to extract one full wave cycle from ECG signals consisting of QRS complexes. The time when R peaks occurred was denoted 0.0 s. The starting point window at 0.2 s before and 0.4 s

Fig. 6.4 Example of waveform after segmentation

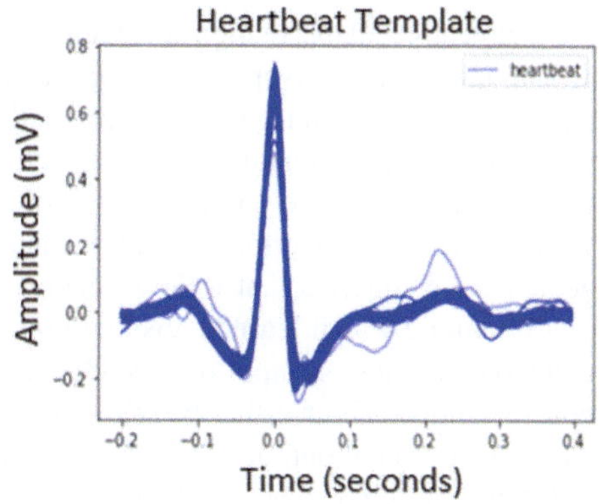

after the time of 0.0 s was extracted. A window of 0.6 s in total was finally obtained. An example of the targeted waveform is shown in Fig. 6.4. Lastly, the median wave of the extracted waveform was determined and selected.

Implementation of CNN

A CNN generally consists of an input and an output layer and in between those two layers are multiple hidden layers. Hidden layers of a CNN typically consist of a series of convolutional layers that convolve with multiplication or other dot products. The activation function is commonly a ReLU layer and usually followed by a subsampling (pooling) layer and one or more fully connected layers referred to as hidden layers because their inputs and outputs are masked by the activation function and final convolution. The full general structure of the convolutional neural network is presented in Fig. 6.5.

The objective of the convolution operation is to extract high-level features from the input image. The CNN need not be limited to only one convolutional layer. The network is locally connected in convolutional layers to extract and convolve features with their associated weights. Weights that constitute parameters of convolutional kernels in each layer are trained by means of the backpropagation error algorithm.

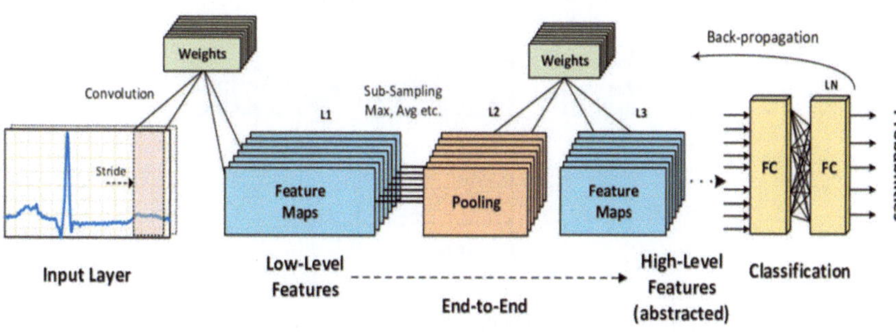

Fig. 6.5 General structure of the CNN [39]

The architecture adapts to high-level features with added layers. Similar to the convolutional layer, max or average pooling is added to decrease the computational power required to process data and reduce the spatial size of the convolved feature. Furthermore, extracting dominant features, which are rotational- and positional-invariant, is important in effectively training the model.

Rectified linear function instead of the sigmoidal activation function is used as the activation function that follows a convolutional layer. The neural network fails to differentiate which learned abstract representations are relevant to the particular input when an unseen input occurs. One neuron represents a given learned abstract representation and can either be relevant or irrelevant. If it is irrelevant, then it fails to contribute to the output of CNN. Thus, using a non-negative activation function for CNN is preferred. The rectified linear function is a commonly used approach and a neuron that uses it is called rectified linear unit (ReLU), $f(x) = \text{argmax}(0, x)$.

Dropout layer is a mask that nullifies the contribution of some neurons towards the next layer without modifying the remaining neurons. We can either apply a dropout layer to the input vector or hidden layer. The dropout layer nullifies some features when the input vector is used but nullifies some hidden neurons when the hidden layer is utilised. Dropout layers are important in training CNNs because they prevent overfitting in training data. If these layers are absent, then the first batch of training samples influences the learning in a disproportionately high manner. A 27-layer CNN architecture was designed to perform the classification task. The results of the median wave selection were fed into the network as input data. The architecture of the CNN model used in this project is illustrated in Fig. 6.6.

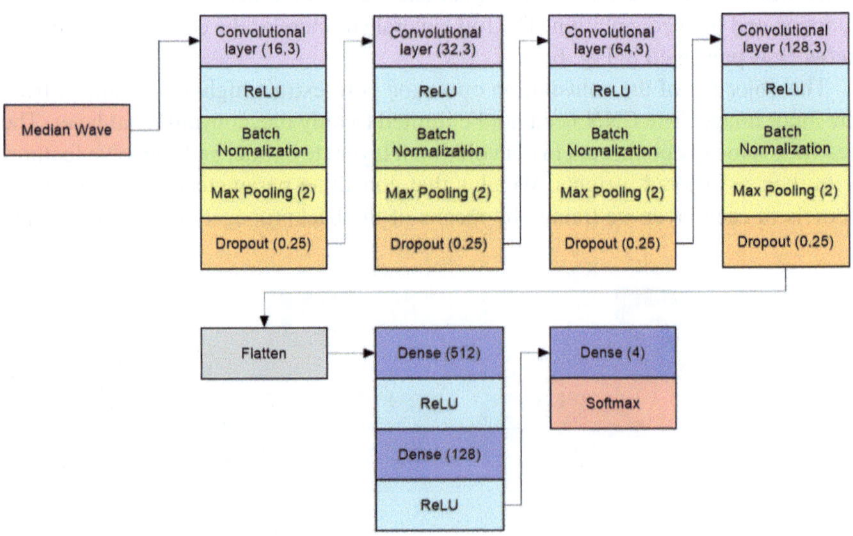

Fig. 6.6 Architecture of the proposed CNN model

The network comprises of four convolutional blocks in which each block includes a 1-D convolution layer, a ReLU activation function, a batch normalisation layer, a max-pooling layer of pool size equal to 2 and a dropout layer with a rate of 0.25.

The rectified linear activation function and batch normalisation were applied after each convolutional layer. Batch normalisation stabilises the learning process and eases the learning process. The max pooling layer was used after each batch normalisation layer to reduce the input image size by the factor of 2. The dropout layer with a rate of 0.25 was also utilised between convolutional layers and after the max-pooling layer.

The output of four convolutional blocks was passed through a flattened layer for conversion into a 1-D array to ensure that it can be sent as the input for the next dense layer. The output shape was reduced by passing the array through two dense layers with the ReLU activation function. The last fully connected layer and softmax activation produced a distribution over the four output classes that have been targeted which were normal rhythm, AF rhythm, other rhythms and noise rhythm.

Implementation of CNN–LSTM

The hybrid model of CNN with LSTM was proposed in this project. The CNN layer functions as a feature extraction layer and the LSTM layer interprets the sequence of subsequences. The LSTM network is a type of recurrent neural network (RNN) capable of managing a series of chronologically ordered data. Therefore, the time-distributed layer adds an additional 'time' dimension in each layer.

Time-distributed layers were required to wrap all layers before the LSTM layer because LSTM was required to work with convoluted signals in this project. Input data were reshaped from three dimensions to four dimensions (samples, subsequences, sequence and features) and four subsequences were assigned in this project. Figure 6.7 shows the architecture of the proposed CNN–LSTM model.

Implementation of the Hybrid CNN–biLSTM Model

The hybrid CNN–biLSTM model was also proposed apart from the hybrid CNN–LSTM model. The architecture of the CNN–biLSTM and CNN–LSTM models is the same, as shown in Fig. 6.7. However, a bidirectional LSTM (biLSTM) layer is used to replace the unidirectional LSTM layer. The biLSTM is an extension of the unidirectional LSTM that can improve model performance. The principle of biLSTM splits neurons of neural networks into two parts. The first part is responsible for the positive time direction whereas the second part is assigned to the negative time direction. The performance of the hybrid CNN–biLSTM of this project was evaluated and then compared with that of the CNN and CNN–LSTM models.

Setting Parameters of Models

EarlyStopping callback in Keras was utilised to stop early training and prevent overfitting. Loss on the validation dataset (val_loss) must be monitored. Training usually halts when val_loss stops improving. The number of epochs for the training process was set to 100 at the beginning. A delay of 20 epochs was assigned in which the training will only stop in the absence of val_loss improvement for 20 continuous

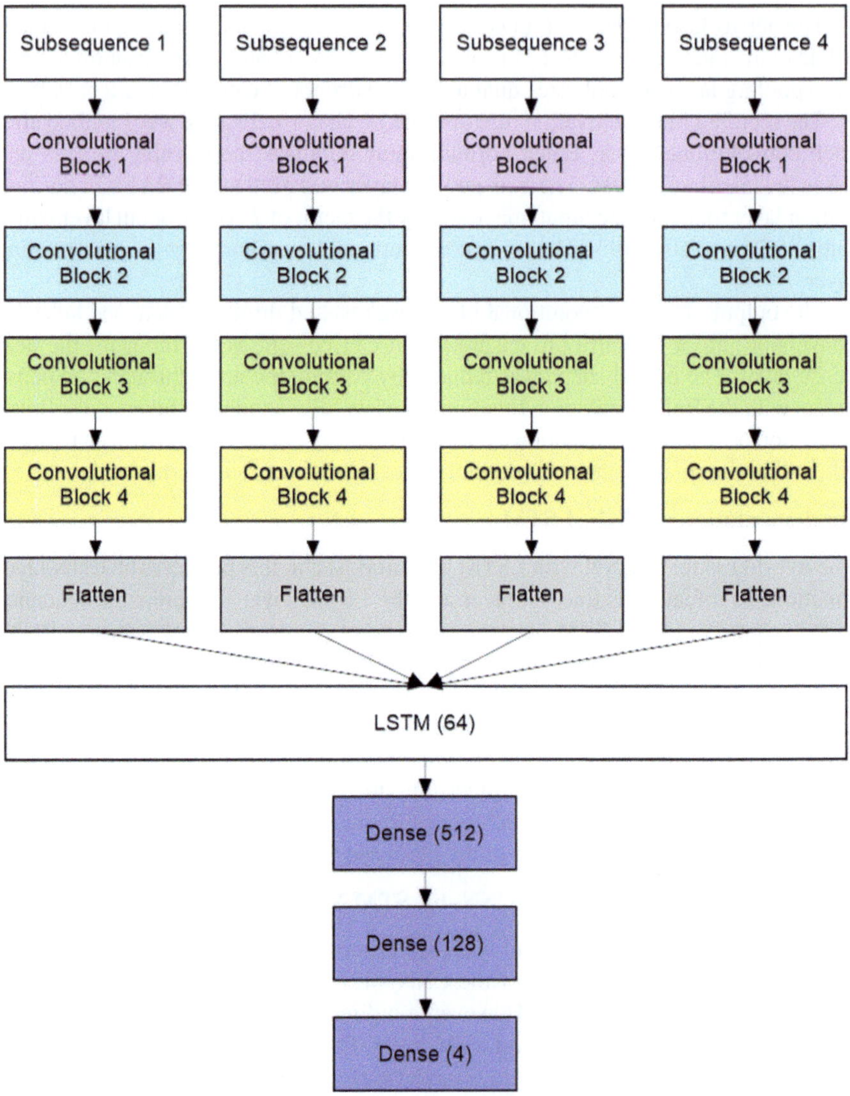

Fig. 6.7 Architecture of the proposed CNN–LSTM model

epochs. An experiment was carried out between 'Adam' and 'SGD' optimisers to determine the most suitable optimiser on the basis of their performance. Evaluation metrics, including accuracy and F1 score, were compared using different optimisers to train the proposed 1-D CNN model with the same input data and number of epochs five times.

Table 6.2 Location of the TP, TN, FP and FN in the prediction method

		True label	
		+	–
Predicted label	+	True positive (TP)	False positive (FP)
	–	False negative (FN)	True negative (TN)

Performance Evaluation

Numerous data were trained and tested using a single-lead ECG dataset to optimise the arrhythmia classification model. Few metrics were used in this study to evaluate the classification performance of the model. Accuracy (Acc), specificity (SP), sensitivity (SE), positive predictive value (PPV) and negative predictive value (NPV) are calculated using true positive (TP), true negative (TN), false positive (FP) and false negative (FN) [7]. The location of TP, TN, FP and FN in the prediction method is presented in Table 6.2.

Accuracy (Acc) is the ratio of correctly classified instances to that of the total number of instances and expressed as follows:

$$\mathrm{Acc} = \frac{\mathrm{TP} + \mathrm{TN}}{\mathrm{TP} + \mathrm{TN} + \mathrm{FP} + \mathrm{FN}} \tag{6.1}$$

Sensitivity (SE), also known as the true positive rate, is calculated as follows:

$$\mathrm{SE} = \frac{\mathrm{TP}}{\mathrm{TP} + \mathrm{FN}} \tag{6.2}$$

Specificity (SP), also known as the true negative rate, is calculated as follows:

$$\mathrm{SP} = \frac{\mathrm{TN}}{\mathrm{TN} + \mathrm{FP}} \tag{6.3}$$

Positive (PPV) and negative (NPV) predictive values are expressed as follows:

$$\mathrm{PPV} = \frac{\mathrm{TP}}{\mathrm{TP} + \mathrm{FP}} \tag{6.4}$$

$$\mathrm{NPV} = \frac{\mathrm{TN}}{\mathrm{TN} + \mathrm{FN}} \tag{6.5}$$

The F1 score is the metric that represents the average of individual F1 scores for the normal heartbeat (N), AF (A), other rhythms (O) and noise rhythms (~) [7]. The overall F1 measurement is expressed as follows:

$$F1 = \frac{1}{4}\left(\frac{2 \times N_{truepositive}}{\sum N_{groundtruth} + N_{predicted}} + \frac{2 \times A_{truepositive}}{\sum A_{groundtruth} + A_{predicted}} + \frac{2 \times O_{truepositive}}{\sum O_{groundtruth} + O_{predicted}} + \frac{2 \times \sim_{truepositive}}{\sum \sim_{groundtruth} + \sim_{predicted}}\right) \tag{6.6}$$

6.4 Results and Discussion

Preprocessing output

An ECG summary that contains the output of filtered ECG, R-peak location indices, instantaneous heart rate and extracted heartbeat templates is illustrated with the help of the *BioSPPy* toolbox. Figure 6.8 shows an example of the ECG summary output.

Figure 8a clearly shows that all 8528 raw signals, which are 30–60 s long, are cut into similar 30 s windows. Purple lines in Fig. 8b denote R-peak locations. Figure 8c presents the instantaneous heart rate waveform. Figure 8d illustrates the templates of a full waveform containing QRS complexes. These templates are saved in a folder named 'feature' and then subjected to median wave selection. Figure 6.9 depicts an example of the final template after median wave selection of the waveform. These templates are ready to be extracted and imported into the neural network model as input data.

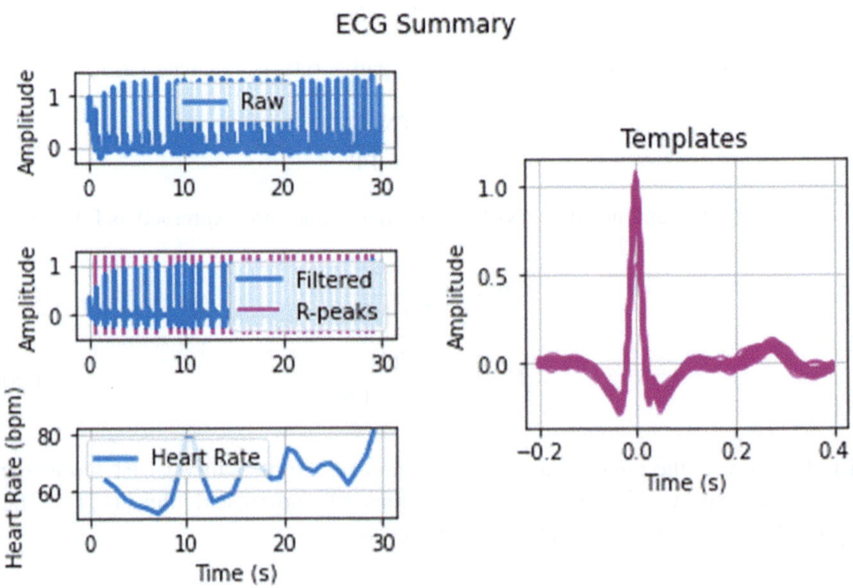

Fig. 6.8 Example of ECG output summary after preprocessing

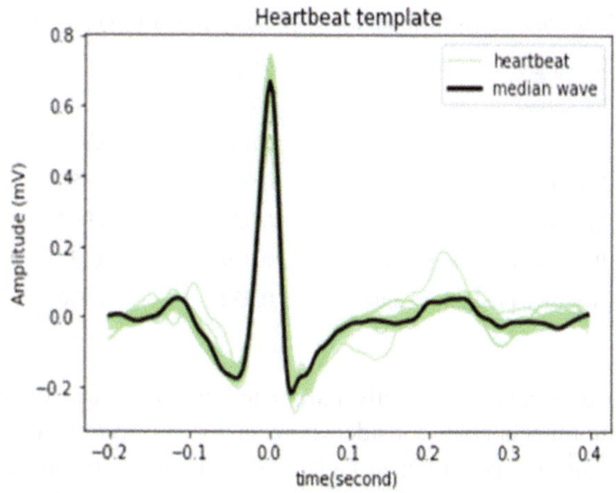

Fig. 6.9 Example of the waveform after median wave selection

Determine the number of epochs and optimiser

The training process is executed with the specified *EarlyStopping* callback five times with the number of epochs equal to 100 and then stops at an average of 75 epochs. This phenomenon indicated that the loss in validation data stops improving at an average of 55 epochs. Therefore, the number of epochs is finalised at 50 for the training of both the CNN and CNN–LSTM models.

The performance of the two optimisers are compared. This experiment aims to select the suitable optimiser and obtain satisfactory results. Evaluation metrics, including accuracy and the F1 score, are compared using different optimisers for training the proposed 1-D CNN model with the same input data and number of epochs. The training and testing of the CNN model are repeated five times and the average is calculated. The performance results of Adam and SGD optimisers on the proposed 1-D CNN model are listed in Table 6.3.

As shown in Table 6.3, both the accuracy and F1 score of the Adam optimiser are significantly higher than those of the SGD optimiser. The average accuracy of the Adam optimiser is 21.06% higher than that of the SGD optimiser. The F1 score of the Adam optimiser is 23.94 higher than that of the SGD optimiser.

Stochastic gradient descent maintains a single learning rate for all weight updates, and the learning rate remains the same throughout the training process. However,

Table 6.3 Accuracy and F1 score results of Adam and SGD optimisers

Optimiser	Metrics	1	2	3	4	5	Average
Adam	Accuracy (%)	90.00	87.00	91.67	90.33	89.67	89.73
	F1 score	88.40	85.14	90.17	89.15	88.59	88.29
SGD	Accuracy (%)	70.33	68.00	68.67	68.00	68.33	68.67
	F1 score	65.81	63.61	63.95	65.03	63.33	64.35

Table 6.4 Classification results of the proposed 1-D CNN model

Accuracy	91.67%			
F1 Score	90.17			
	Normal	AF	Others	Noise
Sensitivity	0.953	0.880	0.829	1.000
Specificity	0.927	0.992	0.991	0.963
Positive predictive value	0.929	0.957	0.967	0.750
Negative predictive value	0.952	0.976	0.950	1.000

Adam adapts not only parameter learning rates on the basis of the average first moment but also considers the average of second moments of gradients because Adam combines advantages of adaptive gradient algorithm (AdaGrad) and root mean square Propagation (RMSProp), which are extensions of the stochastic gradient descent [40]. Hence, the Adam optimiser is utilised in the 1-D CNN, 1-D CNN–LSTM and 1-D CN–biLSTM models to improve results.

Performance Evaluation of the 1-D CNN Model

The trained 1-D CNN is tested using validation data with 50 epochs. The maximum accuracy and F1 score are 91.67% and 90.17, respectively. The minimum accuracy and F1 score are 87.00% and 85.14, respectively. Table 6.4 shows the optimal output results of the proposed 1-D CNN classifier.

Confusion matrixes are created to evaluate the output quality of the classifier with a 4×4 square with labels N (normal rhythm), A (AF rhythm), O (other rhythms) and ~(noise rhythm). Diagonal elements are presented in dark shades and represent the number of points the predicted label is equal to the true label, whilst off-diagonal elements denote the number of points mislabelled by the classifier. High diagonal values of the confusion matrix indicate many correct predictions. Figure 10a shows the normalised confusion matrix. The performance at label A is focused at 0.88, thereby indicating a correct prediction of 88%. Values of 0.06, 0.02 and 0.04 of A are predicted as N, O and ~ , respectively. Some aAF rhythms are erroneously identified as the normal sinus rhythm. A portion of this finding is predicted due to the ambiguous location of the exact onset and offset of the AF in the ECG record. Another common error occurs between other and normal sinus rhythms at a value of 0.11 although a negative P wave occurs every three to four waveforms. This phenomenon can be subtle and difficult to detect, especially when the P wave presents a small amplitude or noise is present in the signal.

Apart from the confusion matrix, accuracy and loss curves are plotted to visualise changes of accuracy and loss as the epoch increases. The accuracy curve plots accuracy against epoch whilst the loss curve presents the graph of loss against epoch. Figure 10b shows the accuracy curve of the 1-D CNN classifier. Figure 10c illustrates the loss curve of the model. The accuracy curve presents a satisfactory fit when the gap is small and overfitting is low. The gap between training and validation accuracy is a clear indication of overfitting. An acceptable fit loss curve demonstrates the

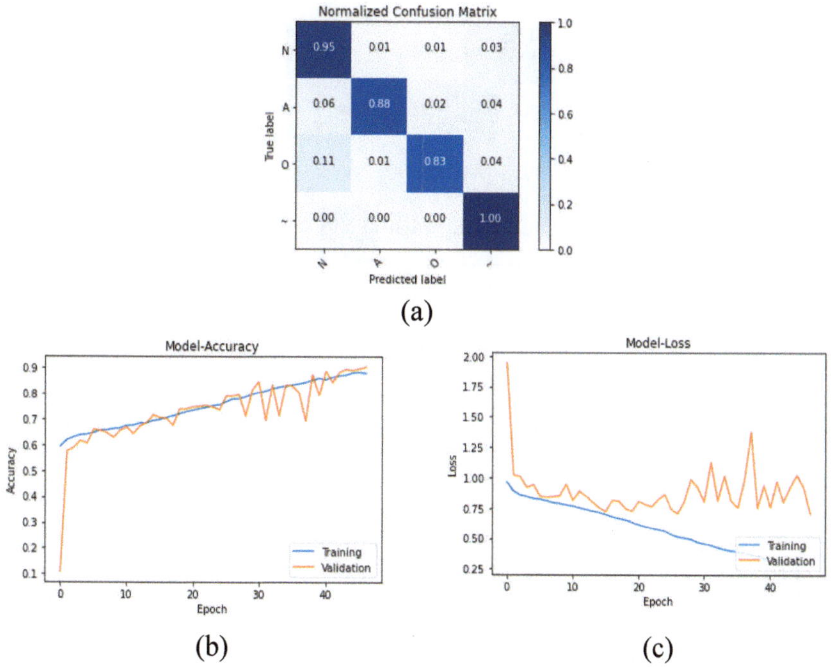

Fig. 6.10 **a** Normalised confusion matrix of the CNN model, **b** accuracy curve of the 1-D CNN classifier and **c** loss curve of the CNN model

initial decrease of training and validation loss and then stable training and validation loss after a certain point. Meanwhile, Fig. 10c shows minimal overfitting because the validation loss gradually stabilises after 15 epochs whilst the training loss continues to decrease. This finding indicated that the model starts sticking too much to the training set and then loses its generalisation power.

Performance Evaluation of 1-D Hybrid CNN–LSTM Models

The LSTM layer transforms the vector sequence into a single vector that contains information about the entire sequence. The total number of parameters and total trainable parameters decrease when the same structure as the 1-D CNN model is used but with an additional LSTM layer before fully connected layers. The maximum accuracy and F1 score are 82.33% and 80.00, respectively. Figure 11a shows the normalised confusion matrix. We can clearly see that only normal and noise rhythms obtain a high percentage of correct prediction. Other rhythms and AF, which is important in this project, only obtained correct predictions of 0.64 and an AF of 0.24 was predicted as normal rhythm. This value is excessively high. If this model were implemented in real life, then 24% of AF patients will be diagnosed as normal. Accuracy and loss curves are shown in Figs. 11b and c, respectively.

Although the loss is very large at epoch 1, it decreases with the increase of epochs because optimisation by the optimiser occurs and the average is reset and computed

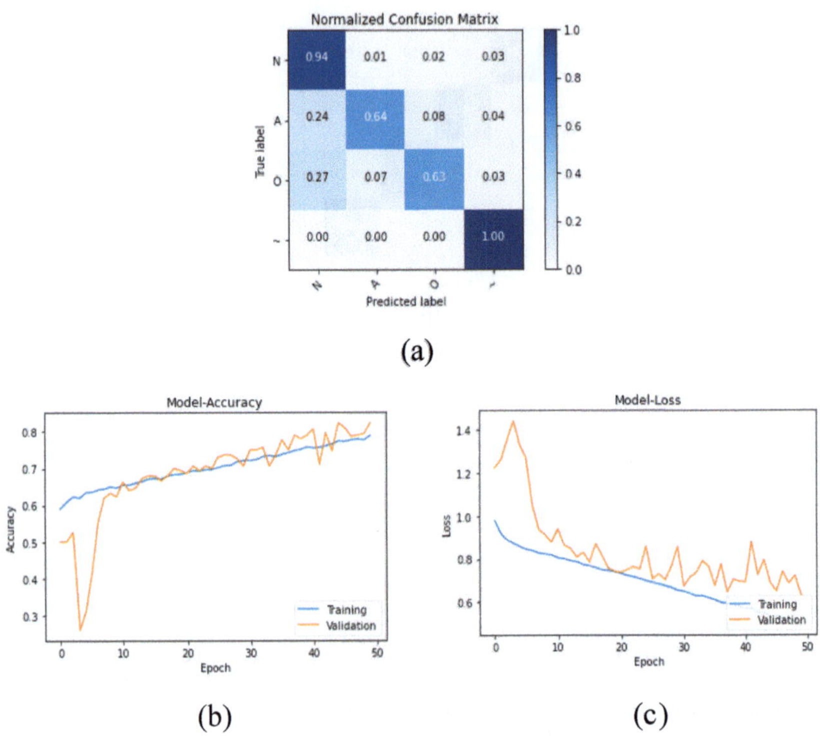

Fig. 6.11 **a** Normalised confusion matrix of the CNN–LSTM model, **b** accuracy curve of the 1-D CNN–LSTM classifier and **c** loss curve of the CNN–LSTM model

again for all the following epochs once epoch 2 starts. Although the accuracy is low, its accuracy curve still shows a satisfactory fit because the gap between training and validation accuracies is small. However, training and validation losses decrease continuously until the end of the plot. This finding indicated that the model is underfit, capable of further learning and that the training process is halted prematurely.

Therefore, the number of epochs is increased to 100 and the CNN–LSTM model is trained again. The unidirectional LSTM layer is replaced with a bidirectional LSTM layer. Table 6.5 shows the optimal output results of the latest 1-D CNN–biLSTM classifier.

The results showed that the proposed 1-D CNN–biLSTM model outperforms the CNN and CNN–LSTM models with the highest accuracy of 94.67% and F1 score of 92.98. Figure 12a presents the normalised confusion matrix. The percentage of correct prediction was higher than that of the CNN–LSTM model. Sensitivity increased from 64 to 94% for AF and from 63 to 90% for other rhythms. Mislabelling also decreased significantly, with the maximum mislabelling at only 4%. The performance of the model at each epoch is analysed by observing the accuracy and loss curve. Accuracy and loss curves of the CNN–biLSTM model are illustrated in Fig. 12b and c, respectively.

Table 6.5 Classification results of the proposed 1-D CNN–biLSTM model

Accuracy	94.67%			
F1 Score	92.98			
	Normal	AF	Others	Noise
Sensitivity	0.960	0.940	0.900	1.000
Specificity	0.980	0.996	0.991	0.963
Positive predictive value	0.980	0.979	0.969	0.750
Negative predictive value	0.961	0.988	0.970	1.000

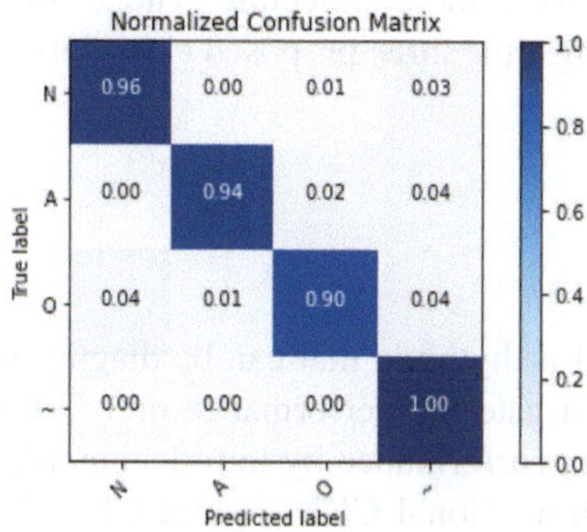

(a)

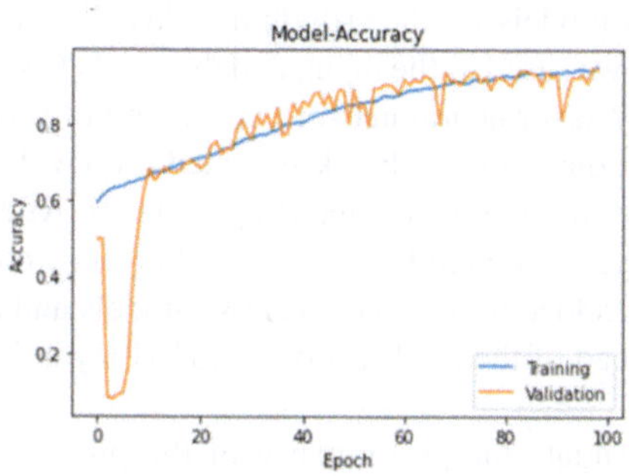

(b)

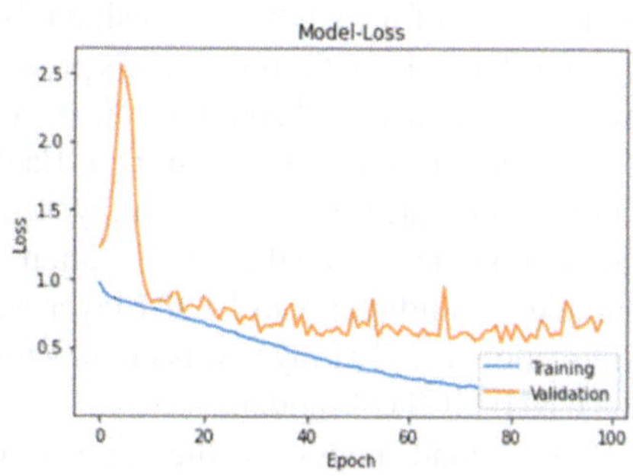

(c)

Fig. 6.12 **a** Normalised confusion matrix of the CNN–biLSTM model, **b** accuracy curve of the 1-D CNN–biLSTM classifier and **c** loss curve of the CNN–biLSTM model

The accuracy curve shows a satisfactory fit because the gap between training and validation accuracies is small. Moreover, both training and validation accuracy lines gradually flatten with the increase of epochs. This finding indicated that the model is not underfit because the number of epochs increases from 50 to 100. The model can be optimally trained. The loss for the model on both training and validation sets reduces over time as the algorithm learns. However, loss of the validation dataset

Table 6.6 Optimal results of 1-D CNN, 1-D CNN–LSTM and 1-D CNN–biLSTM models

Classifier	No. of epochs	SE	SP	Overall F1	Result accuracy
1-D CNN	50	0.880	0.992	90.17	91.67%
1-D CNN–LSTM	50	0.640	0.976	80.00	82.33%
1-D CNN–biLSTM	100	0.940	0.996	92.98	94.67%

stops decreasing from the 40th epoch. The results and evaluation metrics of all three classifiers are listed in Table 6.6. In conclusion, the proposed 1-D CNN–biLSTM classifier obtains the most accurate results compared with 1-D CNN and 1-D CNN–LSTM classifiers under the same architecture. The 1-D CNN–LSTM presents the worst performance amongst the three proposed classifiers.

6.5 Conclusions

AF is a common type of arrhythmia that can be diagnosed using an ECG pattern. This study aims to investigate the performance of 1-D CNN for arrhythmia classification and improve its performance by introducing a hybrid approach based on LSTM approach. One-dimensional CNN, hybrid CNN–LSTM and hybrid CNN–biLSTM models are developed and evaluated in this study to classify ECG signals into (1) normal rhythm, (2) AF rhythm, (3) other rhythms and (4) noisy signal. The first module of the study is to design CNN models for the arrhythmia classification system. The 1-D ECG signal in this project was used as the input, and three 1-D CNN models were designed and developed. A 27-layer neural network consisting of four convolutional blocks was designed. Each convolutional block included a convolutional layer, batch normalization layer, max-pooling layer, and dropout layer. After the fourth convolutional block, a flatten layer and three fully connected layers were applied. A unidirectional LSTM layer was added to the CNN–LSTM models and a bidirectional LSTM layer was chosen instead of the unidirectional LSTM layer for the CNN–biLSTM model.

The second module of the study to evaluate the performance of the proposed 1-D CNN models in classifying the ECG signal into normal rhythm, AF heartbeat, other rhythms and noise rhythm. The performance of all three proposed classifiers is compared. The architecture of models is nearly the same, with the only difference of an additional LSTM layer in the CNN–LSTM model and an additional bidirectional LSTM layer in the CNN–biLSTM model. All models use the 1-D convolutional layer and 1-D input signals. Moreover, these models are trained and tested with the same sets of training and validation data. Experimental results showed that the CNN model presents minimal overfitting compared to the hybrid CNN–LSTM model. This is likely due to the CNN classifier contains more parameters at 690,020 whilst the hybrid CNN–LSTM model only contains 182,372 parameters. The difference between them is fourfold. The CNN model with more parameters is highly susceptible to overfitting compared with the CNN–LSTM model. The increase of model parameters increases the model complexity to ensure that it can tightly fit data in training.

The performance of the developed CNN model achieved an overall accuracy of 91.67% and F1 score of 90.17. The CNN–LSTM model demonstrated the worst performance amongst the three models with an accuracy of 82.33% and F1 score of 80.00. The hybrid CNN–biLSTM model achieved the maximum accuracy of 94.67% and maximum F1 score of 92.98. The performance of the CNN–biLSTM model is better than the CNN model because LSTM preserves the information from inputs that already passed through it using the hidden state. Meanwhile, CNN only exploits the 'spatial correlation' in data and CNN–LSTM uses the output of feature extraction on input signals from the CNN to support the sequence prediction by LSTM. Unidirectional LSTM only preserves information of the past, whereas the bidirectional LSTM runs inputs in two ways, namely, (1) from the past to the future and (2) from the future to the past. This feature can provide additional context to the neural network and result in fast learning.

As a conclusion, these findings indicated that the prediction and classification of arrhythmia with 1-D ECG using the median wave extraction method and the hybrid CNN–biLSTM model are promising to be used to diagnose AF. The sensitivity of the CNN–biLSTM model that correctly predicts AF patients as positive and specificity of the model that correctly predicts non-AF patients as negative outperforms that of the two other models, especially the CNN–LSTM model. The experiment result was also successfully showed that Adam optimizer is the most suitable optimizer to be employed in the proposed model compared to the SGD optimizer. It was discovered that Adam optimizer can result in much higher specificity and sensitivity.

For the future work, further observation based on balance database will be investigated rather than solely employed from the Physionet Cinc Challenge 2017 Database for the experimental data. In this study, the normal sinus rhythm recordings are more dominant with 5154 recordings, which is more than a half of the total number of recordings compared to the AF rhythms that of 771 recordings in the database. Thus, other AF dataset can be combined for more challenging classification. Apart from that, we also observed the implementation of the deep learning approach requires a high memory requirement. Although, in this study, the data is separated to be trained with 3000 iterations at one time, 5.3 GB of RAM is still required. By implementing a large amount of data for future arrhythmia classification system, high memory consumption and longer processing time will be expected. Therefore, a transfer learning is suggested as this approach can provide high classification accuracies with a relatively small amount of data, rather than performing training from scratch.

Acknowledgements This work was sponsored and supported by Universiti Sains Malaysia for Research University Grant (1001.PELECT.8014057).

Appendix 1

The structure and output of the 1-D CNN classifier

Layer (type)	Kernel size/rate	Output shape	Param #
conv1d_1 (Conv1D)	(16, 3)	(None, 178, 16)	64
batch_normalization_1 (BatchNormalization)	–	(None, 178, 16)	64
max_pooling1d_1 (Maxpooling)	2	(None, 89, 16)	0
dropout_1 (Dropout)	0.25	(None, 89, 16)	0
conv1d_2 (Conv1D)	(32, 3)	(None, 87, 32)	1568
batch_normalization_2 (BatchNormalization)	–	(None, 87, 32)	128
max_pooling1d_2 (Maxpooling)	2	(None, 43, 32)	0
dropout_2 (Dropout)	0.25	(None, 43, 32)	0
conv1d_3 (Conv1D)	(64, 3)	(None, 41, 64)	6208
batch_normalization_3 (BatchNormalization)	–	(None, 41, 64)	256
max_pooling1d_3 (Maxpooling)	2	(None, 20, 64)	0
dropout_3 (Dropout)	0.25	(None, 20, 64)	0
conv1d_4 (Conv1D)	(128, 3)	(None, 18, 128)	24,704
batch_normalization_4 (BatchNormalization)	–	(None, 18, 128)	512
max_pooling1d_4 (Maxpooling)	2	(None, 9, 128)	0
dropout_4 (Dropout)	0.25	(None, 9, 128)	0
Flatten_1 (Flatten)	–	(None, 1152)	0
Dense_1 (Dense)	512	(None, 512)	590,336
Dense_2 (Dense)	128	(None, 128)	65,664
Dense_3 (Dense)	4	(None, 4)	516
conv1d_1 (Conv1D)	(16, 3)	(None, 178, 16)	64
Total params			690,020
Trainable params			689,540
Non-trainable params			480

Appendix 2

The structure and output of the 1-D CNN-LSTM classifier

Layer (type)	Kernel size/rate	Output shape	Param #
conv1d_1 (TimeDistributed Conv1D)	(16, 3)	(None, 4, 43, 16)	64

(continued)

(continued)

Layer (type)	Kernel size/rate	Output shape	Param #
batch_normalization_1 (TimeDistributed BatchNormalization)	–	(None, 4, 43, 16)	64
max_pooling1d_1 (TimeDistribute Maxpooling)	2	(None, 4, 22, 16)	0
dropout_1 (TimeDistributed Dropout)	0.25	(None, 4, 22, 16)	0
conv1d_2 (TimeDistributed Conv1D)	(32, 3)	(None, 4, 20, 32)	1568
batch_normalization_2 (TimeDistributed BatchNormalization)	–	(None, 4, 20, 32)	128
max_pooling1d_2 (TimeDistributed Maxpooling)	2	(None, 4, 10, 32)	0
dropout_2 (TimeDistributed Dropout)	0.25	(None, 4, 10, 32)	0
conv1d_3 (TimeDistributed Conv1D)	(64, 3)	(None, 4, 8, 64)	6208
batch_normalization_3 (TimeDistributed BatchNormalization)	–	(None, 4, 8, 64)	256
max_pooling1d_3 (TimeDistributed Maxpooling)	2	(None, 4, 4, 64)	0
dropout_3 (TimeDistributed Dropout)	0.25	(None, 4, 4, 64)	0
conv1d_4 (TimeDistributed Conv1D)	(128, 3)	(None, 4, 2, 128)	24,704
batch_normalization_4 (TimeDistributed BatchNormalization)	–	(None, 4, 2, 128)	512
max_pooling1d_4 (TimeDistributed Maxpooling)	2	(None, 4, 1, 128)	0
dropout_4 (TimeDistributed Dropout)	0.25	(None, 4, 1, 128)	0
flatten_1 (TimeDistributed Flatten)	–	(None, 4, 128)	0
lstm_5 (LSTM)	64	(None, 64)	49,408
dense_1 (Dense)	512	(None, 512)	33,280
dense_2 (Dense)	128	(None, 128)	65,664
dense_3 (Dense)	4	(None, 4)	516
Total params			182,372
Trainable params			181,892
Non-trainable params			480

Appendix 3

The structure and output after the biLSTM classifier

Layer (type)	Kernel size/rate	Output shape	Param #
flatten_1 (TimeDistributed Flatten)	–	(None, 4, 128)	0
bidirectional_lstm_1 (Bidirectional LSTM)	64	(None, 128)	98,816
dense_1 (Dense)	512	(None, 512)	66,048
dense_2 (Dense)	128	(None, 128)	65,664
dense_3 (Dense)	4	(None, 4)	516
Total params			264,548
Trainable params			264,068
Non-trainable params			480

References

1. What is Atrial Fibrillation (AFib or AF). Available from https://www.heart.org/en/health-topics/atrial-fibrillation/what-is-atrial-fibrillation-afib-or-af. Accessed 10 Dec 2020
2. American Dental Association. Guidelines for the Use of Conscious Sedation, Deep Sedation and General Anesthesia for Dentists 2005. House of Delegates, American Dental Association
3. Goodacre, S., Irons, R.: ABC of clinical electrocardiography: atrial arrhythmias. BMJ Clin. Res. Ed. **324**(7337), 594–597 (2002)
4. Marinucci, D., Sbrollini, A., Marcantoni, I., Morettini, M., Swenne, C.A., Burattini, L.: Artificial neural network for atrial fibrillation identification in portable devices. Sensors **20**(12), 3570 (2020)
5. Padmavathi, K., Sri Ramakrishna, K.: Classification of ECG signal during atrial fibrillation using autoregressive modeling. Procedia Comput. Sci. **46**, 53–59 (2015)
6. Rai, H.M., Trivedi, A.: ECG signal classification using wavelet transform and back propagation neural network. In: 5th International Conference on Computers and Devices for Communication (CODEC), pp. 1–4 (2012)
7. Xiong, Z., Nash, M.P., Cheng, E., Fedorov, V.V., Stiles, M.K., Zhao, J.: ECG signal classification for the detection of cardiac arrhythmias using a convolutional recurrent neural network. Physiol. Meas. **39**(9), 094006 (2018)
8. Pourbabaee, B., Roshtkhari, M.J., Khorasani, K.: Deep convolutional neural networks and learning ECG features for screening paroxysmal atrial fibrillation patients. IEEE Trans. Syst. Man Cybern. Syst. **48**(12), 2095–2104 (2018)
9. Shchutskaya, V.: Deep learning: strengths and challenges. InData Labs (2018). https://indatalabs.com/blog/deep-learning-strengths-challenges
10. AI vs. Machine Learning vs. Deep Learning vs. Neural Networks: What's the Difference? (2020) IBM Cloud Education. https://www.ibm.com/cloud/blog/ai-vs-machine-learning-vs-deep-learning-vs-neural-networks
11. Clifford, G.D., Liu, C., Moody, B., Li-wei, H.L., Silva, I., Li, Q., Johnson, A.E., Mark, R.G.: AF classification from a short single lead ECG recording: the PhysioNet computing in cardiology challenge 2017. In: 2017 IEEE Computing in Cardiology (CinC), pp. 1–4 (2017)

12. Mitchell, T.: Machine learning. McGraw Hill, New York, ISBN 0-07-042807-7. OCLC 36417892 (1997)
13. Turakhia, M.P., Hoang, D.D., Zimetbaum, P., Miller, J.D., Froelicher, V.F., Kumar, U.N., Xu, X., Yang, F., Heidenreich, P.A.: Diagnostic utility of a novel leadless arrhythmia monitoring device. Am. J. Cardiol. **112**(4), 520–524 (2013)
14. KannelW, B., Kannel, C., Paffenbarger, R.S., Cupples, L.A.: Heart rate and cardiovascular mortality: the Framingham study. Am. Heart J. **113**(6), 1489–1494 (1987)
15. Mason, J.W., Ramseth, D.J., Chanter, D.O., Moon, T.E., Goodman, D.B., Mendzelevski, B.: Electrocardiographic reference ranges derived from 79,743 ambulatory subjects. J. Electrocardiol. **40**(3), 228–234 (2007)
16. Dhinakaran, S., Tamilanban, T., Vellapandian, C.: Arrhythmia's: types, pathophysiology and therapy: a review. Int. Res. J. Pharm. **10**, 23–30 (2019)
17. Kher, R.: Signal processing techniques for removing noise from ECG signals. J. Biomed. Eng. **1**, 1–9 (2019)
18. Gopinathannair, R., Olshansky, B.: Management of tachycardia. F1000prime Rep **7**, 60 (2015)
19. Guzik, T.J., Mohiddin, S.A., Dimarco, A., Patel, V., Savvatis, K., Marelli-Berg, F., Madhur, M.S., Tomaszewski, M., Maffia, P., D'Acquisto, F., Nicklin, S.A., Marian, A.J., Nosalski, R., Murray, E.C., Guzik, B., Berry, C., Touyz, R.M., Kreutz, R., Wang, D.W., Bhella, D., McInnes, I.B.: COVID-19 and the cardiovascular system: implications for risk assessment, diagnosis, and treatment options. Cardiovasc Res **116**(10), 1666–1687 (2020)
20. Guan, H., Liu, J., Ding, J., Liu, W., Feng, Y., Bao, Y., Li, H., Wang, X., Zhou, Z., Chen, Z.: Arrhythmias in patients with coronavirus disease 2019 (COVID-19) in Wuhan, China: incidences and implications. J. Electrocardiol. **65**, 96–101 (2021)
21. Underlying Cause of Death, 1999–2018.: Centers for Disease Control and Prevention, National Center for Health Statistics
22. Walczak, S., Cerpa, N.: Artificial neural networks. Encycl. Phys. Sci. Technol. 631–645 (2003)
23. Sadiq, R., Rodriguez, J., Mian, H.R.: Empirical models to predict disinfection by-products (DBPs) in drinking water: an updated review. Encycl. Environ. Health 324–338 (2019)
24. Feng, J., Shengnan, L.: Performance analysis of various activation functions in artificial neural networks. J. Phys: Conf. Ser. **1237**, 022030 (2019)
25. Fernández-Cabán, P.L., Masters, F.J., Phillips, B.M.: Predicting roof pressures on a low-rises structure from freestream turbulence using artificial neural networks. Front. Built Environ. **4**, 68 (2018)
26. Fukushima, K.: Neocognitron: a self organizing neural network model for a mechanism of pattern recognition unaffected by shift in position. Biol. Cybern. **36**(4), 193–202 (1980)
27. Ullah, A., Anwar, S.M., Bilal, M., Mehmood, R.M.: Classification of arrhythmia by using deep learning with 2-D ECG spectral image representation. Remote Sens. **12**(10), 1–14 (2020)
28. Cecotti, H., Gräser, A.: Convolutional neural networks for P300 detection with application to brain-computer interfaces. IEEE Trans. Pattern Anal. Mach. Intell. **33**(3), 433–445 (2011)
29. Piczak, K.J.: Environmental sound classification with convolutional neural networks. In: IEEE 25th International Workshop on Machine Learning for Signal Processing (MLSP), pp. 1–6 (2015)
30. Ravisutha, S.S.: Understanding 1D convolutional neural networks using multiclass time-varying signals. All Theses: 2911 (2018)
31. Clifford, G.D., Liu, C., Moody, B., Silva, I., Li, Q., Johnson, A.E.W., Mark, R.G.: AF classification from a short single lead ECG recording: the Physionet computing in cardiology challenge. Comput. Cardiol. **44** (2017)
32. Hannun, A.Y., Rajpurkar, P., Haghpanahi, M., Tison, G.H., Bourn, C., Turakhia, M.P., Ng, A.Y.: Cardiologist-level arrhythmia detection and classification in ambulatory electrocardiograms using a deep neural. Cardiologist-level arrhythmia detection with Convolutional Neural Networks. Nat. Med. **25**(1), 65–69 (2019)
33. Fernando, A., Oliver, C., Marco, A.F.P., Adam, M., Maarten, D.V.: Comparing feature based classifiers and convolutional neural networks to detect arrhythmia from short segments of ECG. Comput. Cardiol. **44**, 1–4 (2017)

34. Goldberger, A.L., Amaral, L.A., Glass, L., Hausdorff, J.M., Ivanov, P.C., Mark, R.G., Mietus, J.E., Moody, G.B., Peng, C.K., Stanley, H.E.: PhysioBank, PhysioToolkit, and PhysioNet: components of a new research resource for complex physiologic signals. Circulation **101**(23), E215–E220 (2000)
35. Behar, J., Andreotti, F., Zaunseder, S., Li, Q., Oster, J., Clifford, G.D.: An ECG simulator for generating maternal-foetal activity mixtures on abdominal ECG recordings. Physiol. Meas. **35**(8), 537–1550 (2014)
36. Mathunjwa, B.M., Lin, Y.T., Lin, C.H., Abbod, M.F., Sadrawi, M., Shieh, J.S.: ECG recurrence plot-based arrhythmia classification using two-dimensional deep residual CNN features. Sensors **22**(4), 1660 (2022)
37. Billeci, L., Costi, M., Lombardi, D., Chiarugi, F., Varanini, M.: Automatic detection of atrial fibrillation and other arrhythmias in ECG recordings acquired by a smartphone device. Electronics **7**(9), 199 (2018)
38. Hamilton, P.S., Limited, E.P.: Open source ECG analysis software documentation. (2002). http://www.eplimited.com/
39. Murat, F., Yildirim, O., Talo, M., Baloglu, U., Demir, Y., Acharya, U.R.: Application of deep learning techniques for heartbeats detection using ECG signals-analysis and review. Comput. Biol. Med. **120**, 103726 (2020)
40. Kingma, D.P., Ba, J.: Adam: a method for stochastic optimization. CoRR (2015). abs/1412.6980

Chapter 7
Polyp Segmentation with Deep Ensembles and Data Augmentation

Loris Nanni, Daniela Cuza, Alessandra Lumini, Andrea Loreggia, and Sheryl Brahman

Abstract Globally, colorectal cancer is one of the leading causes of mortality. Colonoscopies and the early removal of polys significantly increase the survival rate of this cancer, but this intervention depends on the accurate detection of polys in the surrounding tissues. Missing a poly has serious consequences. One way to guard against human error is to develop automatic polyp detection systems. Deep learning semantic segmentation offers one approach to solving the problem of poly detection. In this work, we propose an ensemble of ensembles composed of two deep convolutional neural networks (DCNNs): DeepLabV3+ and HarDNet. Diversity among the single classifiers is enforced on the data level using different data augmentation approaches and on the classifier level with two DCNNs: DeepLabV3+ and HardNet, each using an encoder-decoder unit. In addition, ensembles of DeepLabV3+ are built using fifteen loss functions. Our best ensembles are tested on a large dataset composed of samples taken from five polyp benchmarks. Ensembles are assessed and compared with the best method reported in the literature and shown to produce state-of-the-art results. The source code, the dataset, and the testing protocol used in this study are freely available at https://github.com/LorisNanni.

Keywords Machine learning · Data augmentation · Deep learning · Ensembles · Polyp segmentation

---

L. Nanni · D. Cuza
Department of Information Engineering, University of Padua, viale Gradenigo 6, 35122 Padua, Italy
e-mail: loris.nanni@unipd.it

A. Lumini
Department of Computer Science and Engineering, University of Bologna, Via dell'università 50, 47521 Cesena, Italy
e-mail: Alessandra.lumini@unibo.it

A. Loreggia
Department of Legal Studies, University of Bologna—Via Zamboni, 33—40126 Bologna, Italy

S. Brahman (✉)
Missouri State University, 901 South National Avenue, Springfield, MO 65804, USA
e-mail: SBrahnam@MissouriState.edu

© The Author(s), under exclusive license to Springer Nature Switzerland AG 2023

C.-P. Lim et al. (eds.), *Artificial Intelligence and Machine Learning for Healthcare*, Intelligent Systems Reference Library 228,
https://doi.org/10.1007/978-3-031-11154-9_7

7.1 Introduction

One of the most widespread cancers globally is colorectal cancer: it is the second most prevalent cancer affecting women and the third most affecting men [1]. The first possible indicator of colorectal cancer is the presence of polyps, growths on the lining of the colon or large intestine, common in people over 50. Most polyps are harmless, but some can become malignant. Accurate identification of polyps increases the chances of removing colorectal cancer in the early stages, which significantly increases patient survival.

The standard method for identifying and removing cancer-causing polyps is colonoscopy, the accuracy of which hovers around 70–80%, with a miss rate of polyp detection up to 30% [1]. Locating polyps in a video colonoscopy (which numbers about 50,000 frames with a frame rate of about 25–30 frames per second) is highly difficult, as a polyp might only be visible for a few frames [2]. The hit rate is often represented by the ADR (Adenoma detection rate), a quality benchmark acknowledged by companies working in the industry. ADR is the proportion of patients with at least one histologically proven adenoma or carcinoma [2]. The higher the hit rate, the lower the chance of cancer [3].

The high detection error rate is mainly due to two factors: (1) the presence of blind spots (a problem somewhat solvable with wide-angle colonoscopy [4]) and (2) the existence of various classes of polyps (adenomatous, serrated, hyperplastic, tubulovillous adenoma, and inflammatory) whose edges and color are similar to the surrounding mucosa tissue. Among these five classes, adenomas are the most dangerous and difficult to detect. Human factors must also be taken into consideration when discussing high detection error rates: the doctor's experience and skill in detecting polyps, which can vary widely, and the physical and psychological conditions of the doctors, which decrease as workload stresses increase [5], have a significant impact. One way to reduce human errors is to position another expert observer alongside the first. However, the inclusion of a second expert does not always guarantee the detection of every dangerous poly [4]. Developing real-time high-performance automatic polyp recognition systems can offset some of the causes of human error. This is where deep learning and neural networks come into play.

Deep learning is a branch of machine learning that is part of the broader world of artificial intelligence. Deep learning networks aspire to achieve the human brain's functionality with its massive interconnections of 86 billion neurons by building models that interlink highly specialized networks. Despite its long history and thanks to the sharp rise in available data and cheap GPUs, deep neural networks have demonstrated their discriminative power across a wide range of applications in the last decade and now dominate the field of machine learning. Deep learning models like Convolutional Neural Networks (CNNs) are currently the mainstay in image classification, having usurped the position of traditional classifiers like the Support Vector Machine. This trend appears to be happening in polyp classification: a study reported in [6], for instance, showed that a CNN could significantly outperform standard classifiers in certain situations, and the CNN system in [7] won the first and second awards in the 2017 and 2018 Gastrointestinal Image ANAlysis (GIANA) contests.

There are, however, some problems training deep learners, one of the foremost being the issue of overfitting, which occurs when the system produces a better performance on the training dataset than on the testing set. Overfitting makes the learner ineffective when evaluated on any new dataset [8]. What is sought is generalizability, the ability of a network to obtain the same performance on both the training and testing datasets [8].

Many strategies have been developed to avoid overfitting: some of the best include dropout, batch normalization, and image augmentation [7]. Dropout is a stochastic regularization technique [9] that incorporates various neural network architectures. The main idea behind dropout is to randomly remove neurons from the network while training so that no information flows through the dropout neurons. Another regularization technique is batch normalization, which is typically used to train very deep neural networks. This strategy normalizes the output of the activation functions. As a result, the speed of training increases with the outlying large weights. Normalization produces a network that is more stable.

Data augmentation is a technique that generates artificial images by manipulating images in the training set. A larger dataset reduces overfitting. Common augmentations include geometric transformations, distortions, the addition of noise and blur, kernel filters (the application of a matrix to modify images by adding different kinds of blur, sharpening, etc.), mixing images, random erasing (by randomly selecting a rectangular region within an image and replacing its pixels with random values), and by changing the levels of saturation, brightness, or contrast of the images [8].

An additional advantage to using data augmentation for polyp recognition is that training deep learners with augmented images increases the network's ability to discern polyps in real-world scenarios. Although there are many polyp datasets (such as CVC-ClinicDB, ETIS-Larib, CVC-Colon dataset, Kvasir-Seg, and CVC-ClinicVideoDB), the images in these collections are relatively pristine and fail to reflect the true complexity encountered in the clinic. Most images in these benchmarks are of high quality and contain polyps similar in size and shape; polyps in the clinic are far more diverse, lower in quality, and often obscured by motion blurs [2].

Among the techniques available for locating and analyzing objects within an image, one of the most common is semantic segmentation, which has proven itself in many fields, such as scene understanding, autonomous driving, and robotic navigation [10]. Semantic segmentation divides images into regions of interest (ROIs) that are easy to analyze and interpret. For every ROI, each pixel is assigned a label intended to identify specific objects (such as a polyp) by highlighting its borders or edges [3], which in the case of polyp segmentation means distinguishing them from the surrounding mucosa [3].

In this chapter, we take an approach to semantic segmentation based on techniques for building ensembles. Ensembles are sets of classifiers whose individual decisions are aggregated into a single prediction model. The classifiers can be of one type or many; what is crucial is that there be sufficient diversity among them to learn something different from the training data.

In this study, we develop ensembles using a method for semantic segmentation called DeepLabV3+ [11] (described in Sect. 7.2, where the polyps identified by each instance of DeepLabV3+ are not allowed to overlap with any of the others. Diversity is injected by varying the loss functions and augmentation methods used to expand the training set. We also combine sets of DeepLabV3+ with HarDNet [12], another method for semantic segmentation that is likewise trained on different sets of augmentations.

The main contributions of this study are the following:

1. We develop an ensemble of ensembles of deep learners for semantic segmentation using DeepLabV3+ and HarDNet.
2. We show that diversity can be enforced by varying the loss functions of these models and by employing a set of data augmentation techniques.
3. We provide an extensive empirical analysis demonstrating the power of our approach on the task of colon polyp segmentation.
4. Our results are verified by comparing our best ensemble model with state-of-the-art methods based on both CNN approaches and transfer learning. Our best ensembles are shown to outperform the state-of-the-art.

It should be noted that there is one significant shortcoming using our proposed approach: the ensemble we develop here is classical, thus requiring considerable computation time when training.

7.2 Related Methods

Semantic segmentation aims at identifying objects in an image and determining their boundaries. This technology is essential for many practical applications, ranging from medical diagnosis [13] to autonomous vehicles [14]. As noted in the introduction, semantic segmentation assigns a class label at the pixel level to each object in an image.

As far as deep semantic segmentation goes, an early Deep CNN (DCNN) for semantic segmentation is the Fully Convolutional Network (FCNs), which solves the problem of semantic segmentation by replacing the last fully connected layer of a CNN architecture with a fully convolutional layer so that the network can make pixel-level predictions [15]. Since the method proposed in this work is based on DCCN, the discussion that follows will focus on DCCN semantic segmentation methods. For image segmentation with other deep learning models (e.g., recurrent neural networks and attention and generative models), the reader is referred to [16].

By adding an autoencoder unit into FCN, it becomes possible to design and train deconvolutional networks. An autoencoder is a unit composed of an encoder network (typically a pretrained CNN, such as VGG or ResNet) followed by a decoder network.

The task of the encoder is to extract features to produce a latent image, while that of the decoder is to reconstruct the image.

A popular autoencoder developed for semantic segmentation is U-Net [17]. The autoencoder in U-Net downsamples the image while simultaneously increasing the input feature size and resolution of the image for segmentation. Another common autoencoder for semantic segmentation is SegNet [18], where the encoder network is VGG [19], and the input of the decoder is not the expected output of the encoder. Instead, each layer of the decoder in SegNet is fed the max pool indices of the corresponding encoder layer. This design allows SegNet to consume less memory and better handle segmentation.

Some other deep segmentation methods are based on the transformer [20], a deep approach that was initially designed for text comprehension and summarization. Interestingly, the framework of the transformer appears to replicate the vision process in the human brain. It was an easy step, therefore, to apply this segmentation method to computer vision.

The transformer is based on the autoencoder units but adds a self-attention mechanism that considers information in the input with the greatest detail simultaneously with the remaining information.

The training phase is a two-step process [16]:

Step 1: the model is trained on a large dataset to set the weights so that the model generalizes to a more extensive solution space than it would have otherwise.

Step 2: the model is finetuned on a smaller dataset so as better to fit the task at hand better.

Because the complexity of the attention operator is quadratic, some reduction of the input size is necessary, which is accomplished by initially dividing the image into patches [21], a common practice in computer vision. Once the image is divided, linear transformation and position embeddings are applied. The result is the input to the transformer encoder.

An excellent example of this segmentation method applied in the medical domain is TransFuse [22], which combined the power of CNN kernels to capture local information with the transformer to represent information at a higher level. Another approach based on considering information on both the local and global level is UACANet [23], which employs U-Net combined with a parallel axial attention encoder and decoder.

DeepLab [24] is a family of evolving networks produced by Google that has an established track record in semantic segmentation. With DeepLab, an atrous convolution process upsamples the output of the last convolution layer by applying a dilation rate to increase the window of filters while simultaneously sustaining the computational effort. The performance gains obtained by the DeepLab family of segmentators [11] are primarily due to the following:

- The dilated convolution produces more resolution despite pooling and stride effects;
- Atrous Spatial Pyramid Pooling retrieves information at different scales;

- CNNs, in combination with probabilistic graphical models, improve the localization of object boundaries.

DeepLabV3 improves DeepLab in two ways: (1) it combines cascade and parallel units for convolutional dilation and (2) includes batch normalization and 1×1 convolutions in Atrous Spatial Pyramid Pooling. DeepLabV3+ [11] adds to DeepLabV3 a decoder with point-wise convolutions that operate on the same channel but at different locations and depth-wise convolutions that work at the same location but on different channels.

Another DCCN, HarDNet-MSEG [12] (hereafter abbreviated HarDNet), was developed explicitly for polyp segmentation. The backbone of HarDNet is a CNN with an encoder-decoder called HarDNet68 [25] that has established a good track record on many computer vision problems. The decoder in HarDNet was motivated by the Cascaded Partial Decoder [26], which is known for its speed in accurately detecting salient objects. Before the output of the encoder is passed to the decoder, a Receptive Field Block [27] strengthens the features by adding different receptive fields.

Provided in this section is a description of the proposed method, as well as the mathematical definitions of the loss functions and metrics used in this study.

7.2.1 Overview of the Propose System

As noted in the introduction, we build ensembles (with decisions combined via sum rule) at the data level using data augmentation and at the classifier level by combining ensembles of DeepLabV3+ [11] and HarDNet [12] trained on different sets of data augmentations (see Sect. 7.3). The CNN for the encoder part in DeepLabV3+ is ResNet101 [28], a well-known CNN that learns a residual function with reference to the block input (for a comprehensive list of CNN structures, see [29]).

With DeepLabV3+ , each augmentation set is trained on a set of ResNet101s built using fifteen different loss functions (see Sect. 2.2). The loss function used with the HarDNet encoder is the same as that in the original paper [12].

Transfer learning in the form of pretrained encoders is another viable choice when designing models and ensembles; we chose instead to focus this study on changing the loss function. On the VOC segmentation dataset (see Sect. 4.1), however, we used a pretrained network, finetuning it with the parameters suggested at https://github.com/matlab-deep-learning/pretrained-deeplabv3plus.

To avoid overfitting, none of the following were modified:

- initial learning rate = 0.01;
- number of epoch = 10;
- momentum = 0.9;
- L2Regularization = 0.005;
- Learning Rate Drop Period = 5;
- Learning Rate Drop Factor = 0.2;

- Shuffle training images: every-epoch;
- Optimizer: SGD (Stochastic Gradient Descent).

We also tested the Adam optimizer, but the network failed to converge properly.

For specific details on how each set of ensembles was built and which were combined, see the experimental analysis in Sect. 3.2.

7.2.2 *Loss Functions*

One of the most widely used loss functions in semantic segmentation is pixel-wise cross-entropy loss. Classification with this loss function simply compares a prediction at the pixel level with the factual label. A significant drawback with this loss function is that it treats each pixel equally, which becomes a problem when the dataset is unbalanced. Solutions for handling such datasets are many. For a review of loss functions in semantic segmentation, see [30].

As noted before, we employ different loss functions to add diversity to ensembles. The loss functions tested here are those proposed in [31]:

- Dice Loss [32]
- Tversky Loss [33]
- Three Cross-Entropy variants (Binary Cross-Entropy, Focal Loss [34], and Focal Tversky Loss [35])
- Log-Cosh Dice Loss and Log-Cosh Binary Cross-Entropy Loss [31]
- Focal Generalized Dice Loss [31]
- Log-Cosh Tversky Loss [31]
- Log-Cosh Focal Tversky Loss [31]
- SSIM Loss [36]
- $\text{Comb}_{1,2,3}$ [31]
- Neighbor Loss [37]

7.2.2.1 Dice Loss

Dice Loss is a popular loss function in semantic segmentation models. It is based on the Sørensen-Dice coefficient, which determines the degree of similarity between two images in the range [0, 1].

The Generalized Dice Loss (L_{GD}) between the predictions Y and the training targets T was developed for the multiclass problem [32] and is defined as:

$$L_{GD}(Y, T) = 1 - \frac{2 * \sum_{k=1}^{K} w_k * \sum_{m=1}^{M} Y_{km} * T_{km}}{\sum_{k=1}^{K} w_k * \sum_{m=1}^{M} (Y_{km}^2 + T_{km}^2)} \tag{7.1}$$

$$w_k = \frac{1}{(\sum_{m=1}^{M} T_{km})^2} \tag{7.2}$$

where M is the number of pixels, K is the number of classes, w_k is a weighting factor that focuses the network on a small region inversely proportional to the frequency of the labels of a given class k.

7.2.2.2 Tversky Loss

Similar to Dice Loss is Tversky Loss [33], which adds another weighting factor to overcome a common problem in image segmentation: the dominance of one class over another. Tversky Loss comes from the Tversky Index and its two weighting factors α and β that handle a give-and-take between false positives and false negatives. When $\alpha = \beta = 0.5$, the Dice Similarity coefficient and the Tversky Index are the same. In this work, $\alpha = 0.3$ and $\beta = 0.7$, values which emphasizes false negatives as can be observed in Eq. 7.3.

The Tversky Index TI_k between predictions Y and ground truth T for a given class k is:

$$TI_k(Y,T) = \frac{\sum_{m=1}^{M} Y_{pm}T_{pm}}{\sum_{m=1}^{M} Y_{pm}T_{pm} + \alpha \sum_{m=1}^{M} Y_{pm}T_{nm} + \beta \sum_{m=1}^{M} Y_{nm}T_{pm}} \tag{7.3}$$

where p is the positive class, n the negative class, and M the total number of pixels.

The formula of the Tversky Loss (L_T) is:

$$L_T(Y,T) = \sum_{k=1}^{K}(1 - TI_k(Y,T)) \tag{7.4}$$

where K is the number of classes.

7.2.2.3 Cross-Entropy Variants: Binary Cross-Entropy, Focal Loss, and Focal Tversky Loss

Cross-entropy is a distribution-based loss function that minimizes the difference between two probability distributions. There is no bias between large and small regions with Cross-entropy. Two well-known cross-entropy variants include Binary Cross-Entropy and Focal loss [34]. Binary Cross-Entropy is a version of cross-entropy designed to handle binary classification problems. Focal loss focuses the model on the hardest samples to classify by down-weighting examples that are easier to classify.

Focal loss adds a modulating factor $\gamma > 0$ to cross-entropy that gives it the ability to handle a high imbalance between foreground and background classes. Focal loss is not the only loss function utilizing the modulating factor to learn hard examples. Both Focal Tversky Loss [35] and Exponential Logarithmic Loss [38] do the same.

The relation between Focal Loss (L_F) and Tversky Loss (L_T) can be defined as

$$L_{FT}(Y,T) = L_T(Y,T)^{\frac{1}{\gamma}} \tag{7.5}$$

As the name suggests, Focal Tversky Loss uses the Tversky Index to realize a good trade-off between recall and precision.

7.2.2.4 Focal Generalized Dice Loss

Focal Generalized Dice Loss [31] adds the modulating factor γ to Dice Loss (set here to 4/3) by down-weighting common examples and focusing on small ROIs.

Focal Generalized Dice Loss (L_{FGD}) is defined as

$$L_{FGD}(Y,T) = L_{GD}(Y,T)^{\frac{1}{\gamma}} \tag{7.6}$$

7.2.2.5 Log-Cosh Dice Loss

Log-Cosh Dice Loss is a variant of Dice Loss that applies the Log-Cosh function common in regression problems for smoothing the curve, which is approximately $x^2/2$ for small x and $|x| - \log(2)$ for large x.

$$\begin{aligned}&\text{Log} - \text{Cosh Generalized Dice Loss } (L_{lcGD}) \text{ is defined as}\\ &L_{lcGD}(Y,T) = \log(\cosh(L_{GD}(Y,T)))\end{aligned} \tag{7.7}$$

7.2.2.6 Log-Cosh Binary Cross-Entropy Loss, Log-Cosh Tversky Loss, and Log-Cosh Focal Tversky Loss

Influenced by Log-Cosh Dice Loss, the smooth loss function curve was applied in [31] to generate Log-Cosh Binary Cross-Entropy Loss, Log-Cosh Tversky Loss, and Log-Cosh Focal Tversky Loss. The only difference between these loss functions is the addition of the Log-Cosh term, as shown here for the Log-Cosh Focal Tversky Loss (L_{lcFT}) :

$$L_{lcFT}(Y,T) = log(\cosh(L_{FT}(Y,T))) \tag{7.8}$$

7.2.2.7 Neighbor Loss

The recently proposed Neighbor Loss [37] function is akin to the weighted cross-entropy but considers the spatial correlation in the neighborhood. The weight of each pixel in Neighbor Loss depends on its eight neighbors, specifically on the number of neighbors with a different prediction from the center. Neighbor Loss also tries to deal with difficult samples by using a threshold t and a binary indicator function $1\{\cdot\}$ that drops some easily classified pixels.

Although included in the set of loss functions in [37] and tested in this study, it is not reported in the analysis as its performance was too low to be included.

7.2.2.8 SSIM Loss

SSIM Loss [36], more commonly used to estimate image quality, derives from the Structural Similarity (SSIM) index [39].

SSIM Loss can be defined as

$$SSim(x, y) = \frac{(2\mu_x\mu_y + C_1)(2\sigma_{xy} + C_2)}{(\mu_x^2 + \mu_y^2 + C_1)(\sigma_x^2 + \sigma_y^2 + C_2)} \tag{7.9}$$

where μ_x, μ_y, σ_x, σ_y, and σ_{xy} are the local means, the standard deviations, and the cross-covariance for images x and y. The terms C_1, C_2 are regularization constants.

The SSIM Loss between image Y and the corresponding ground truth T is

$$L_S(Y, T) = 1 - SSim(Y, T) \tag{7.10}$$

7.2.2.9 Comb$_{1,2,3}$

Comb$_{1,2,3}$, proposed in [31], combines loss functions to obtain the best results for a specific concern. In applications with unbalanced data, for example, a serious risk would be to achieve high precision but low recall, highly undesirable in applications like the early detection of cancer.

The first combination, Comb$_1$, tries to overcome a limitation with the Dice Loss function that concerns the fact that it is a harmonic mean of FPs and FNs. To ensure the location of each lesion, there needs to be some flexibility in balancing FPs and FNs. Experts weigh FNs higher than FPs.

Comb$_1$ focuses the model on hard examples while incorporating the benefits of both Focal Generalized Dice Loss and Focal Tversky Loss and is defined as

$$Comb_1(Y, T) = L_{FGD}(Y, T) + L_{FT}(Y, T) \tag{7.11}$$

The second combination, Comb$_2$, down-weights samples easy to classify by mixing Log-Cosh Dice Loss, Focal Generalized Dice Loss, and Log-Cosh Focal Tversky Loss. The nonconvex nature of the curve is controlled by applying the Log-Cosh approach.

Comb$_1$ is defined as

$$Comb_2(Y,T) = L_{lcGD}(Y,T) + L_{FGD}(Y,T) + L_{lcFT}(Y,T) \tag{7.12}$$

Finally, the combination, $Comb_3$, combines SSIM Loss and Generalized Dice Loss:

$$Comb_3(Y,T) = L_S(Y,T) + L_{GD}(Y,T) \tag{7.13}$$

7.3 Data Augmentation

The classification enhancement of three nontrivial image augmentation techniques is investigated here. The goals are to increase the size of the starting dataset and produce a more robust system that can handle noisy, "dirty" data. Performance gains should result. Both shape and color transformation are explored here. With shape-based transformations, the augmentation is applied to the training images and their labels. Augmentation is only applied on the training sets.

7.3.1 Shadows

A shadow is randomly applied either to the left or the right of the original image to obtain a new image. The intensities of the columns are multiplied by as follows:

$$y = \begin{cases} \min\{0.2 + 0.8\sqrt{\frac{x}{0.5}}, 1\} direction = 1 \\ \min\left\{0.2 + 0.8\sqrt{\frac{1-x}{0.5}}, 1\right\} direction = 0 \end{cases}$$

where shadow $direction = 1$ is applied to the right and $direction = 0$ to the left.

7.3.2 Contrast and Motion Blur

As the name of this augmentation indicates, two techniques are applied: first, the contrast of the original image is adjusted by either increasing or decreasing it; second, a motion filter simulating camera movement is applied. In the code, we implement two different contrast functions; only one chosen randomly between the two is actually applied to the image.

The first contrast function is defined as

$$y = \frac{(x - \frac{1}{2})\sqrt{1 - \frac{k}{4}}}{\sqrt{1 - k(x - \frac{1}{2})^2}} + 0.5, k \leq 4$$

where k controls the contrast: contrast increases when $k < 0$ and decreases when $0 < k \leq 4$. When $k = 0$, the image undergoes no contrast. Parameter k is chosen randomly in the following ranges:

- $\mathcal{U}(2.8, 3.8) \rightarrow$ Hard decrease in contrast.
- $\mathcal{U}(1.5, 2.5) \rightarrow$ Soft decrease in contrast.
- $\mathcal{U}(-2, -1) \rightarrow$ Soft increase in contrast.
- $\mathcal{U}(-5, -3) \rightarrow$ Hard increase in contrast.

The second contrast function is defined as

$$y = \begin{cases} \frac{1}{2}\left(\frac{x}{0.5}\right)\alpha 0 \leq x < \frac{1}{2} \\ 1 - \frac{1}{2}\left(\frac{1-x}{0.5}\right)\alpha \frac{1}{2} \leq x \leq 1 \end{cases}$$

where α controls the contrast: contrast increases when $\alpha > 1$ and decreases when $0 < \alpha < 1$. When $\alpha = 1$, the image undergoes no contrast. Parameter α is chosen randomly the following ranges:

- $\mathcal{U}(0.25, 0.5) \rightarrow$ Hard decrease in contrast.
- $\mathcal{U}(0.6, 0.9) \rightarrow$ Soft decrease in contrast.
- $\mathcal{U}(1.2, 1.7) \rightarrow$ Soft increase in contrast.
- $\mathcal{U}(1.8, 2.3) \rightarrow$ Hard increase in contrast.

In order to simulate the motion blur caused by camera jitter, the MATLAB function fspecial('motion', len, theta) is applied.

7.3.3 Color Mapping

Color mapping requires two images: the input sample A and another sample B that is randomly selected from the remaining images in the training set. Three methods of color normalization from the Stain Normalization toolbox by Nicholas Trahearn and Adnan Khan (https://warwick.ac.uk/fac/cross_fac/tia/software/sntoolbox/ accessed 2/21/22) are then applied: (1) RGB Histogram spedification, (2) Reinhard, and (3) Mcenko.

7.4 Experimental Results

7.4.1 Data and Testing Protocol

Our ensembles and the state-of-the-art were evaluated on training/testing datasets composed of five well-known colon benchmarks:

- Kvasir-SEG [40] (**Kvasir**): this is a dataset that contains 1000 polyp images acquired by a high-resolution electromagnetic imaging system: 90% of the images formed the testing set and 10% the training set.
- CVC-ColonDB [41] (**ColDB**): this dataset contains 380 images of size 574 × 500 representing fifteen types of polyps;
- EndoScene-CVC300 (**CVC-T**): this dataset is the test set belonging to a large dataset [42];
- ETIS-Larib Polyp DB [43] (**ETIS**): this dataset contains 196 high-resolution images of size 1225 × 966, extracted from frames in colonoscopy videos (annotations were made by expert video endoscopists);
- CVCClinic DB [44] (**ClinDB**): this dataset contains 612 images of size 384 × 288 extracted from frames in colonoscopy videos (annotations were made by expert video endoscopists);

The testing protocol for this study includes a training set of 1450 images (900 from Kvasir and 550 from ClinDB) and the following five testing sets:

1. The remaining100 images in Kvasir
2. The remaining 62 images in ClinDB
3. All 380 images in ColonDB
4. All 196 images in ETIS
5. All 60 images in CVC-T

The training and testing sets are available on GitHub[1] [12]. The training images were reduced in size to 352 × 352 or 513 × 513.

Before data augmentation, images were reduced to 352 × 352 in cases where another size is not specified in Sect. 3.2 (sometimes images were resized to fit the input of the model). Predicted masks were always resized back to the original dimensions, and performance was evaluated on the original size of the masks. No methods were evaluated here on models using different sizes of images.

The following metrics were used to evaluate performance.

Dice: twice the overlap area of the predicted and ground-truth masks divided by the total number of pixels (Dice and F1score are the same for binary masks, or a weighted average of recall and precision).

Mathematically, Dice is defined as

$$F1score = Dice = \frac{|A \cap B|}{|A| + |B|} = \frac{2 \cdot TP}{2 \cdot TP + FP + FN} \tag{7.14}$$

[1] https://github.com/james128333/HarDNet-MSEG.

Intersection over Union (IoU): the area shared between predicted mask A and ground truth map B, divided by the area of the union between the two maps.

Mathematically, IoU is defined as

$$IoU = \frac{|A \cap B|}{|A \cup B|} = \frac{\text{TP}}{\text{TP} + \text{FP} + \text{FN}} \tag{7.15}$$

where, in a bi-class problem (foreground/background), TP, TN, FP, and FN refer to the true positives, true negatives, false positives, and false negatives, respectively.

7.4.2 Experiments

Two different data augmentation approaches are evaluated:

- DA1, base data augmentation consisting of a horizontal and vertical flip (90° rotation);
- DA2, where the following eleven operations are performed:

  Displacement of the image to the right or to the left.
  Displacement of the image either up or down.
  Rotation of the image by an angle randomly selected from the range [0° 180°].
  Application of horizontal or vertical shear by with the function randomAffine2d.
  Application of horizontal or vertical flip.
  Alteration of the brightness levels by adding the same value to each RGB channel.
  Alteration of the brightness levels by adding different values to each RGB channel.
  Addition of speckle-noise using the function imnoise.
  Application of the technique "Contrast and Motion Blur," described previously.
  Application of the technique "Shadows," described previously.
  Application of the technique "Color Mapping," described previously.

Some artificial images in the DA2 approach contain only background pixels. To discard them, we deleted all images belonging to the class polyp that were less than 10 pixels.

An example of data augmentation starting from an original image is provided in Fig. 7.1.

The first set of experiments compares the following approaches:

- ELoss101: an ensemble of 10 networks (combined by sum rule) with backbone Resnet101 trained using different loss functions: $2 \times L_{GD} + 2 \times L_T + 2 \times$ Comb1 $+ 2 \times$ Comb2 $+ 2 \times$ Comb3;
- ELoss101_15: the same as ELoss101 but trained for 15 epochs;

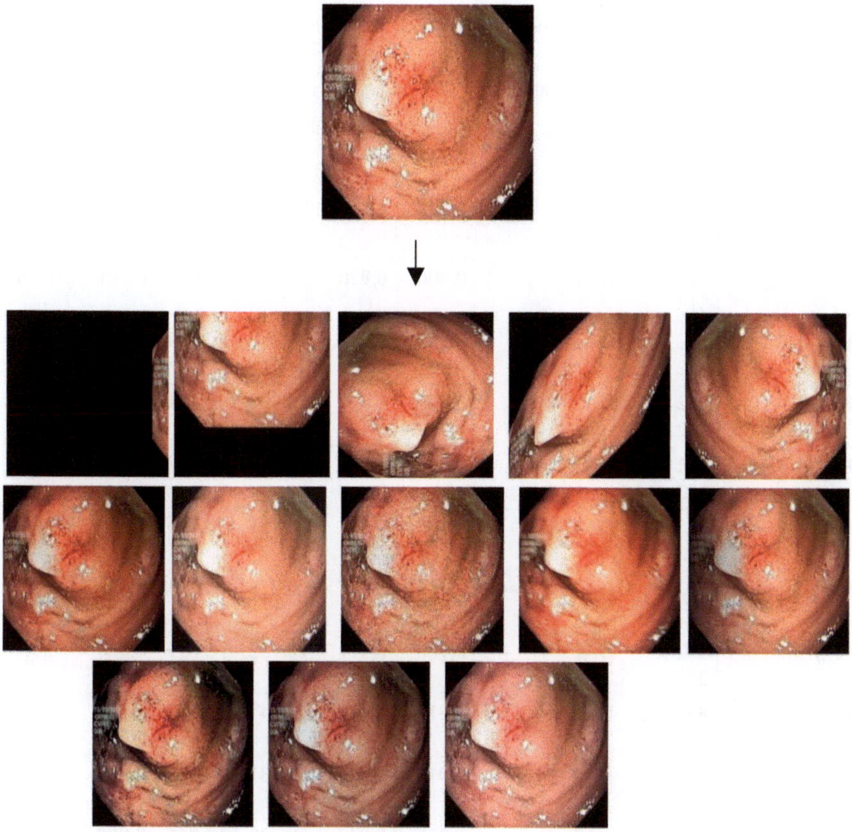

Fig. 7.1 An example image (top) that has undergone DA2 augmentation

- Eloss101-Mix: similar to ELoss101 but based on both DA1 and DA2-15 epochs: sum rule among $L_{GD} + L_T$ + Comb1 + Comb2 + Comb3 (DA1) and $L_{GD} + L_T$ + Comb1 + Comb2 + Comb3 (DA2 - 15 epochs);
- H_S and H_A: experiments using HardNet trained by SGD and Adam optimizers (using the code shared by the authors);
- FH: sum rule between H_A and H_S;
- FH(2): sum rule between two H_A and two H_S;
- Eloss101-Mix + FH: the fusion of 10 × FH + ELoss101(10); the weight of FH is ten since ELoss101(10) is the sum rule among ten networks and FH is the sum rule of two HardNets;
- Eloss101-Mix + FH(2): the fusion of 5 × FH(2) + ELoss101(10); the weight of FH(2) is five since ELoss101(10) is the sum rule among ten networks and FH is the sum rule of 4 HardNets.

Examining the results reported in Table 7.1, we draw the following conclusions:

Table 7.1 Performance of the proposed ensembles

	Training Image size	Data Augmentation	Kvasir	ClinDB	ColDB	ETIS	CVC-T	Avg
Eloss101	352 × 352	DA1	0.912	0.927	0.763	0.719	0.891	0.843
Eloss101	513 × 513	DA1	0.905	0.923	0.746	0.673	0.879	0.825
Eloss101_15	513 × 513	DA1	0.906	0.926	0.745	0.674	0.881	0.826
Eloss101	352 × 352	DA2	0.904	0.916	0.789	0.714	0.869	0.838
Eloss101_15	352 × 352	DA2	0.909	0.926	0.792	0.724	0.863	0.843
Eloss101-Mix	352 × 352	DA1/DA2	0.907	0.929	0.789	0.748	0.880	0.851
H_A	352 × 352	DA1	0.906	0.924	0.751	0.716	0.903	0.840
H_A	352 × 352	DA2	0.896	0.927	0.778	0.774	0.893	0.854
H_S	352 × 352	DA1	0.908	0.911	0.752	0.639	0.868	0.816
H_S	352 × 352	DA2	0.914	0.944	0.747	0.727	0.901	0.847
FH	352 × 352	DA2	0.919	**0.948**	0.781	0.746	0.903	0.859
FH(2)	352 × 352	DA2	0.918	0.947	0.778	**0.756**	**0.909**	**0.862**
Eloss101-Mix + FH	352 × 352	DA1/DA2	0.920	0.947	**0.787**	0.750	0.908	**0.862**
Eloss101-Mix + FH(2)	352 × 352	DA1/DA2	0.918	0.944	0.784	**0.756**	**0.909**	**0.862**

- Training with 15 epochs boosts the performance of Eloss101 when coupled with DA2; the performance is similar to that obtained by Eloss101 when combined with DA1;
- DA2 boosts the performance of H_A and H_S;
- Eloss101-Mix outperforms Eloss101. Using different data augmentation improves the performance of the ensemble;
- Eloss101-Mix + FH outperforms both Eloss101-Mix and FH; the performance of Eloss101-Mix + FH(2) is similar to that obtained by FH(2).
- Eloss101 does not perform very well when trained on images that are 513 × 513, even when Eloss101 is pretrained with images of that size.

In Table 7.2, we report the performance of the best state-of-the-art approaches evaluated using both Dice and IoU as the performance indicators. It will be noted

Table 7.2 Comparison of our best approaches with the literature

Method	Kvasir (100)		ClinicalDB (62)		ColonDB (380)		ETIS (196)		CVC-T (60)		Average	
	IoU	Dice	IoU	Dice	IoU	Dice	IoU	Dice	IoU	Dice	IoU	Dice
Eloss101-Mix + FH	**0.871**	**0.920**	**0.903**	**0.947**	**0.720**	**0.787**	0.681	0.750	0.845	0.908	**0.804**	**0.862**
Eloss101-Mix + FH(2)	0.868	0.918	0.900	0.944	0.719	0.784	**0.688**	**0.756**	0.846	0.909	**0.804**	**0.862**
FH(2)	0.867	0.918	**0.903**	**0.947**	0.713	0.778	0.687	**0.756**	0.846	0.909	0.803	**0.862**
[31]	**0.871**	0.917	0.886	0.931	0.697	0.769	0.663	0.740	0.829	0.901	0.790	0.852
HarDNet-MSEG [45]	0.857	0.912	0.882	0.932	0.66	0.731	0.613	0.677	0.821	0.887	0.767	0.828
PraNet [45]	0.84	0.898	0.849	0.899	0.64	0.709	0.567	0.628	0.797	0.871	0.739	0.801
SFA[45]	0.611	0.723	0.607	0.700	0.347	0.469	0.217	0.297	0.329	0.467	0.422	0.531
U-Net + + [45]	0.743	0.821	0.729	0.794	0.41	0.483	0.344	0.401	0.624	0.707	0.570	0.641
U-Net [45]	0.746	0.818	0.755	0.823	0.444	0.512	0.335	0.398	0.627	0.710	0.581	0.652
SETR [41]	0.854	0.911	0.885	0.934	0.69	0.773	0.646	0.726	0.814	0.889	0.778	0.847
TransUnet [42]	0.857	0.913	0.887	0.935	0.699	0.781	0.66	0.731	0.824	0.893	0.785	0.851
TransFuse [21]	0.870	**0.920**	0.897	0.942	0.706	0.781	0.663	0.737	0.826	0.894	0.792	0.855
UACANet [22]	0.859	0.912	0.88	0.926	0.678	0.751	0.678	0.751	**0.849**	**0.910**	0.789	0.850
[46]	0.847	0.904	0.859	0.916	0.670	0.753	0.654	0.750	0.815	0.888	0.769	0.842
[47]	0.862	0.907	0.879	0.921	0.678	0.755	0.664	0.719	0.807	0.869	0.778	0.834

that the ensembles proposed in this work produce superior results, even when compared with methods based on transformers (such as TransFuse and TransUnet). The drawback in applying our solution is the computational time required to train the ensembles, which is much higher than the stand-alone approaches.

7.5 Conclusions

Crucial technology for medical image analysis is semantic segmentation. Therapies depend on the identification and boundary circumscription of anomalies in the human body, especially in the early stages of a disease. This study develops ensembles of deep networks for semantic segmentation. Ensemble diversity is ensured by varying the loss functions of the internal networks.

Ensembles with several loss functions are evaluated on polyp segmentation, a real-world problem. An in-depth empirical analysis that includes a comparison of recent state-of-the-art models, including transformer-based approaches, confirms that the method proposed here obtains competitively good results across many benchmarks.

Future studies will focus on reducing the complexity of the ensembles by experimenting with pruning, distillation, quantization, and low-rank factorization, among other techniques.

Moreover, we want to validate the main findings of this work in other datasets:

- Eloss101-Mix outperforms Eloss101, i.e., to apply different data augmentation improves the ensemble performance;
- HardNet works better with large data augmentation (i.e., DA2);
- FH(2) outperforms FH; FH outperforms stand-alone HardNet; thus, HardNet seems well suited for building ensembles;
- Eloss101-Mix + FH(2) obtains a performance that is similar to FH(2);
- Eloss101-Mix + FH(2) and FH(2) obtain state-of-the-art performance, even outperforming recent approaches based on a transformer.

Acknowledgements Through their GPU Grant Program, NVIDIA donated the TitanX GPU that was used to train the CNNs presented in this work.

Data Availability Code for all experiments is publicly available at https://github.com/LorisNanni.

References

1. Jha, D. et al.: Kvasir-seg: a segmented polyp dataset. In: International Conference on Multimedia Modeling, pp. 451–462. Springer (2020)
2. Repici, A., et al.: Efficacy of real-time computer-aided detection of colorectal neoplasia in a randomized trial. Gastroenterology **159**(2), 512–520 (2020)

3. Corley, D.A., et al.: Adenoma detection rate and risk of colorectal cancer and death. N. Engl. J. Med. **370**(14), 1298–1306 (2014). https://doi.org/10.1056/NEJMc1405329
4. Luo, Y., et al.: Artificial intelligence-assisted colonoscopy for detection of colon polyps: a prospective, randomized cohort study. J. Gastrointest. Surg. **25**(8), 2011–2018 (2021). https://doi.org/10.1007/s11605-020-04802-4
5. Ma, Y., Chen, X., Cheng, K., Li, Y. and Sun, B.: LDPolypVideo benchmark: a large-scale colonoscopy video dataset of diverse polyps. In: International Conference on Medical Image Computing and Computer-Assisted Intervention (MICCAI 2021), vol. LNCS 12905, pp. 387–396. Springer, Cham (2021). https://doi.org/10.1007/978-3-030-87240-3_37
6. Thambawita, V. et al.: The medico-task 2018: disease detection in the gastrointestinal tract using global features and deep learning. arXiv Prepr. (2018). arXiv:1810.13278
7. Guo, Y.B. and Matuszewski, B.: GIANA polyp segmentation with fully convolutional dilation neural networks. In: 14th International Joint Conference on Computer Vision, Imaging and Computer Graphics Theory and Applications (VISIGRAPP), Prague, Czech Republic, pp. 632–641. SCITEPRESS-Science and Technology Publications (2019)
8. Shorten, C., Khoshgoftaar, T.M.: A survey on image data augmentation for deep learning. J. Big Data **6**(60), 1–48 (2019)
9. Srivastava, N., Hinton, G., Krizhevsky, A., Sutskever, I., Salakhutdinov, R.: Dropout: a simple way to prevent neural networks from overfitting. J. Mach. Learn. Res. **15**(1), 1929–1958 (2014)
10. Lumini, A., Nanni, L. and Maguolo, G.: Deep ensembles based on stochastic activation selection for polyp segmentation. arXiv Prepr. (2021). arXiv:2104.00850
11. Chen, L.C., Zhu, Y., Papandreou, G., Schroff, F. and Adam, H.: Encoder-decoder with atrous separable convolution for semantic image segmentation. In ECCV (2018)
12. Huang, C.H., Wu, H.Y. and Lin, Y.L.: Hardnet-mseg: a simple encoder-decoder polyp segmentation neural network that achieves over 0.9 mean dice and 86 fps. arXiv Prepr. (2021). arXiv:2101.07172
13. Brandao, P., et al.: Towards a computed-aided diagnosis system in colonoscopy: automatic polyp segmentation using convolution neural networks. J. Med. Robot. Res. **03**(02), 1840002 (2018). https://doi.org/10.1142/s2424905x18400020
14. Feng, D., et al.: Deep multi-modal object detection and semantic segmentation for autonomous driving: datasets, methods, and challenges. IEEE Trans. Intell. Transp. Syst. **22**(3), 1341–1360 (2021). https://doi.org/10.1109/TITS.2020.2972974
15. Long, J., Shelhamer, E. and Darrell, T.: Fully convolutional networks for semantic segmentation. In: 2015 IEEE Conference on Computer Vision and Pattern Recognition (CVPR), pp. 3431–3440 (2015)
16. Minaee, S., Boykov, Y.Y., Porikli, F., Plaza, A.J., Kehtarnavaz, N. and Terzopoulos, D.: Image segmentation using deep learning: a survey. IEEE Trans. Pattern Anal. Mach. Intell. (2021)
17. Ronneberger, O., Fischer, P. and Brox, T.: U-Net: convolutional networks for biomedical image segmentation. In: Presented at the MICCAI 2015 LNCS (2015)
18. Badrinarayanan, V., Kendall, A., Cipolla, R.: SegNet: a deep convolutional encoder-decoder architecture for image segmentation. IEEE Trans. Pattern Anal. Mach. Intell. **39**, 2481–2495 (2017)
19. Simonyan, K., Zisserman, A.: Very deep convolutional networks for large-scale image recognition. Cornell University (2014). arXiv:1409.1556v6
20. Khan, S., Naseer, M., Hayat, M., Zamir, S.W., Khan, F.S. and Shah, M.: Transformers in vision: a survey. ACM Comput. Surv. (CSUR) (2021)
21. Dosovitskiy, A. et al.: An image is worth 16x16 words: transformers for image recognition at scale. arXiv Prepr. (2020). arXiv:2010.11929
22. Zhang, Y., Liu, H. and Hu, Q.: Transfuse: fusing transformers and cnns for medical image segmentation. In: International Conference on Medical Image Computing and Computer-Assisted Intervention, pp. 14–24. Springer (2021)
23. Kim, T., Lee, H. and Kim, D.: UACANet: uncertainty augmented context attention for polyp segmentation. In: Proceedings of the 29th ACM International Conference on Multimedia, pp. 2167–2175 (2021)

24. Chen, L.-C., Papandreou, G., Kokkinos, I., Murphy, K., Yuille, A.: DeepLab: semantic image segmentation with deep convolutional nets, atrous convolution, and fully connected CRFs. IEEE Trans. Pattern Anal. Mach. Intell. **40**, 834–848 (2018)
25. Chao, P., Kao, C.-Y., Ruan, Y.-S., Huang, C.-H., Lin, Y.-L.: Hardnet: a low memory traffic network. In: Proceedings of the IEEE/CVF International Conference on Computer Vision, pp. 3552–3561 (2019)
26. Wu, Z., Su, L. and Huang, Q.: Cascaded partial decoder for fast and accurate salient object detection. In: Proceedings of the IEEE/CVF Conference on Computer Vision and Pattern Recognition, pp. 3907–3916 (2019)
27. Liu, S. and Huang, D.: Receptive field block net for accurate and fast object detection. In: Proceedings of the European Conference on Computer Vision (ECCV), pp. 385–400 (2018)
28. He, K., Zhang, X., Ren, S. and Sun, J.: Deep residual learning for image recognition. In: Presented at the 2016 IEEE Conference on Computer Vision and Pattern Recognition (CVPR), Las Vegas, NV (2016)
29. Khan, A., Sohail, A., Zahoora, U., Qureshi, A.S.: A survey of the recent architectures of deep convolutional neural networks. Artif. Intell. Rev. **53**(8), 5455–5516 (2020)
30. Jadon, S.: A survey of loss functions for semantic segmentation. In: 2020 IEEE Conference on Computational Intelligence in Bioinformatics and Computational Biology (CIBCB), pp. 1–7. IEEE, (2020)
31. Nanni, L., Cuza, D., Lumini, A., Loreggia, A. and Brahnam, S.: Deep ensembles in bioimage segmentation. arXiv Prepr. (2021). arXiv:2112.12955
32. Sudre, C.H., Li, W., Vercauteren, T., Ourselin, S. and Jorge Cardoso, M.: Generalised dice overlap as a deep learning loss function for highly unbalanced segmentations. In: Deep learning in medical image analysis and multimodal learning for clinical decision support, pp. 240–248. Springer (2017)
33. Salehi, S.S.M., Erdogmus, D. and Gholipour, A.: Tversky loss function for image segmentation using 3D fully convolutional deep networks. In: International Workshop on Machine Learning in Medical Imaging, vol. LNCS 1054, pp. 379–387. Springer (2017). https://doi.org/10.1007/978-3-319-67389-9_44
34. Lin, T.Y., Goyal, P., Girshick, R., He, K. and Dollár, P.: Focal loss for dense object detection. In: Proceedings of the IEEE International Conference on Computer Vision, pp. 2980–2988 (2017)
35. Abraham, N. and Khan, N.M.: A novel focal Tversky loss function with improved attention u-net for lesion segmentation. In: 2019 IEEE 16th International Symposium on Biomedical Imaging (ISBI 2019), pp. 683–687. IEEE (2019)
36. Qin, X., Zhang, Z., Huang, C., Gao, C., Dehghan, M. and Jagersand, M.: Basnet: boundary-aware salient object detection. In: Proceedings of the IEEE/CVF Conference on Computer Vision and Pattern recognition, pp. 7479–7489 (2019)
37. Yuan, W., Xu, W.: Neighborloss: a loss function considering spatial correlation for semantic segmentation of remote sensing image. IEEE Access **9**, 75641–75649 (2021)
38. Wong, K.C., Moradi, M., Tang, H. and Syeda-Mahmood, T.: 3D segmentation with exponential logarithmic loss for highly unbalanced object sizes. In: International Conference on Medical Image Computing and Computer-Assisted Intervention, vol. LNCS 11072, pp. 612–619. Springer (2018).https://doi.org/10.1007/978-3-030-00931-1_70
39. Wang, Z., Bovik, A.C., Sheikh, H.R., Simoncelli, E.P.: Image quality assessment: from error visibility to structural similarity. IEEE Trans. Image Process. **13**(4), 600–612 (2004). https://doi.org/10.1109/TIP.2003.819861
40. Jha, D., et al.: Real-time polyp detection, localization and segmentation in colonoscopy using deep learning. IEEE Access **9**, 40496–40510 (2021)
41. Bernal, J., Sánchez, J., Vilarino, F.: Towards automatic polyp detection with a polyp appearance model. Pattern Recogn. **45**(9), 3166–3182 (2012). https://doi.org/10.1016/j.patcog.2012.03.002
42. Vázquez, D. et al.: A benchmark for endoluminal scene segmentation of colonoscopy images. J. Healthc. Eng. 2017 (2017). https://doi.org/10.1155/2017/4037190

43. Silva, J., Histace, A., Romain, O., Dray, X., Granado, B.: Toward embedded detection of polyps in wce images for early diagnosis of colorectal cancer. Int. J. Comput. Assist. Radiol. Surg. **9**(2), 283–293 (2014). https://doi.org/10.1007/s11548-013-0926-3
44. Bernal, J., Sánchez, F.J., Fernández-Esparrach, G., Gil, D., Rodríguez, C., Vilariño, F.: WM-DOVA maps for accurate polyp highlighting in colonoscopy: validation vs. saliency maps from physicians. Comput. Med. Imaging Graph. **43**, 99–111 (2015). https://doi.org/10.1016/j.compmedimag.2015.02.007
45. Nanni, L., Lumini, A., Ghidoni, S. and Maguolo, G.: Stochastic selection of activation layers for convolutional neural networks. Sensors (Basel, Switz), **20**(6) (2020).https://doi.org/10.3390/s20061626
46. Wei, J., Hu, Y., Zhang, R., Li, Z., Zhou, S.K., Cui, S.: Shallow attention network for polyp segmentation. In: Medical Image Computing and Computer Assisted Intervention—MICCAI 2021, vol. LNCS 12901, Springer (2021)
47. Zhao, X., Zhang, L. and Lu, H.: Automatic polyp segmentation via multi-scale subtraction network. In: International Conference on Medical Image Computing and Computer-Assisted Intervention, pp. 120–130. Springer (2021)

Chapter 8
Autistic Verbal Behavior Parameters

Daniela López De Luise, Federico Hertzulis, Jesica Peralta, Pablo Pescio, Ben Raúl Saad, and Tiago Ibacache

Abstract When patients suffer ASD (Autism Spectrum Disorder), they experience severe difficulties in speech and socializing. Even a simple sentence and facial expressions are hard to understand for them. Biotech is a research project to get new alternates to help these individuals to communicate. The main goal here is to provide advances and tuned tools through audio and video real-time processing. Part of the previous work in this research stated the basis to understand that every individual has its own natural language expressed in ways of Robert Berwicks' verbal communications. Rather than only consider a one way approach on traditional PECS, the contribution of the entire research is to articulate some kind of feedback based on the way the patient reacts upon each event. This makes it possible to get the inner feeling of the individual. This paper is focused on the performance and evaluation of head bouncing and can be extended to some other movements during interactions recorded in diverse circumstances with ASD patients. A short tracking and lightweight processing approach is presented, and applied to a small video test set. Results are validated against manually detected movements. A workflow for processing stimmings and collecting relevant meta data is presented. It applies Machine Learning, and represents a model for tuning the tracking process. Preliminary results show that precision is good enough for detecting the main patient's behavior and for collecting information about the set of specific individual's autistic verbal behavior.

Keywords Autistic spectrum disorder · Linguistics · Segmentation · Sound processing

D. López De Luise (✉)
CI2S Lab—IEEE, Buenos Aires, Argentina
e-mail: mdldl@ci2s.com.ar

D. López De Luise · F. Hertzulis · J. Peralta
CAETI-Centro de Altos Estudios en Tecnología Informática, Universidad Abierta Interamericana, Buenos Aires, Argentina

P. Pescio · B. R. Saad · T. Ibacache
IDTI Lab, Facultad de Ciencia Y Tecnología, UADER, Concepción del Uruguay, Argentina

© The Author(s), under exclusive license to Springer Nature Switzerland AG 2023

C.-P. Lim et al. (eds.), *Artificial Intelligence and Machine Learning for Healthcare*, Intelligent Systems Reference Library 228,
https://doi.org/10.1007/978-3-031-11154-9_8

8.1 Introduction

Autistic Spectrum Disorder (ASD) is a neuro-developmental disorder that might present different degrees of severity reaching to the impossibility of language development [22]. Patients can present stereotyped behaviors associated with restricted interests, and social interaction disorder [8]. It affects any aspect of the individual's life. Since it presents a wide variety of clinical and behavioral expressions it is hard to detect. Every person manifests multi-factorial developmental dysfunctions of the central nervous system [10].

ASD symptoms have differences in timing of symptoms, severity, and nature [3]. This paper focuses on the cases of altered verbal language where the patient has a complete impossibility of speech.

Both treatment and detection rely on a wide range of alternatives. From the technical perspective, both goals derive in different types of proposals. Among the studies for detection, one in [4] uses an accelerometer and maps samplings on orthogonal subspaces, to populate a database that is used for a clustering. The sets are considered representative signals. It is quite frequent in ASD visual attention alteration. There are studies that evaluate which aspects of attention are affected and how much [13, 24]. Eye tracking (ET) and discriminant analysis can be used to differentiate Typically Developing (TD) children from Autistic Spectrum Disorder [27]. It could be used when other better diagnostic approaches are not available, for the early detection of ASD. In some cases the use of Machine Learning and Eye-Tracking derive in a too optimistic perspective when it is used for predicting Autism [2, 6]: a patient with these symptoms are already in the hard road of autism. There is no prediction.

Regarding the technical proposals for treatment, in [21] authors present an emotionally directed interactive agent. It requires the participation of the parents. The interaction consists in the representation of different moods (angry, sad, happy or scared) that must be evaluated by the children. Other authors define eight parameters to track the evolution and severity of the disorder [5]: age, non-verbal IQ matching, verbal IQ matching, motion, social content, ecological validity, audio input and attention bids. But the paper has a misconception using verbal in place of vocal activity, instead of the original Berwick's definition [9]. Furthermore, every parameter needs a more rigorous definition. The list of proposals is large and involves diverse technologies like video-games, robots and augmented reality [12, 15]. Table 8.1 is a very short summary of these authors and some others. The total production in this field is too large to reproduce here and the references here are just a brief introduction to some of the main approaches.

This paper aims to apply simple algorithms to track movements and to analyze which stimming is present. This will be complemented with a similar processing performed on the audio of the same recording (see [18], and associated with specific stimulus.

The rest of this paper organizes as follows: Sect. 8.2 presents some of the state of the art, Sect. 8.3 introduces the proposal, materials and methods, Sect. 8.4 describes

Table 8.1 Some approaches in the ASD field

Author	Device	Approach	Goal
Cheol-Hong and Ahmed	Accelerometer	Clustering	Detect focus of attention
Koldewyn et al. Señor, Shulman, and Di Lavore	Camera	Multiple Object Tracking	Detect focus of attention
Wan et al.	Camera	Discriminant analysis	Differenciate typically developing children
Cilia et al. Bjørklund et al.	Camera	Deep learming	ASD prediction
Mower et al.	PC	Interactive agent	Treatment
Chita-Tegmark	Sound recorded	Verbal IQ matching	Severity evaluation tracking of evolution
Krans *Zachary Warren*	Humanoid robot	Mimic game	Treatment
Khowaja et al.	Several	Augmented reality	Treatment
López de Luise, Azor and Párraga	Sound recorded	Machine learning	Communication semantics
Denise Dador	PC + VR device	Virtual reality	Treatment
D. K. Oller et al.	Sound recordings	Vocal analysis	Diagnostic
J. Lozano-Martínez, S. Alcaraz-García	PC	Gamification	Treatment

a testing protocol, Sect. 8.5 is a detailed analysis of sound recordings of a use case, and Sect. 8.6 has conclusions and future work.

8.2 Estate of the Art

The DSM-V [1] of the American Psychiatric Association, establishes a classification guide, a coding used by much of the scientific community to diagnose different mental disorders. According to the authors [20] those who suffer from ASD experience a series of symptoms based on Wing's triad, these disorders refer to social interaction, communication and lack of flexibility in reasoning and behavior. In turn, there are classifications of different degrees in the guides and manuals, which leads specialists [20] to affirm that despite Wing's classification, no person suffering from ASD is similar to another in terms of their observable characteristics.

People who are diagnosed with Autism Spectrum Disorder ASD have deficiencies in communication and social interaction. The DSM-V guide determines the level of ASD on a three-grade scale:

- Grade 1: Needs help. Without on-site help, deficiencies in social communication cause major problems. Restricted and repetitive behaviors, behavioral inflexibility and difficulty alternating activities.
- Grade 2: Needs Notable Help. Notable deficiencies in verbal and non-verbal social communication skills. Reduced response or abnormal responses to the social openness of other people. Restricted and repetitive behaviors. Behavioral inflexibility.
- Grade 3: Needs Very Notable Help. Severe deficits in verbal and nonverbal social communication skills. Restricted and repetitive behaviors. Behavioral inflexibility, intense anxiety/difficulty in changing focus of action.

DSM-V refers to verbal and non-verbal social communication, when indicating one of the problems that patients with ASD present. Skinner [25] carried out studies on verbal behavior, indicating that vocal language is only a part or subset, arguing that the emission of sounds or certain actions such as gestures are verbal even though they are not part of an organized language, since they provoke a reaction in the listener or observer similar to the emission of vocal language and therefore must be part of the verbal behavior.

Repetitive and stereotyped behaviors are considered an important symptom of autism spectrum disorders (ASD). Jumping, turning, and other rhythmic body movements were described in the first patients originally described in Kanner's series [14, 28]. Leo Kanner conducted an evaluation in the case study with 8 boys and 3 girls, describing various repetitive movements such as: rhythmic jumping, clapping, sucking sounds, walking on tiptoe, not looking directly at the face, continuous repetition of words and/or phrases. Later, in 1979, Wing and Gould [28] determined that people with Autism Spectrum Disorder have problems in three areas: (a) they cannot develop skills in reciprocal social interaction, (b) they have difficulties in their verbal and non-verbal communication and (c) they have restricted patterns of behavior and interests. These symptoms are known as the Wing Triad.

8.3 Proposal, Materials and Methods

Decreased interaction performance is not due to deficits in dynamic attention but instead to a diminished capacity to select and maintain attention on multiple targets [13]. Certain expressions of autism spectrum are often called stimmings, a self-stimulatory behavior characterized by the repetition of physical movements, sounds, words, or moving objects. This section introduces a proposal that intends to determine typical reactions that might be part of the patient stimming. Every person with ASD present a unique selection of possible manifestations. For that reason it is important to collect the verbal responses of the patient to certain stimuli in order detect the context and be able to infer a kind of "semantic" assigned to them.

Table 8.2 Summary of videos processed

ID	MB	Re	I	Fmt	FPs	Sc	N	S	m	St	x	y
v1_	7.33	480 × 360	1	mp4	30	1.2	10	10,10	10	0.75	2	1
v2_	9.76	480 × 360	2	mp4	29.97	1.2	10	10,10	10	0.75	8	5
v3_	11.5	480 × 360	3	mp4	29.97	1.2	10	10,10	10	0.75	3	3
v4_	24.8	480 × 360	2	mp4	29.97	1.2	10	10,10	10	0.75	20	15
v5_	70.8	1280 × 720	2	mp4	30	1.2	10	10,10	10	0.75	17	16
v6_	22	480 × 360	2	mp4	29.97	1.2	10	10,10	10	0.75	12	8
v7_	130.1	1280 × 720	2	mp4	30	1.2	10	10,10	10	0.75	24	12
v8_	86.8	1280 × 720	2	mp4	30	1.2	10	10,10	10	0.75	22	12
v9_	5.05	480 × 360	1	mp4	29.97	1.2	10	10,10	10	0.75	2	1
v10_	45.2	1280 × 720	2	mp4	30	1.2	10	10,10	10	0.75	8	4
v11_	35.2	720 × 480	1	mp4	29,97	1.09	10	10,10	10	0.75	0	2
v12_	25.9	720 × 480	1	mp4	29,97	1.04	7	15,15	10	0.75	4	2
v13_	35.8	720 × 480	1	mp4	29,97	1.05	4	15,15	10	0.75	36	26
v14_	18.3	720 × 480	1	mp4	29,97	1.07	5	15,15	10	0.75	6	4
v15_	31.8	720 × 480	1	mp4	29,97	1.01	7	15,15	10	0.75	78	76
v16_	14.8	480 × 360	1	mp4	30	1.02	7	15,15	10	0.75	42	40
v17_	11.2	480 × 360	1	mp4	29,97	1.12	4	15,15	10	0.75	36	95

The rest of this section presents the set of videos used for a general purpose testing and a specific use case that shows specific concerns that arise during tracking in the context of stimming detection.

General testing

The set of videos used for the testing were collected from the Internet. In all cases there is an autistic individual just playing or in therapy. Table 8.2 is a summary of the dataset.

The size is in megabytes (MB), then there is the resolution (Re), the number of individuals (I), the format (Fmt), scale reduction factor from the original size to accelerate the processing (Sc), number of hits in neighborhood (N), minimum number of frames by movement (m), size of of the box (S), maximum seconds in the same frame (St), number of stimmings in x(x) and y(y) orientation. Note that videos v11 to v17 required different values in parameters in order to work properly. This is due to the recording's quality, focus and illumination.

Since videos v1 to v10 are with the best quality and results, the testing analysis is performed just with them. The routines used to perform the tracking are traditional Cascade Object Detector with Python (c). An extra algorithm was implemented to infer when a movement is stimming or not. Figure 8.1 shows the histogram of detected head, eyes and brow (marked with h, e, and b) and stimmings in x and y

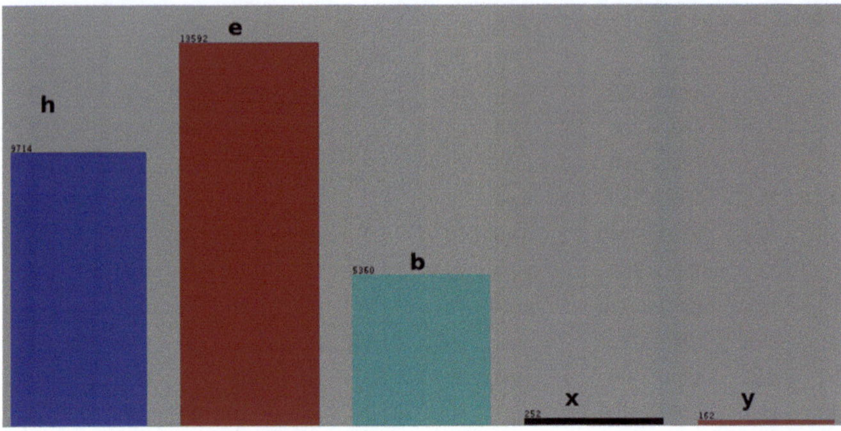

Fig. 8.1 Movements and stimmings detected

directions (denoted with x and y). As can be seen, there are many movements but autistic behavior is a reduced subset.

The use case

A video that was filmed in a session of the work of a therapist with a patient diagnosed with severe ASD is analyzed while they carry out tasks of identification, concentration, pointing, etc. The video has a total duration of 22:00 min, in order to identify sounds and movements, the different actions of the patient were recorded in an online Google spreadsheet called videos.xls.

The first sheet of the worksheet was divided into the following columns: Time, Action, Characteristics, Comments. Figure 8.2 shows an example of the original spreadsheet, considered for data collection.

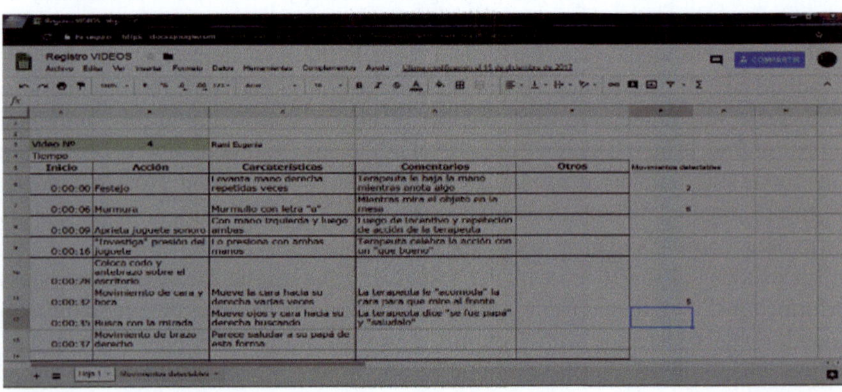

Fig. 8.2 Data collection spreadsheet

Afterwards, the worksheet is corrected to add to the time column, two new columns where the time before the start of the movement/listening and the time after it are recorded. In the Action column, the detectable movements according to the list prepared are recorded; A brief description of these movements is recorded in the Characteristics column and finally, in the Comments column, the actions and expressions that the therapist performs at each opportunity are recorded. Later this sheet is corrected again taking each column with the exact time of occurrence (see Table 8.3).

The registration has been traditionally performed manually according to the actions of the patient and the indications of the therapist. The actions are those that are described in the introduction section and that are added to the capture protocol. The list of detectable movements (see an excerpt in Table 8.4) was taken from the work of Riviere [23] and modified according to the description of each of the movements by the author and the therapists.

8.4 Testing Protocol

The audio of the Use-case video was used to identify moments when vocal sounds or clapping of the patient are heard. Then the sounds identified were used to validate Table 8.1 findings, and processed. The resulting is a reduced number of 4 typical stimmings expressed after determined stimuli, and related to specific body movements. In this paper, this matching with video is proposed as an automatic task based on simple and stackable procedures.

Modeling the problem with metadata

Figure 8.3 shows the basic steps of the processing. The routines performs a typical processing while recording a log reporting the coordinates of the frame with the position of heads and eyes. This information is used to derive metadata that helps determine evidence of repetitive movements like bouncing or clapping.

The key part is the processing parameter's tuning with Machine Learning in order for the model to keep the ability of detecting and tracing movements of the patient with good precision.

Every recording is processed with several parameters configurations generating a database with the resulting log. There is also a file that summarizes main data of every running against data.

(1) Data collected for ***VIDEO_params*** are:

1. filename = the name of the video under processing
2. FRAME_RATE = number of images per second in the file
3. SIZE x = size in pixels in x dimension
4. SIZE y = size in pixels in y dimension
5. total size in k-bytes = size of the file in kilobytes
6. RESOLUTION = final resolution of images before being processed

Table 8.3 Time-sheet of stimulus upon every sound slice detected

ID	$time_1$	$time_2$	$time_3$	$time_4$	$time_5$	$time_6$	$time_7$
Slice 1	0:00:00	2:31:00	3:58:00	4:18:00	5:17:00	6:52:00	7:25:00
Label: iuuu		He moved or was someone in the room, before he had lost focus	The book is given	The therapist stood up	Most of the time she is standing behind him + sound uuuuu	A vehicle is heard (background) while passing the pages of book	Got bored reading the book a second time and turning the pages seemed
Time Slice 1							
Slice 2	1:57:00	2:07:00	2:19:00	2:52:00	3:18:00	7:03:00	8:20:00
Label: Aaaa	Won the token + timer beep + eye contact + gives him yellow toy	Token arrangement	Points to card and the therapist congratulates him + gives him red toy	Buenisimooooooo (good)	He gives him yellow ball, (Biennnn Excellentee)	Wait for the stimulation of the therapist to turn the page	Look at the floor, he gets bored of waiting
Slice 4	3:40:00	10:30:00	16:25:00	16:30:00	18:10	19:09:00	
Clapping Sound 4	Given the lack of attention to him, the therapist takes a long time in his notes	Asks for silence, takes him a glass and plate and touches his mouth. Seems eager to play and win the lollipop	Sneezing and health	Sneezing and health	They clean his nose	He's bored now, he makes many new movements, he stretches, he wants to finish now	

Table 8.4 ASD typical behavior

Movement	Description
Rhythmic jumps	The body sitting/standing, the patient facing the front, performs vertical stentorian movements with/without arm movements
Clapping	It is the action of clapping the palms of the hands together repeatedly as a sign of both approval (joy) and, sometimes, rejection
Sucking sounds	It is the effect of producing a sound similar to the sucking of the bottle or the mother's breast when drinking milk
Walk on tiptoe	It is the action of walking on the balls of the feet without contact between the heels and the ground. It hits both feet at the same time
Do not look to the face directly	The patient, seen from the front, does not direct his gaze towards us but appears skewed, to the right (more frequently) or to the left
The list continues…	

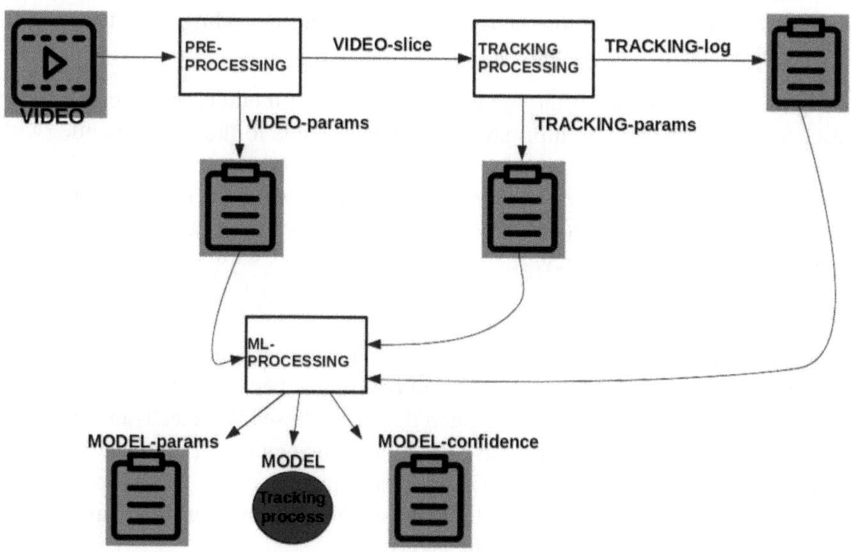

Fig. 8.3 Workflow

7. total marks = number of marks detected during file's processing. Marks are described in (2). This indicates the number of "element" and "start" in the log, which is a combination denoting the times of starting end ending of a stimming
8. SCALE_FACTOR = how much the image size is reduced at each image scale. 1.05 is a good possible value for this, which means a small resizing, i.e. reduce

size by 5%. This increases the chance of a matching size with the model for detection.
9. MIN_NEIGHBORS = number of neighbors each candidate rectangle should have to retain it. This parameter affects the quality of the detected faces. Higher value results in less detections but with higher quality.
10. MIN_MOVEMENT_FRAMES = minimum number of frames considered for movement detection. It is strongly recommended to use an even number.
11. MIN_SIZE = Minimum possible object size. Objects smaller than that are ignored.

(2) Data collected for ***TRACKING_params*** are:

1. time = timestamp, second since the beginning of the video
2. R, G, B = red, green and blue balance value in the image.
3. x, y = x and y coordinates of the box once an element is segmented
4. wx, wy = size in of both sides of the box
5. element = denotes what part of the body is in movement. Is one of the following: { eye | head | nose | mouth | hand | arm | leg}. The list could be extended in future tests
6. mark = indicates that this image is the beginning or ending of a stimming. It could be one of {start | end}

Figure 8.4 shows part of the log built with tracking module, and Fig. 8.5 is the Cascade Object Detector's information that corresponds to the same test file (with ID = v1).

The next step is to process this information extracted from the entire database of videos and to derive with Machine Learning the best parameter configuration to improve the algorithm efficacy.

Wavelets

To detect a stimming, this project splits sound from images and processes each of them with different approaches. Fourier transform has been largely used for signal processing but it has many limitations and this project uses Wavelet Transform with better results for sound. Findings also apply Morphosyntactic Linguistic Wavelets (MLW) for in-depth information [17], that provides excellent results to examine reasoning process related to linguistic expressions [16] and verbal behavior [26], detecting verbal activities with specific audios.

Verbal behavior is very used in ASD therapies [7] for tracking evolution and onto-genetics of development, which are specific for every individual [11]. Octave functions implement algorithms that read audios and derive proper metadata saved in csv format. As shown in previous publications, the results are good enough to detect most of the stimming but there are some extra detections that need to be filtered out with the video processing help [19].

time	element	x	y	w	h	mark
0:3.40	head	517	273	620	376	start
0:3.43	head	515	270	621	376	start
0:3.47	head	514	267	623	376	start
0:3.47	eyes	514	267	623	376	start
0:3.50	head	514	267	623	376	start
0:3.50	eyes	514	267	623	376	start
0:3.50	eyes	514	267	623	376	start
0:3.53	head	514	265	625	376	start
0:3.53	eyes	514	265	625	376	start
0:3.53	eyes	514	265	625	376	start
0:3.57	head	515	265	624	374	start
0:3.57	eyes	515	265	624	374	start
0:3.57	eyes	515	265	624	374	start
0:3.60	head	514	264	625	375	start
0:3.60	eyes	514	264	625	375	start
0:3.63	head	515	263	627	375	start
0:3.63	eyes	515	263	627	375	start
0:3.67	head	518	263	626	371	start
0:3.67	eyes	518	263	626	371	start
0:3.70	head	519	263	627	371	start
0:3.70	eyes	519	263	627	371	start
0:3.73	head	519	262	628	371	start
0:3.73	eyes	519	262	628	371	start
0:3.77	head	518	260	630	372	start
0:3.80	head	519	257	634	372	start
0:3.83	head	520	257	635	372	start

Fig. 8.4 Tracking log for ID-v1

8.5 Analysis of Tests

As mentioned previously, videos v1 to v10, are considered for the present analysis. The main goal now here is to determine if the meta-data generated during tracking are good enough to describe each patient's behavior. If so, it is possible to use them to automatically determine the unique trace's characteristics. Therefore every ASD has a set of metadata with certain values representing a typical movement of the individual.

The 29,080 records extracted from V1 to v10 trace, have distributions as shown in Table 8.5.

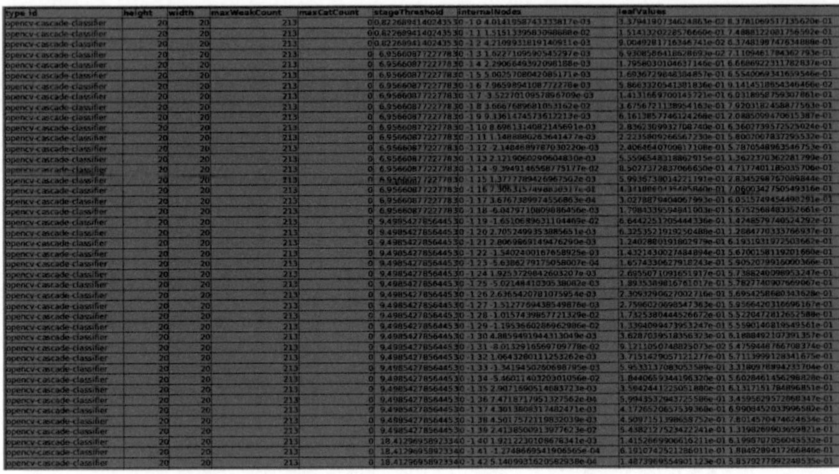

Fig. 8.5 COD for ID = v8

Table 8.5 Instances in each video

ID	Count
v1	1048
v2	3033
v3	490
v4	3059
v5	3958
v6	2777
v7	6742
v8	4540
v9	105
v10	3328

Every record have the metadata indicating position (x, y), size of the box enclosing certain part of the body (eyes, nose, mouth, or head), and the mark, a code denoting the type of movement (starting or ending of a stimming). These data are classified with WEKA, in order to determine the whether it is possible to automatically infer the mark using the other variables. Table 8.6 shows every heuristic used for modeling and quality metrics in each case.

The summary shows that any of the heuristics is able to infer the individual activity using the set of meta-data proposed. Kappa statistics keeps high in every case and relative squared error as well. The details about every heuristics can be found in [29].

Table 8.6 Summary of inference heuristic tested

Heuristic	Detail	%OK	Kappa	SQE
Hoeffding tree	An incremental, anytime decision tree induction algorithm that is capable of learning from massive data streams, assuming that the distribution generating examples does not change over time	74.78	0.71	65.0
J48	Generates a pruned or unpruned C4.5 decision tree. Created by Ross Quinlan (1993)	99.76	0.99	7.41
LMT tree	Classifier for building 'logistic model trees', which are classification trees with logistic regression functions at the leaves	99.82	0.99	6.04
Random forest	Builds a forest of random trees According to Leo Breiman (2001)	99.92	0.99	4.36
Random tree	A forest of random trees, according to Leo Breiman (2001)	99.77	0.99	7.21
REP tree	Fast decision tree learner, based on a decision/regression tree using information gain/variance and prunes it using reduced-error pruning (with backfitting)	99.42	0.99	10.87
Hrip	A propositional rule learner, Repeats Incremental Pruning to Produce Error Reduction (RIPPER), which was proposed by William W	99.49	0.99	10.65

8.6 Conclusions and Future Work

This paper introduces the main characteristics of patients with ASD, and the relevance of having a good tool to understand their verbal behavior. It is possible to determine several repetitive movements and sounds, known as stimmings. The use case presented here shows how stimuli can be related to very specific movements. The results obtained with sound processing were manually validated with expert's records.

Sounds can be considered as part of the stimming, with a pattern complemented with body attitudes. In order to evaluate this, a workflow with standard tracking algorithms was introduced. Tests results have high Kappa values (0.99 in most of the cases) and excellent percentage of correctly classified instances (over 99.42) when inferring the patient's ID from the collected stimmings and movements.

Among the pending activities are: improve tracking by training the Neural Networks with low quality videos, associate tags to movements, and to cross body stimmings with sounds.

References

1. American Psychiatric Association: DSM-V Encoding update. Supplement to the Diagnostic and Statistical Manual of Mental Disorders. 5th edn (2014)
2. Bjørklund, G., Meguid, N.A., El-Ansary, A., El-Bana, M.A., Dadar, M., Aaseth, J., Hemimi, M., Osredkar, J., Chirumbolo, S.: Diagnostic and severity-tracking biomarkers for autism spectrum disorder. J. Mol. Neurosci. **66**, 492–511 (2018)
3. Bustamante, P., Lafalla, A., Coria, N., Agüero, M., López De Luise, D., Parra, C., Azor, R., Moya, J., Cuesta. M.: Protocol for evaluation of somatic and oral behavior to sound stimuli in patients with autism spectrum. University of Burgos (2020)
4. Cheol-Hong, N., Ahmed H.: Novel pattern detection in children with autism spectrum disorder using iterative subspace identification. Department of electrical and computer engineering university of Minnesota, USA. 978-1-4244-4296-6/10. IEEE ICASSP, pp. 2266–2269 (2010)
5. Chita-Tegmark, M.: Social attention in ASD: a review and meta-analysis of eye-tracking studies. PMID: 26547134 (2015). https://doi.org/10.1016/j.ridd.2015.10.011
6. Cilia, F., Carette, R., Elbattah, M., Dequen, G., Guérin, J.L., Bosche, J., Le Driant, B.: Computer-aided screening of autism spectrum disorder: eye-tracking study using data visualization and deep learning. JMIR Hum. Factors **8**(4), e27706 (2021)
7. Greer, R.D.: The ontogenetic selection of verbal capabilities: contributions of skinner's verbal behavior theory to a more comprehensive understanding of language. Int. J. Psychol. Ther. **8**(3), 363–386 (2008)
8. Filipek, P.A., Accardo, P.J., Ashwal, S.: Parameter practice: detection and autistic diagnose. Neurology **55**, 468–479 (2000). https://doi.org/10.1212/wnl.55.4.468
9. Friederici, A.D., Chomsky, N., Berwick, R.C.: Language, mind and brain. Nat. Hum. Behav. **1**, 713–722 (2017). https://doi.org/10.1038/s41562-017-0184-4
10. Greer, R.D.: The comprehensive application of behavior analysis to schooling. CABAS®. Behav. Soc. Issues. **7**(1) (1997)
11. Greer, R.D.: The wide application of behavior analysis to schooling behavior. CABAS®. Behav. Soc. Matter. (1997)
12. Khowaja, K., Banire, B., Al-Thani, D., Sqalli, M.T., Aqle, A., Shah, A., Salim, S.S.: Augmented reality for learning of children and adolescents with autism spectrum disorder (ASD): a systematic review. IEEE Access **8**, 78779–78807 (2020). https://doi.org/10.1109/ACCESS.2020.2986608
13. Koldewyn, K., Weigelt, S., Kanwisher, N., Jiang, Y.: Multiple object tracking in autism spectrum disorders. J. Autism Dev. Disord. **43**(6), 1394–1405 (2013). https://doi.org/10.1007/s10803-012-1694-6
14. Kanner, L.: Autistic disturbances of affective contact. Nervous Child. N2, (217250). Translated by Teresa Sanz Vicario. Published in the Spanish Journal of Intellectual Disability Siglo Cero (1943)
15. Krans, B.: Small humanoid robot helps children with ASD. Healthline News (2013). Obtained from http://www.healthline.com/healthnews
16. De Luise, D.L.: Morphosyntactic linguistic wavelets for knowledge management. InTechOpen **8**, 167–189 (2012). https://doi.org/10.5772/35438
17. De Luise, D.L., Hisgen, D., Cabrera, A., Morales Rins, M.: Modeling dialogs with linguistic Wavelets. Theory Pract. Mod. Comput. **1**, 11–13 (2012)
18. de Luise, D.L., Azor, J., Párraga, C.: Autistic verbal behavior. Automated model of the patient profile—audio. Spanish Academic Edit. ISBN 978-3-659-07183-6 (2015)
19. De Luise, D.L., Saliwonczyk, C., Pescio, P., Saad, B., Ibacache, T., Soria, L.: Autistic verbal behavior parameters. Handbook of Research on New Investigations in Artificial Life, AI, and Machine Learning (2021)
20. Ministry of Science and Innovation Spain: Clinical practice guide for the management of patients with autism spectrum disorders in primary care. Nipo: 477-09-052-8 ISBN 978-84-451-3244-9. Estilo Estugraf Impresores (2009)

21. Mower, E., Black, M.P., Flores, E., Williams, M., Narayanan, S.: Design of an emotionally targeted interactive agent for children with autism. University of Southern California (USC), ISSN 978-1-61284-350-6/11 (2011)
22. Palau, M., Valls Santasusana, A., Salvadó, B.: Neurolinguistic disorders of ASD. Neuro Anat. Funct. Basis **50**, 69–76 (2010)
23. Riviere, A., Martos, J.: The little boy with autism. ISBN 9788460702610 (2000)
24. Señor, C., Shulman, C., Di Lavore, P.: Regression and loss of speech in ASD TruM specification. Mag. Child. Psycol. Psyichiatry. **45**(5), 93655 (2004)
25. Skinner, B.F.: Verbal Conduct. Translation by Rubén Ardilla, Edit. Trillas Mexico, ISBN 968-24-0987-X (1981)
26. Sundberg, M.: A brief overview of a behavioral approach to language assessment and intervention for children with autism association for behavior analysis. ASD Newsletter **30**(3) (2007)
27. Wan, G., Kong, X., Sun, B., Yu, S., Tu, Y., Park, J., Lang, C., Koh, M., Wei, Z., Feng, Z., Lin, Y., Kong, J.: Applying eye tracking to identify autism spectrum disorder in children. PMID: 30097760 (2019). https://doi.org/10.1007/s10803-018-3690-y
28. Wing, L.: The definition and prevalence of autism: a review. Euro. Child Adolesc. Psychiatry **2**, 61–74 (1993)
29. Witten, I.: Data mining. Practical machine learning tools and techniques. 4th edn. Elsevier, eBook ISBN 9780128043578 (2016)

Chapter 9
Advances in Modelling Hospital Medical Wards

P. Landa, M. Resta, E. Tànfani, and A. Testi

Abstract The growth of elder population in Italy increased the access to Internal medicine wards and generated overcrowding issues with doctors treating patients with larger clinical complexity and needs. The patients in medical wards exhibit multiple pathologies, with a burden of activities, risks, and costs for health systems, mining their sustainability. Internal Medicine Departments play an important role in the care of those patients that access the hospital for not-surgical treatments. In this study we focus on the use of unsupervised learning algorithms (namely Self-organizing Maps -SOMs- combined to K-means clustering) to group patients belonging to specific Diagnosis Related Groups (DRGs) and to examine how the SOM can help to find the main features of the clusters, to provide a more effective grouping methodology with respect to resource utilization.

Keywords Medical wards · Complexity · Big data · Frail patients · Self-organizing maps

---

P. Landa
Département d'opérations et Systèmes de Décision, Université Laval, Pavillon Palasis-Prince, 2325, Rue de la Terrasse, Québec, QC G1V 06, Canada
e-mail: paolo.landa@fsa.ulaval.ca

M. Resta (✉) · E. Tànfani · A. Testi
Department of Economics, School of Social Sciences, University of Genova, Via Vivaldi 5, 16126 Genova, Italy
e-mail: marina.resta@economia.unige.it

E. Tànfani
e-mail: etanfani@economia.unige.it

A. Testi
e-mail: testi@economia.unige.it

P. Landa
Centre Hospitalière Universitaire (CHU) de Québec—Université Laval, 1050 Chemin Ste-Foy, Québec, QC G1S 4L8, Canada

© The Author(s), under exclusive license to Springer Nature Switzerland AG 2023

C.-P. Lim et al. (eds.), *Artificial Intelligence and Machine Learning for Healthcare*, Intelligent Systems Reference Library 228,
https://doi.org/10.1007/978-3-031-11154-9_9

Acronyms

APR-DRG	All Patient Refined Diagnosis Related Group
ASL	Local Health Authority
CCI	Charlson Comorbidity Index
DRG	Diagnosis Related Groups
DRG 087	Pulmonary oedema and respiratory failure
DRG 089	Pneumonia and pleuritis with complications
DRG 090	Pneumonia and pleuritis >17-year-old patients
DRG 127	Heart failure and shock
DRG 576	Sepsis without medical ventilation
EPR	Electronic Patient Record
HDED	Hospital Discharge Episodes Database
ICD	International Classification of Diseases
IMW	Internal Medicine Ward
LEA	Essential Health Care Levels
LOS	Length of Stay
SOM	Self-Organizing Maps

9.1 Introduction and Problem Addressed

Patients admitted in medical wards mostly exhibit multiple-pathologies and frailty, with a burden of activities, risks, and costs for health systems, mining their sustainability [24]. The problem is mostly related to over 65 patients, especially those admitted in hospital with an average of 2.7 chronic diseases requiring medical care for an acute transient condition, i.e., an infection, that triggers a decompensation of chronic condition or acute decompensated heart failure, and/or a complication such as diabetes onset [7]. Furthermore, the clinical complexity is increased by functional and cognitive decline. These patients, often called frail, require urgent organizational changes to address their health needs appropriately [3, 4]. Furthermore, patients should be admitted to different wards depending on the prevalent clinical problem, such as cardiology, respiratory diseases, gastroenterology, geriatrics, etc., gemmated from Internal Medicine [1]. As a matter of fact, however, patients with similar conditions are often admitted in various departments [13, 16], hence receiving different care with different costs associated to them. A proper grouping criterion of those patients could help to give more information about clinical and epidemiological characteristics related with the resource consumption.

Overall, the framework we have depicted suggests the existence of a great deal of information and complexity to be managed which is suitable for the application of clustering and segmentation methods. The number of applications of cluster analysis in health care raised in the international literature of the last decade [2, 20, 22, 23, 27, 28]. This research stream benefits of an increasing number of contributions, since the analysis of Big Data is now more feasible, hence accomplishing the larger need to understand large, complex, information inside data sets [6, 11]. This rise of interest led to more than one million articles, and the quantity of data produced exceeded 40 Zetabytes [9]. An interesting review is presented in [12], where the Big Data analytics are evaluated focusing on four main characteristics: levels, techniques, application, domains. A systematic review on data mining application in healthcare is presented in [10]. The study presented by Hong et al. [9] provides an extended literature review on application and challenges on Big Data in health care, with details on Hospital Information Systems. The study developed by Lefèvre et al. [18] applies multivariate clustering techniques to health data looking for potential associations between user features and patterns of healthcare demand. Another study proposed by Tseng et al. [25] applies clustering methods to explore variations in input and output service volumes to investigate resource allocation and health care service efficiency in district hospitals in Taiwan.

With these premises, we use the Self-Organizing Map (SOM) [14, 15] nested to K-Means clustering [8] to group patients and to evaluate the impact of this grouping criterion with respect to resource utilisation.

The chapter is organized as follows: in Sect. 9.2, we present the case study and the data under examination. The results of the unsupervised clustering techniques are discussed in Sect. 9.3. In Sect. 4 conclusions and future direction of the research are reported.

9.2 Case Study and Data Analysis

The case study refers to a Ligurian Local Health Authority (ASL5) located in the La Spezia province (Italy). It provides, directly or through accredited public and private subjects, several facilities including: (i) Essential Health Care Levels (LEA) facilities in the form of district assistance and hospital care health services, (ii) high social and health integrated assistance, and (iii) emergency health services. The catchment area contains 217,507 inhabitants, 27.4% of which is over 65. About 8500 people are frail and at risk of disability, while 8300 have a declared disability.

Administrative data from the Hospital Discharge Episodes Database (HDED) and medical data from the Electronic Patient Record (EPR) have been observed and collected over a whole year. The dataset includes administrative data, as well as the date of admission and discharge, the transfers of the patient between wards, the diagnosis, and the assigned Diagnosis Related Groups (DRG). Data from EPR contain all the tests and consultations (blood transfusion, specialist visits, diagnostic tests, laboratory tests, and other tests) performed to the patient during the hospital stay. The cost of these specialist and diagnostics services were provided by the Italian National Health System official fees list. Other data were collected by the Hospital management accounting service.

The work uses the data already employed in [17] and it is focused on the six medical wards reported in Table 9.1, two of them (Internal Medicine 1 and Internal

Table 9.1 Number of patients admitted for each DRG and ward

Ward	087	089	090	127	576	Total
Cardiology	71	1	2	140	5	219
Geriatrics	64	83	14	155	61	377
Infectious diseases	–	21	15	1	97	134
Internal medicine 1	199	52	36	129	109	525
Internal medicine 2	566	37	16	163	351	1133
Respiratory medicine	266	40	27	3	3	339
Total	1166	234	110	591	626	2727

Medicine 2) are generic, while the remaining four are specialist wards. With reference to the pathology, the analysis focused on five DRGs covering on average 70% of the total cases (DRG 087: Pulmonary oedema and respiratory failure, DRG 089: Pneumonia and pleuritis with complications, DRG 090: Pneumonia and pleuritis >17-year-old patients, DRG 127: Heart failure and shock, DRG 576: Sepsis without medical ventilation).

All DRGs are treated within each of the six wards. Although the patients should be distributed based on the prevailing condition, as a matter of fact this is not always true, with a portion of patients distributed among the wards in a more "erratic way". For instance, specialist wards, as cardiology and infectious diseases, admit patients with heart failure and sepsis, respectively, but also with respiratory problems. Internal Medicine Wards (IMWs) treat patients belonging to the five DRGs. This situation, in turn, requires different tests and interventions with different length of stay and average cost of treatment for each patient at the parity of the DRG (see Tables 9.2 and 9.3). For instance, Heart failure has a Length of Stay (LOS) ranging from 5.9 in the specialist ward Cardiology to 9.4 days in Internal Medicine 1. There is also a large variability across wards: for instance, Internal Medicine 1 has a larger average LOS for all the DRGs, while Internal Medicine 2 has on average three days less.

Demographic, and clinical data summarized in Tables 9.4 and 9.5 show large variability in the complexity of patients addressing different wards. Complexity is assessed by three features drawn from HDED: (i) age, sex; (ii) comorbidity status

Table 9.2 Average patient length of stay (in days) for each DRG and ward of admission

Ward	087	089	090	127	576	Average
Cardiology	7.3	5.0	5.5	5.9	16.0	6.6
Geriatrics	8.7	9.5	8.2	8.9	9.5	9.1
Infection and immunology	–	11.6	6.9	7.0	15.7	14.0
Internal medicine 1	10.2	11.3	8.2	9.4	12.9	10.5
Internal medicine 2	7.4	6.7	5.6	6.5	7.8	7.3
Respiratory medicine	9.6	7.9	6.3	6.7	2.7	9.0
Average	8.4	9.3	7.1	7.6	10.1	8.7

Table 9.3 Average number of tests and interventions for each DRG and ward of admission

Ward/DRG	087	089	090	127	576	Average
Cardiology	71	1	2	140	5	43.8
Geriatrics	64	83	14	155	61	75.4
Infection and immunology	–	21	15	1	97	33.5
General medicine by internal medicine 1	199	52	36	129	109	105
General medicine by internal medicine 2	566	37	16	163	351	226.6
Respiratory medicine	266	40	27	3	3	67.8
Average	233.2	39	18.33	98.5	104.33	

Table 9.4 Number of patients for age class, sex, and charlson comorbidity index

Ward	Age			Sex		Charlson comorbidity index-CCI-			
	≤65	>65 and ≤80	>80	Male	Female	0	1–2	3–4	≥5
Cardiology	22	65	132	109	110	161	48	9	1
Geriatrics	–	47	330	113	264	123	192	51	11
Infection and immunology	50	59	25	72	62	90	27	11	6
Internal medicine 1	52	151	322	267	258	222	249	35	19
Internal medicine 2	69	258	806	513	620	417	592	104	20
Respiratory medicine	88	147	104	188	151	127	195	8	9
Total	281	727	1719	1262	1465	1140	1303	218	66

Table 9.5 Severity conditions and mortality risk: number of patients for each ward and APR code

Ward	APR severity class				APR mortality risk				
	1	2	3	4	1	2	3	4	Total
Cardiology	99	115	5	0	42	146	31	0	219
Geriatrics	63	212	94	0	51	186	120	20	377
Infection and Immunology	33	52	42	8	54	34	30	16	134
Internal medicine 1	114	350	55	7	115	247	147	16	525
Internal medicine 2	101	642	357	6	103	396	536	98	1133
Respiratory medicine	33	260	46	33	103	158	78	0	339
Total	443	1631	599	54	468	1167	942	150	2727

(measured by the Charlson Comorbidity Index (CCI); (iii) severity condition and mortality risk (APR-DRG classes). For what is concerning the CCI, it is a method to categorize comorbidities of patients based on the International Classification of Diseases (ICD) diagnosis codes reported in administrative data. We computed it following the study developed by [5]; the higher is the score, the more likely the predicted outcome will result in mortality or higher resource use. On the other hand, the All Patient Refined Diagnosis Related Group (APR-DRG), is an inpatient classification system that assigns a Diagnostic Related Group value, a Risk of Mortality subclass and a Severity of Illness subclass ranging from 1 to 4 in ascendant order of risk and severity [19].

Large variability is also observed in Table 9.3 with regards to the average number of tests and interventions for each DRG (blood transfusion, specialist visits, diagnostic tests, laboratory tests, and other tests).

The variability depends on the clinical pathway (DRG), requiring different bundle of services, as well as on the set of other patients' characteristics such as the demographic features and the comorbidity status that are shown in Table 9.4, and the severity conditions, i.e., severity class and mortality risk which are reported in Table 9.5.

Internal medicine wards have the largest quantity of patients covering about 70% of the overall sample, while the smallest units in terms of patient treated are Cardiology and Infection diseases wards. More than half (63%) of overall patients is over 80 while the patients in ages 65 and 80 and the patients with less than 65 years 27% and 10% of the cohort, respectively. Most of the patients have a CCI of 1–2 (48%) and 0 (42%). Patients with a CCI of 3–4 and larger than 5, are 8% and 2%, respectively A larger quantity of CCI 3–4 is in the Geriatric unit (14%).

The most frequent APR severity class is 2 (60%), where in Internal Medicine 1 and Respiratory Medicine has a maximum of 67% and 77%, respectively. The 16% and 22% of patients have a severity class of 1 and 3, respectively, while only the 2% has a severity class of 4. The most frequent APR mortality risk is 2 (43%), where in Cardiology and Geriatric units has a maximum of 67% and 49%, respectively. The 17% and 35% of patients have a mortality risk of 1 and 3, respectively, while only the 5% has a mortality risk of 4. Infection and Immunology ward treat patients with higher APR values (both severity class and mortality risk). Geriatrics, Immunology, and Internal Medicine 1 and 2 have at least the 30% of patients with a high risk of mortality (3 or 4). Different combinations of complexity characteristics for each Clinical Pathway (represented by the DRG) define groups of patients that should be homogeneous with respect to the resource use and cost.

9.3 Methodology and Results

As widely known, the Self-Organizing Map–SOM [14, 15] is a type of Artificial Neural Network which follows an unsupervised learning approach and it is trained through a competitive learning algorithm, according to the "winner takes all" (takes the most) mantra.

The way SOMs work can be easily described. Assume to denote by $\mathbf{x}(t) \in \mathbb{R}^d$ the pattern extracted from the input space X at time t, and by M a rectangular or hexagonal lattice with elements being arrays whose components (weights) number is the same as in the inputs. Then:

Step 0. All the weights are initialized at random.

Step 1. Set t varying from 1 to T.

Step 2. Extract x(t) from X.

Step 3. Find the winner neuron at step t as the neuron satisfying:

$$i_t^* = \arg\min_{i \in M} \left(\sum_{i \in M} \sum_{j=1}^{n} \left| x_j(t) - m_{ij}(t) \right|^p \right)^{1/p}, p \in \mathbb{N}$$

where p is the distance parameter. More common choices for p include p = 1 (Manhattan or city block distance) and p = 2 (Euclidean distance).

Step 4. Correct map nodes: if $\aleph_{i_t^*}(t)$ is the set of neurons in the map belonging (in a topological sense) to the neighbourhood of i_t^*, then:

$$m_i(t+1) = m_i(t) + h_{ii^*}(t)[x(t) - m_i(t)]$$

where $h_{i;i}$ is the interaction function, governing the way the nodes adjust in relation to the winning neuron on the grid.

Step 5. If t = T, once a proper convergence threshold level is reached, stop the procedure, otherwise repeat Steps 1–4.

In general, it is customary to enhance the results of the SOM by nesting it with an incremental K-means clustering procedure [8], stopping once the lowest average distance between clusters (less within-group distance) is reached. The ending point of the procedure is chosen according to the *elbow point criterion*, as shown in Fig. 9.1: if one plots the percentage of variance explained by the clusters against the number of clusters, the first clusters add considerable information (explain a lot of variance), but at some point, the marginal gain will drop, giving an angle to the graph corresponding to the number of clusters to be chosen, in our case eleven.

Moving accordingly, the SOM was organized into eleven clusters named as resulting in Fig. 9.2.

For each cluster we then performed the same analyses originating Tables 9.1, 9.2 and 9.5. The results are now presented in Tables 9.6, 9.7, 9.8 and 9.9.

By the analysis of the results, it is possible to highlight that the SOM clusters are homogeneous with respect to the age, with similar percentage of patients in the various classes of age. Besides the results are less sparse with respect to the LoS, which is similar among clusters, closer to an average value of 8.77 in contrast to the distribution of observable data among the wards (Table 9.2).

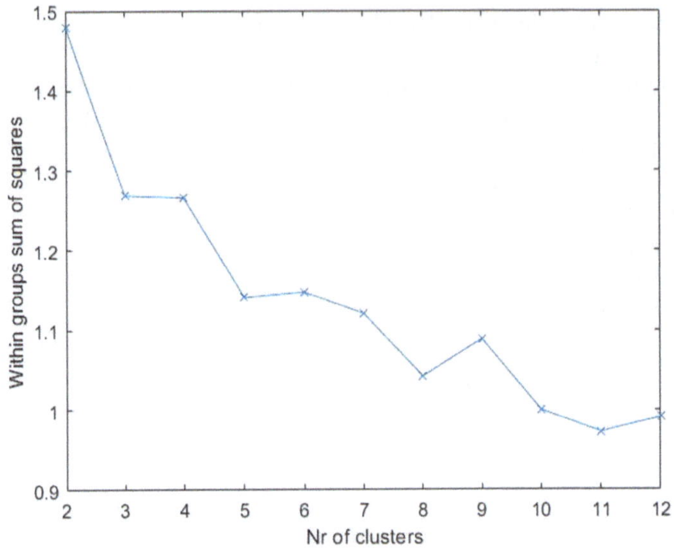

Fig. 9.1 Number of clusters according to the Elbow criterion

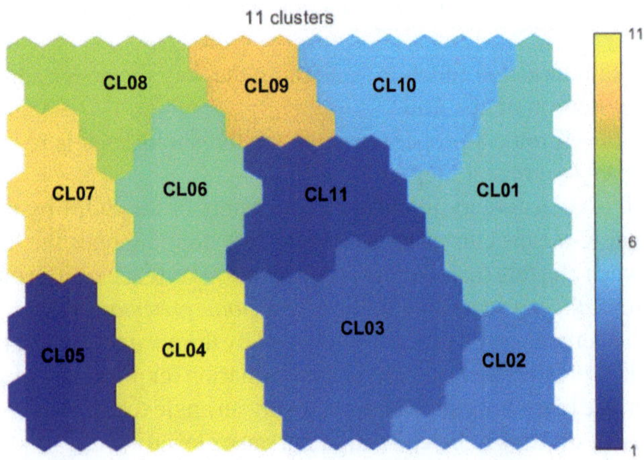

Fig. 9.2 The SOM clusters

Another interesting point concerns the distribution of the patients along the clusters depending on the scores of the Charlson Comorbidity index (CCI) as well as on the APR severity. Consider for instance, values in clusters CL01 and CL07: while the number of patients in cluster CL01 associated to the CCI in the range [3, 4] is 117, the corresponding value in CL07 is notably lower, as it equals to 70. In a similar fashion, the number of patients of CL01 in the APR Severity class 2–3 is 216 whereas

Table 9.6 SOM results

	087	089	090	127	576	Total
CL01	117	29	12	44	65	267
CL02	121	22	4	53	44	244
CL03	198	36	12	82	73	401
CL04	85	9	6	45	38	183
CL05	139	19	8	72	83	321
CL06	122	26	11	81	96	336
CL07	64	20	5	48	53	190
CL08	83	20	12	47	52	214
CL09	48	12	12	28	26	126
CL10	103	23	15	44	56	241
CL11	85	18	13	47	40	203

Number of per cluster (row) patients for each DRG (column)

Table 9.7 SOM results

	087	089	090	127	576
CL01	145.14	35.17	15.09	51.60	80.11
CL02	161.32	30.33	4.90	73.91	57.98
CL03	160.99	29.23	9.53	63.61	59.26
CL04	149.95	16.27	10.20	85.20	66.13
CL05	140.69	17.77	8.62	75.83	82.69
CL06	121.14	25.52	10.58	75.96	94.95
CL07	113.47	33.85	7.65	82.06	93.82
CL08	135.50	31.46	17.86	69.57	76.68
CL09	126.05	29.54	30.86	70.37	70.52
CL10	137.21	29.06	22.06	60.50	77.69
CL11	139.82	28.40	19.97	72.99	61.89

Average cost per patient (in Euro, €) for each DRG (rows) and clusters (columns)

the value in CL07 is 156. This, in turn, impacts on the different number of patients of the examined clusters with Death Probability higher than 0.2.

As preliminary conclusion, then, we may observe that clustering patients with the SOM generates groups that are homogeneous with respect to the LoS which in general is a proper proxy for resource consumption [21, 26]. In contrast, the generated clusters differentiate patients with respect to the complexity (CCI and APR Severity) and impact on the Death Probability as well as on the Number of Tests and Interventions, reported in Table 9.9 and organized per cluster (row) and DRG (column).

Table 9.8 SOM clustering results

		CL01	CL02	CL03	CL04	CL05	CL06	CL07	CL08	CL09	CL10	CL11
Average LoS		9.78	8.46	8.89	8.18	8.80	8.06	9.4	8.55	9.35	9.19	7.82
Age	≤65	11.99%	11.07%	13.22%	8.74%	9.35%	11.01%	9.47%	8.41%	8.73%	13.28%	12.25%
	(65,80]	23.97%	25.82%	23.19%	25.14%	26.79%	25.00%	28.42%	26.17%	28.57%	30.71%	25.98%
	>80	64.04%	63.11%	63.59%	66.12%	63.86%	63.99%	62.11%	65.42%	62.70%	56.02%	61.76%
CCI	0	7	5	2	3	6	8	2	2	1	3	1
	1–2	131	129	205	80	151	171	110	123	74	143	141
	3–4	117	99	166	93	142	137	70	80	49	87	57
	5	12	11	28	7	22	20	8	9	2	8	5
APR severity	<2	50	26	52	24	48	49	31	32	17	35	38
	2–3	216	212	343	154	267	271	156	176	109	201	166
	4	1	6	6	5	6	16	3	6	0	5	0
DeathProb	<0.2	218	223	355	160	284	293	166	180	113	214	172
	[0.2,0.4)	46	20	46	22	37	42	23	34	13	25	31
	[0.4,0.6)	3	1	0	1	0	1	1	0	0	2	1

For each cluster (columns) we analysed the Average LoS, as well as the clusters composition for what is regarding the CCI index, the APR severity, and the Death Probability (DeathProb)

Table 9.9 SOM clustering of Number of tests and interventions. Clusters are in rows, DRG in columns

	087	089	090	127	576	Average
CL01	117	29	12	44	65	53.40
CL02	121	22	4	53	44	48.80
CL03	198	36	12	82	73	80.20
CL04	85	9	6	45	38	36.60
CL05	139	19	8	72	83	64.20
CL06	122	26	11	81	96	67.20
CL07	64	20	5	48	53	38
CL08	83	20	12	47	52	42.80
CL09	48	12	12	28	26	25.20
CL10	103	23	15	44	56	48.20
CL11	86	18	13	47	40	40.80
Average	106	21.27	10	53.72	56.91	

Looking at the Number of Tests and Interventions, it sensitively differs from the values discussed in Table 9.3. On average, the number of tests and interventions per cluster in the groups obtained with the SOM is lower than when patients are distributed depending on the type of wards. This suggests that the cluster organization inferred by the SOM generates a different distribution of patients in terms of both APR severity and the number of interventions which can be therefore considered a proper proxy for resources consumption and costs.

The data-driven approach suggests a patients' organization that from one hand spreads them on a higher number of groups than in the case of the wards (eleven clusters versus six wards), but on the other hand, generates a lower number of tests and interventions and therefore a different resources consumption with respect to a more erratic allocation of the patients.

9.4 Conclusion

This study focuses on a data-driven approach lead by the Self-Organizing Maps (SOMs) nested with K-means clustering in a real case study based on a medium hospital setting.

The main goal of the work was to verify whether the SOM unsupervised clustering methodology offer alternative ways to analyse the complexity of frail patients using a large amount of information. The basic idea was to analyse the groups originated by the SOM in search of distinctive features of the clusters. to create representative groups of patients, with similar characteristics in terms of the intensity level of care and corresponding resources allocation.

The results show that the data-driven model provides a different organization of the patients with the LOS missing its conventional power as proxy of the resource allocation because it is more homogeneous among the clusters, in favour of other determinants. The organization into eleven clusters, in fact, highlighted a different distribution of almost all the variables, such as the APR severity, the Probability of Death, the Charlson Comorbidity Index and the Number of Tests and Interventions whose group values, on average, are lower than those occurring when the patients are managed and organized into "conventional" wards and in a more erratic way.

Nevertheless, at the present stage, this study shows two main limitations. First, we made a limited use of outcome indicators, where other outcomes should be included such as 90-days patient readmission and in-hospital mortality. Second, as the model is based on the hospital data, a sensitivity analysis should be provided to verify the robustness of the results.

Future work will be directed to test the model on a larger dataset, made up of more years of hospital data records.

References

1. Bauer, W., Schumm-Draeger, P.M., Koebberling, J., Gjoerup, T., Garcia Alegria, J.J., Ferreira, F., Higgens, C., Kramer, M., Licata, G., Mittelman, M., O'hare, J., Unal, S.: Political issues in internal medicine in Europe. A position paper. Eur. J. Int. Med. **16**(3), 214–217 (2005)
2. Booth, A., Harris, J., Croot, E., Springett, J., Campbell, F., Wilkins, E.: Towards a methodology for cluster searching to provide conceptual and contextual "richness" for systematic reviews of complex interventions: case study (CLUSTER). BMC Med. Res. Methodol. **13**, 118 (2013)
3. Bruzzi, S., Landa, P., Tànfani, E., Testi, A.: Conceptual modelling of the flow of frail elderly through acute-care hospitals: an evidence-based management approach. Manag. Decis. **56**(10), 2101–2124 (2018)
4. Clegg, A., Young, J., Iliffe, S., Rikkert, M.O., Rockwood, K.: Frailty in elderly people. The Lancet **381**, 752–762 (2013)
5. Deyo, R.A., Cherkin, D.C., Ciol, M.A.: Adapting a clinical comorbidity index for use with ICD-9-CM administrative databases. J. Clin. Epidemiol. **45**(6), 613–619 (1992)
6. Dash, S., Shakyawar, S.K., Sharma, M., Kaushik, S.: Big data in healthcare: management, analysis and future prospects. J. Big Data **6**, 54 (2019)
7. Duckitt, R., Palsson, R., Bosanska, L., Dagna, L., Durusu, T.M., Vardi, M.: CDIME group. Common diagnoses in internal medicine in Europe 2009: a pan-European, multi-centre survey. Eur. J. Int. Med. **21**(5), 449–452
8. Hartigan, J., Wang, M.: A K-means clustering algorithm. J. Royal Stat. Soc. Ser. C (Appl. Stat.) **28**, 100–108 (1979)
9. Hong, L., Luo, M., Wang, R., Lu, P., Lu, W., Lu, L.: Big data in health care: applications and challenges. Data Inf. Manage. **2**(3), 175–197 (2018)
10. Islam, M.S., Hasan, M.M., Wang, X., Germack, H.D., Noor-E-Alam M.: A systematic review on healthcare analytics: application and theoretical perspective of data mining. Healthcare (Basel, Switzerland), **6**(2), 54 (2018)
11. Jothi, N., Rashid, N.A., Husain, W.: Data mining in healthcare—a review. Proced. Comput. Sci. **72**, 306–313 (2015)
12. Kamble, S.S., Gunasekaran, A., Goswami, M., Manda, J.: A systematic perspective on the applications of big data analytics in healthcare management. Int. J. Healthcare Manage. **12**(3), 226–240 (2019)

13. Katsaliaki, K., Mustafee, N.: Applications of simulation within the healthcare context. J. Operat. Res. Soc. **62**(8), 1431–1451 (2011)
14. Kohonen, T.: Self-organized formation of topologically correct feature maps. Biol. Cybern. **43**, 59–69 (1982)
15. Kohonen, T.: Self-Organized Maps. Springer-Verlag, Berlin Heidelberg (1997)
16. La Regina, M., Guarneri, F., Romano, E., Orlandini, F., Nardi, R., Mazzone, A., Fontanella, A., Campanini, M., Manfellotto, D., Bellandi, T., Gussoni, G., Tartaglia, R., Squizzato, A.: What quality and safety of care for patients admitted to clinically inappropriate wards: a systematic review. J. Gen. Intern. Med. **34**, 1314–1321 (2019)
17. Landa, P., La Regina, M., Tanfani, E., Orlandini, F., Campanini, M., Fontanella, A., Manfellotto, D., Testi, A.: Modelling hospital medical wards to address patient complexity: a case-based simulation-optimization approach. Springer Proc. Math. Stat. **316**, 25–39 (2020)
18. Lefèvre, T., Rondet, C., Parizot, I., Chauvin, P.: Applying multivariate clustering techniques to health data: the 4 types of healthcare utilization in the Paris metropolitan area. PLoS ONE **9**(12), e115064 (2014)
19. McCormick, P.J., Lin, H., Deiner, S.G., Levin, M.A.: Validation of the all patient refined diagnosis related group (APR-DRG) risk of mortality and severity of illness modifiers as a measure of perioperative risk. J. Med. Syst. **42**, 81 (2018)
20. Meader, N., King, K., Moe-Byrne, T., Wright, K., Graham, H., Petticrew, M., Power, C., White, M., Sowden, A.J.: A systematic review on the clustering and co-occurrence of multiple risk behaviours. BMC Publ. Health **16**, 657 (2016)
21. Rachoin, J.S., Skaf, J., Cerceo, E., Fitzpatrick, E., Milcarek, B., Kupersmith, E., Scheurer, D.B.: The impact of hospitalists on length of stay and costs: systematic review and meta-analysis. Am. J. Manag. Care **18**(1), e23–e30 (2012)
22. Rivera, E., Corte, C., DeVon, H.A., Collins, E.G., Steffen, A.: A systematic review of illness representation clusters in chronic conditions. Res. Nurs. Health **43**(3), 241–254 (2020)
23. Salazar-Reyna, R., Gonzalez-Aleu, F., Granda-Gutierrez, E.M., Diaz-Ramirez, J., Garza-Reyes, J.A., Kumar, A.: A systematic literature review of data science, data analytics and machine learning applied to healthcare engineering systems. Manag. Decis. **60**(2), 300–319 (2020)
24. Salive, M.E.: Multimorbidity in older adults. Epidemiol. Rev. **35**(1), 75–83 (2013)
25. Tseng, S.F., Lee, T.S., Deng, C.Y.: Cluster analysis of medical service resources at district hospitals in Taiwan, 2007–2011. J. Chin. Med. Assoc. **78**(12), 732–745 (2015)
26. Wachter, R.M., Goldman, L.: Zero to 50,000—The 20th anniversary of the hospitalist. N. Engl. J. Med. **375**, 1009–1011 (2016)
27. Yan, S., Kwan, Y.H., Tan, C.S., Thumboo, J., Low, L.L.: A systematic review of the clinical application of data-driven population segmentation analysis. BMC Med. Res. Methodol. **18**, 121 (2018)
28. Yin, Z., Sulieman, L.M., Malin, B.A.: A systematic literature review of machine learning in online personal health data. J. Am. Med. Inform. Assoc. **26**(6), 561–576 (2019)

Chapter 10
Tracking Person-Centred Care Experiences Alongside Other Success Measures in Hearing Rehabilitation

Gareth Priday, Sonja Pedell, Jessica Vitkovic, and Lauren Story

Abstract Soundfair Australia Ltd collaborated with Swinburne University's Living Lab to create person-centred care measures that are routinely tracked alongside other success measures in hearing rehabilitation. A Living Lab approach was applied. Living Lab projects at their heart apply co-design in real-life contexts involving multiple stakeholders to achieve innovative products and services for the people involved—in this project, patients as well as staff providing the hearing rehabilitation service. To ensure applied innovative design solutions remain focused on the goal and needs of the end-users it is important to measure their impact and revise and improve both the measures and solutions on a regular basis. To come to relevant conclusions, data needs to be collated and interpreted against the original goals over time. This project aimed to develop a dashboard—an artificial intelligence infrastructure—to bring together the data. Here we report on (i) the process to ensure the right patient data was collected and fed into the system to achieve meaningful measures and (ii) the barriers that we faced when collating and interpreting the measures of the dashboard in practice. We suggest the barriers identified are common in the health sector. We advance the discussion of barriers as consideration points to improve and establish implementation of artificial intelligence in the health sector to improve person-centred care.

Keywords Person-centred care · Hearing rehabilitation · Dashboard · Co-design · Evaluation measures · Case study · Artificial intelligence · Health care · Living lab approach

---

G. Priday · S. Pedell (✉)
Centre for Design Innovation, Swinburne University of Technology, Melbourne, VIC, Australia
e-mail: spedell@swin.edu.au

J. Vitkovic · L. Story
Soundfair Australia Ltd., Mount Waverley, VIC, Australia

© The Author(s), under exclusive license to Springer Nature Switzerland AG 2023
C.-P. Lim et al. (eds.), *Artificial Intelligence and Machine Learning for Healthcare*,
Intelligent Systems Reference Library 228,
https://doi.org/10.1007/978-3-031-11154-9_10

10.1 Person-Centred Care in Research and Practice

Person-centred care and patient-centred care continue to receive more and more interest from health practitioners and the research community [1]. There is evidence that both improve patient outcomes [2] as well as other benefits such as increased satisfaction and adherence to treatment, reduced errors and frequency of attendance and lower costs of service provision. This has led to new policies and standards in health care with a focus on the patient. However, research on patient-centred care has received less attention in audiology than in other fields [3] and the elements of care may be different in audiology settings to other healthcare contexts. To address this Grenness et al. [3] developed a model for patient-centred care that focuses on the therapeutic relationship, information exchange and decision making between the audiologist and patient with the aim of developing individualised care. Grenness et al. [3] went on to develop a model for operationalising patient-centred care that included the four core elements of 'therapeutic relationship', 'inform', 'involve', and 'individualise'. In contrast, the Person-Centered Hearing Network (PCHN[1]) has six core principles for person-centred care more concretely focusing on aspects of a therapeutic relationship (aspects 3,5, and 6), but is also stressing the importance of individual needs and preferences (aspect 2). Information generation is a two-way endeavour and even involves other stakeholders to achieve person-centredness (aspects 1 and 4):

1. Involvement of family and friends
2. Understanding of individual preferences
3. Empathy
4. Shared goal setting and decision making
5. Active listening
6. Open ended questions and reflective conversations.

Håkansson et al. [4] literature review of research papers on patient and person-centred care found that most research articles describe the common "goal of person-centred care to be a meaningful life" (p. 8). Given the high-level definition, it is important to understand the care goals of people with hearing conditions to ensure that their needs and preferences are truly at the centre of their care. We prefer the term person-centred care over the term patient-centred care as it considers the whole person incorporating the various dimensions to whole well-being, including a person's context and individual expression, preferences and beliefs [5].

Person-centred care (PCC) has not been traditionally integrated into healthcare quality improvement [2]. While there has been interest in developing person-centred care within audiology, its application is still emerging. Laplante-Lévesque et al. [6] showed that measures of patient-centred care were overall similar to other health settings; however, there were significant differences between private and public or community practices, with the former showing lower scores. Other factors that influence person-centred care include the age of the practitioner and years in practice.

[1] https://idainstitute.com/ida_community/our_partners/person_centered_hearing_network/

Tai et al. [7] demonstrated that students only partially displayed person-centred care skills noting "within the function of decision making, enabling treatment behaviour and responding to emotions were rarely observed" (p. 104). Since person-centred care has been shown to positively influence health outcomes, financial outcomes and patient satisfaction in other healthcare contexts, it is important for hearing health practitioners to understand their performance in the provision of person-centred care, based on the perception of those they serve. However, principles as put forward by PCHN only go as far as guiding audiologists in person-centred care best practice during a consultation, rather than articulating how people with hearing conditions are feeling during their care experiences or their desired outcomes from their interaction and relationship building. To construct a PCC evaluation tool that, in itself, is person-centred, we first need to understand what we should be measuring from the perspective of the person with the hearing condition and create tools based on these insights.

10.1.1 Situated Action—Understanding the Context as a Basis for Meaningful Measures

From a participatory perspective, we recognise that current patients and prospective clients of hearing rehabilitation services can share their experiential knowledge about what they want for their life [8], which is grounded in their knowledge about the context in which they are immersed [9]. However, at the beginning of the journey, many patients do not have any experience with hearing aids and the services around them, and have little, if any, experience with what to expect from the interaction with the hearing rehabilitation provider. As patients do not know much about the potential of hearing rehabilitation and the service provider does not know anything specific about the patients (yet), we need an approach to bridge the knowledge gaps over time to provide the best person-centred care. This includes understanding the experience of the service journey in terms of interacting with the service provider and being able to communicate the goals and needs appropriately. Hence at the beginning, there is a situation where both parties come together without much knowledge of each other, and providers need to understand the client's needs and goals when immersed in different contexts. This concept of situated activities has been described in detail by Lucy Suchman [10]. Suchman's [10] concepts of situated action and thinking about technologies, not as 'smart' but located in a social and material context are helpful when thinking about technologies to create benefits. We suggest this not only applies to technologies, in this case, hearing aids and their associated accessories but the whole service system. To be true to Suchman's notion of situated action [10] and acknowledging that patients are the experts of their life context and staff of health service provision, we decided to follow an approach informed by the principles of participatory design that provides us, as a research team, with the relevant everyday knowledge and goals [11, 12]. Understanding the desired experiences and goals to be achieved through the service and technology helps to derive meaningful measures of person-centred care.

10.1.2 *Situated AI for Achieving High-Quality Person-Centred Care*

From an artificial intelligence (AI) perspective, an infrastructure needs to be created and the right data needs to be collected to be able to draw conclusions from the data and use them for predictions. AI is only as good as the infrastructure behind it [13] and the system can only be as intelligent as the quality of the data fed to the system. Hence a key data management aspect is understanding the data's quality and pedigree [13]. Lawrence's [14] data readiness levels, summarised by Freeman [13] (p. 29) are shown in Table 10.1. They illustrate that data used for meaningful machine learning (ML) (here we include ML as a subset AI) is beyond definitions and data storage standards.

We suggest that the ability to collect AI ready data will depend on the collection tool for the person-centred data and verification that we are measuring what we set out to do.

In health, what patients and providers want are products and services that are relevant to real-life situations as promoted by Suchman [10]. Ognjanović and Šendelj [15] who investigated the potential for AI to promote PCC in neurology settings, emphasised the use of data in processing, making recommendations and monitoring rehabilitation, and that all these services would aim to improve person-centred care rather than *evaluate* person-centred care. In our study, we are interested in evaluation of any measures deemed important to end-users overall and not limited to direct service application or application in hearing aids themselves.

Understanding and designing for different situations where hearing rehabilitation and technology would be used by an individual patient, helps patients to feel in control and their individual needs validated. Hence, we do need to know about the skills, experiences and goals of patients before introducing evaluation measures. We

Table 10.1 Data readiness levels from Freeman [13] p. 29

Level	Quality	Description
Level AAA	Safe	Data are issue free, include integrity checks, have complete provenance information
Level AA	Auto-Analyse	Data supports the automation of bias detection, feature selection, normalisation, and more
Level A	Analyse	Known meta-data and meaningful values to the problem at hand
Level B	Believe	The data have known and correct data types, data pedigree known (data history), and documented missing values
Level C	Conceive	Machine readable data, accessible

therefore applied a participatory approach to understanding the extent to which AI could be used in the context of our participants (who were patients as well as hearing professionals). We utilised a strategy that aimed to maintain the focus on people instead of AI, as suggested by Gyldenkaerne et al. [16] when doing research on AI in healthcare.

10.2 Co-design for Person-Centred Care Measures

Co-design is a method that focuses on real-life contexts, emphasising the importance of realism in the design process and user experience. In our context this extended to adopting a Living Lab approach that applies co-design in real-life contexts involving multiple stakeholders to achieve innovative products and services for the people involved. Co-design is also used within other design processes such as service design [17]. Malmberg [17] notes the alignment between service design and patient-centred care, which includes the importance of the user (patient) as an expert, capturing a holistic view of their life, changing the power dynamic, and value co-creation techniques. The use of design is woven into practice [18], education and promotion [2]. While there is considerable material on co-design and person-centred care generally, there are relatively few co-design or participatory design studies in audiology considering the implications to service models and evaluation. An exception is Ferguson et al. [19] who used participatory design methods to develop e-learning for first time hearing aid users.

Being able to discover, in a participatory way, the individual needs and their measures of effectiveness is central to PCC. As Fig. 10.1 shows many different life contexts outside of the audiology clinical setting will influence the individual goals of the patient. Also, the outcomes of PCC stretch beyond the clinical setting and are individually experienced in everyday life in these contexts. Patients need to feel heard regarding what their needs are and be considered experts in their own life for their hearing to be improved in settings that matter to them. A good relationship between clinic staff and the patient means the patient has the opportunity to describe the time and places where desired impact is most relevant for them. The focus of the treatment should be on the key contexts where the patient wants to see the benefit. One patient might prioritise hearing their partner in noisy social settings while another person wants to avoid embarrassment of mishearing in a professional setting. These types of scenarios are likely to be raised in a clinical context, however higher order contextual factors such as socioeconomic status or cultural background may also interact with the system and the patients' needs and preferences. For instance, it may be important to not feel like a financial burden on their family due to their hearing loss while another would like to overcome the stigma their culture places on people with a hearing disability, yet these scenarios are less often raised in an audiological rehabilitation setting. This stresses the importance of co-design considering different life contexts and a holistic view of user experience to reveal areas where further benefit might be unlocked.

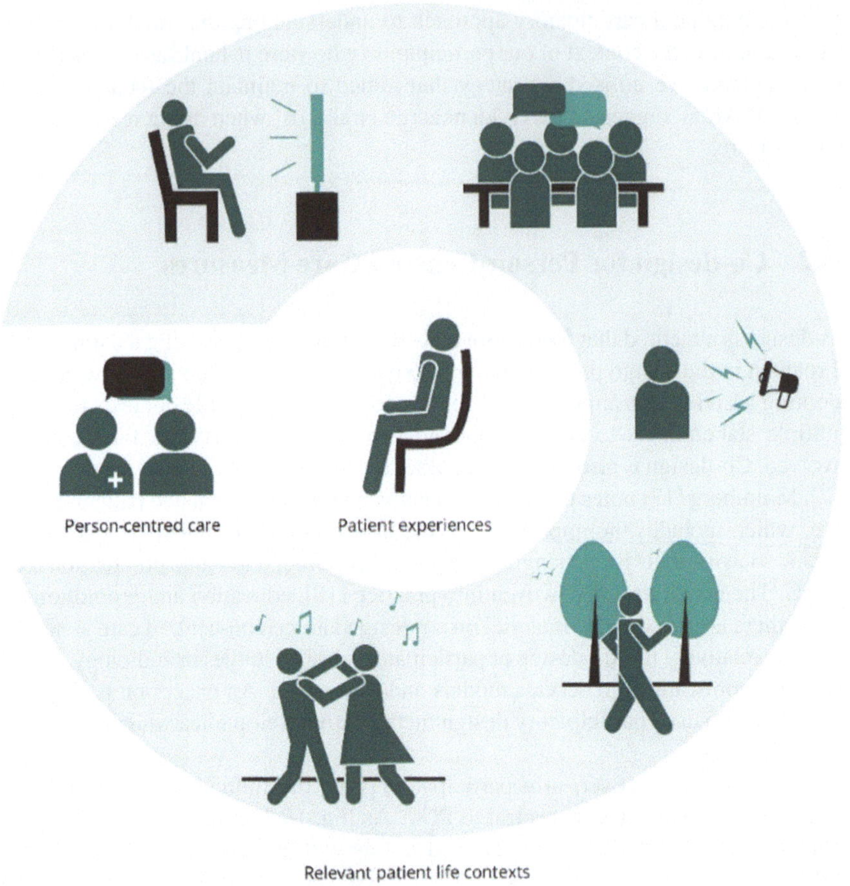

Fig. 10.1 The living experience in different contexts influences the goals and measures for PCC in the audiology clinical setting

While meeting individualised treatment goals is central to PCC, a central dimension of hearing care that requires individualisation is the therapeutic relationship [3]. Yet what constitutes a therapeutic relationship is different for any given individual [3]. Therefore, giving stakeholders a strong voice through a co-design process is important to create PCC tools that are able to measure individualisation in what the patient treatment needs are as much as how they would like feel during their care experiences or their desired outcomes from their interaction and relationship building.

10.2.1 Co-design of Evaluation Instruments

According to Santana et al. [2] "PCC is a model in which health-care providers are encouraged to partner with patients to co-design and deliver personalised care that provides people with the high-quality care they need and improve healthcare system efficiency and effectiveness" (p. 1). Measuring the person-centredness of the care provided by health practitioners is key to improving such care services. Our aim was to co-design a PCC evaluation tool with audiologists and people with hearing conditions. Involving end-users in the development of services and products has been shown to increase quality and acceptance, and ownership of the end outcome [20–22]. Kusunoki [23] advocates for the suitability of design approaches for creating evaluation tools as the problems that are seen in design also relate to the evaluation of different life contexts and understanding of use. Wright et al. [24] suggest that "Evaluation approaches can only do this if they are co-designed with service users who are set to benefit most from the results" (p. 13). Cooper et al. [25] note that co-design methods within existing service or educational contexts are useful because services often change over time.

10.2.2 Artificial Intelligence and PCC

Artificial intelligence used in healthcare settings is a rapidly evolving field with many existing and emerging applications across e-health, internet of things and other sensing technology in clinical and home settings, clinical practice and decision making to name some. There are relatively few papers that have made the connection between AI and its potential impact on person-centred care. Bjerring and Busch [26] argue that AI as "black box medicine" (p. 351) goes against PCC because the patient views and context are not taken into consideration, and the practitioner may not be able to explain why a specific decision was made. Triberti et al. [27] also suggest that there is the possibility that AI will not aid patient outcomes unless there is an implementation of explainable AI. Explainable AI means decisions can be reconstructed and a user-centred design of interfaces exists that support doctors, patients and other stakeholders. Ognjanović and Šendelj [15] highlight a range of opportunities for patient-centred care interventions through patient data and potential diagnostic capabilities. However, the use of PCC evaluation data in broader contexts are not considered.

Living labs are also being used as spaces to research the impact of AI [28, 29]. We believe there is an opportunity to collect person-centred data that can provide information about a patient over time, and be aggregated to a clinic, sector or geographic area. Vollmer et al. [30] "believe that interdisciplinary groups pursuing research and impact projects involving machine learning and artificial intelligence for health would benefit from explicitly addressing a series of questions concerning transparency, reproducibility, ethics, and effectiveness." (p. 1.) and go on to propose 20 critical questions for health-related AI and machine learning projects. These include the following questions that are particularly relevant here as well:

1. What is the health question relating to patient benefit?
2. What evidence is there that the development of the algorithm was informed by best practices in clinical research and epidemiological study design? (p. 3).

Key objectives of the European standard of patient-centred-care demand:

"To ensure that patient participation is included in person-centred research and to ensure patient participation in designing, implementation and evaluation of quality indicators and improvement work at all operational and strategic levels within the healthcare settings." [31]. These considerations influenced our participatory approach to this specific research.

10.3 Case Study: Co-creation of PCC Measures and Dashboard with Hearing Rehabilitation Provider

At the beginning of the COVID-19 pandemic, Swinburne's Future Self and Design Living Lab was approached to conduct a series of stakeholder workshops. Ethics approval was obtained by Swinburne's Human Research Ethics Committee (Project ID 0741). We use this case study to demonstrate the process of creating tools to collect high-quality data, setting up an AI infrastructure and discuss the challenges we have experienced.

Existing measures often focus on the functional aspects of service, e.g., waiting times, functional hearing/audiology outcome measures (e.g., aided receptive speech understanding scores or hearing aid usage time logged in hearing devices). We used an approach that interrogated the quality and emotional aspects of person-centred care experiences. These attributes are quite different from existing questionnaires but Sterling et al. [32] emphasise the importance of emotional factors. They found out that trust and respect are the main influencing factors for a positive experience when patients are interacting in a teleaudiology service environment.

10.3.1 Method

We ran a co-design study with the goal to develop a dashboard to routinely measure the experience of person-centred care against other clinical success measures in hearing rehabilitation. First, two tools to collect high-quality data were developed (i) the Whole-Person Hearing Questionnaire (WPQ) and (ii) the Person-Centred Care Questionnaire (PCCQ). Current literature was incorporated with stakeholder research and direct clinical involvement to produce a whole-person hearing care dashboard, covering three key areas: patient hearing health outcomes, person-centred care (PCC) experiences, and clinic sustainability. The project was broken down into a series of phases which are detailed below.

10.3.1.1 Best Practice Review

The team examined the current literature on areas of interest to the dashboard, including PCC, patient hearing rehabilitation outcomes in cases of adult hearing loss, and dashboard visual and logistical inspiration. This phase presented the opportunity for researchers to examine the current literature around person-centred care and audit tools that have already been created, in and out of audiology, to measure PCC in a clinical setting to develop the PCCQ. An audit on current tools to measure hearing outcomes, participation changes for people with hearing impairment, quality of life, mental health, and general wellbeing was undertaken for the WPQ. Questions from tools were collated and researchers identified key groups of questions present across the literature. As the impacts of hearing impairment are diverse incorporating bio, psycho, social and spiritual aspects of a person, the research team expanded the literature search to identify impacts of hearing loss beyond one's ability to hear sound.

10.3.1.2 Primary Data Collection with Stakeholders

Any questionnaires developed need to be viable and accessible in a clinical setting, meaning patients need the opportunity to fill them out before, during or after their appointment. To map these opportunities, the project officer attended the clinic and observed the patient's journey and experiences from when they arrived at the building, through checking in with reception, waiting in the waiting room, to attending their hearing care appointment and leaving again. The project officer then interviewed the front-of-house staff and clinical staff to establish all the time points at which contact was made between the clinic and the patients. From this data, the project officer generated a map of opportunity timepoints for data collection. The data collection points of interest were the three key inputs for the dashboard; the whole-person outcomes (impact of hearing condition/intervention outcomes captured via the WPQ), delivery of person-centred care (PCC) and sustainability. For example, opportunities for filling out the PCCQ were either during the appointment or after the appointment with a follow-up email or other contact; crucially, as a measure of care given, it cannot be conducted before the appointment.

To understand hearing rehabilitation experiences and goals in more detail two workshops with stakeholders were also conducted (both with participants with hearing impairment and clinicians/managers who work in hearing healthcare clinics). The workshops focused on what the stakeholders valued in adult hearing healthcare, what they felt was important to measure, and how they felt hearing healthcare could be improved by drawing from their own lived experience.

The workshops took a living lab approach with multiple stakeholders present. The workshops were conducted with eight clinicians/clinic managers (the 'clinician group') and seven hearing-impaired clients of audiological rehabilitation (the 'hearing-impaired group') who explored their thoughts and feelings on what should be measured and what would be helpful in a whole-person hearing dashboard. The first set of stakeholder workshops took place via Zoom during the pandemic. The focus of the participatory workshops was on what should be measured, how it should be measured, and what was important to each group to achieve in audiological rehabilitation. The topic areas were the overall patient journey, intervention impact, person-centred care experiences, and sustainability. A particular focus was on how patients would like to/should feel like during the service journey similar to Sterling et al. [32].

Two activities were conducted. The first activity was designed to elicit three different dimensions of a topic: (1) What should care do—the functional components; (2) How should care be—quality components and (3) How should care feel—feeling of emotional components.

In the second activity of the workshop, we ask participants, informed by step one, what data for evaluating care should be collected, when it should be collected and how it should be collected. These questions were asked from the point of view of:

- Clinical intervention (e.g. were hearing needs met)
- Intervention impact for indirect or non-audiological impacts (e.g. mental health, relationships)
- Business sustainability (e.g. consultation times) this was captured for clinicians only
- Patient journey stages (e.g. referral, before arrival, during, after, at follow-up).

10.3.1.3 Iterative Development of Tools and Dashboard

The researchers developed two tools from analysis of the literature and integration with themes from stakeholder workshops to measure whole-person patient outcomes and delivery of PCC. Feedback for these tools from stakeholder workshops (on topics such as clarity, relevance, usability and other issues such as data analysis and anonymity) was integrated into the tools. Each tool underwent two rounds of feedback gathering from patients who filled out the questionnaires at the Soundfair Hearing Centre, and the feedback was integrated into the revised tools. Data input and output options were also discussed and key themes from the workshop were documented for the development phase.

A preliminary dashboard was built. As the dashboard was to be implemented in everyday practice, sustainability measures relevant to that clinic were identified in consultation with the clinical team and incorporated into the dashboard, too. Data from the tools was entered into the dashboard and presented to the clinical team. Feedback from the clinical team on relevance and usability was taken on board and the dashboard was revised accordingly. Due to the government restrictions in place to stop the spread of COVID-19 in Melbourne, few patients were seen in the clinic and thus development of the dashboard was conducted with fewer patient data than planned.

10.4 Results

10.4.1 Stakeholder Workshops—Development of Tools

10.4.1.1 Hearing-Impaired Group

The hearing-impaired group recognised hearing difficulty, mental health and quality of life were important to be measured. They also recognised that these measurements may change over time, so repeat measuring would be helpful.

A key theme of the discussion with the hearing-impaired group was the importance of the relationship between the client and the clinician. This included the trust that formed between the client and the clinician and the trust that was formed with a hearing organisation. They reported that trust could be lost when they feel a 'sales push', as this is perceived to not be in their best interests. Feeling 'heard' was also a key theme, with clients emphasising this was important for building a meaningful relationship with the clinician. They also spoke about the importance of people around them understanding their hearing difficulties, which can be seen as a PCC request by ensuring appropriate involvement of family members and significant others. Other key themes with a strong relationship to how patients wanted to feel included safety and respect. Interestingly these feelings came up again and again across the different measures of PCC and patient outcomes. This means there is a set of feelings that are relevant across different key hearing rehabilitation goals.

For the timing of questionnaire administration, the hearing-impaired group spoke of trust with the clinician, and that any type of measure of their hearing health outcomes would be appropriate to be discussed during the appointment time. As such, they would be happy with completing the WPQ questionnaire before or during the appointment and did not require the scores or results to be kept anonymous. However, this was different to measures specifically on PCC experiences. When asked when the best time would be to fill out a PCCQ, clients responded that they would prefer time to consider and reflect on their experience before giving this rating, so would prefer to be contacted with the PCCQ, but soon after the appointment. There was also a strong motif from the hearing-impaired focus group that they would prefer measures of PCC to be anonymous. This was largely due to a perceived power imbalance with their clinician; they were more likely to be comfortable giving a truthful answer if they were assured that any feedback they gave about their clinician would be anonymous. They reported being more likely to not fill out a questionnaire if it was not anonymous. They also would appreciate a mixture of closed- and open-ended questions to adequately feel heard.

An important part of the workshops was the discussion of the patient journey, and how it contributes to the overall experience an individual would have with an organisation. Metrics to this end included: the waiting period to the appointment, accessibility of the clinic, and comfort with temperature in the waiting room, among others. However, these metrics were deemed beyond the scope of this research as other aspects and brevity of the evaluation tool had higher priority.

10.4.1.2 Clinician Group

Within the clinician group, there was a strong view that hearing care should be tailored towards empowering and validating the patient. They also recognised that the therapeutic relationship goes both ways equally valuing the clinician's and patient's expertise. For example, clinician's wellbeing is an important aspect of preventing workplace stress and burnout. This issue is relevant when discussing sustainability, as the provision of person-centred care must be sustainable for both financial viability and staff wellbeing.

On the topic of anonymity, while resoundingly unanimous in the hearing-impaired group, the clinician group was more conflicted. When discussing measuring PCC, there was much discourse around the usability of the data and what each clinic/clinician would like collected. Clinicians saw value in receiving feedback on their delivery of PCC from their clients to identify what areas they are excelling at and what they need to continue working on. While some clinicians saw the benefit in generalised results across patients to identify areas they could work on, others preferred client-specific results to address any shortcomings more directly. The concern was raised that this measure could be used as a KPI to evaluate the clinician's performance; caution must be taken when interpreting the PCC data as it may not be a direct reflection on the clinician's performance, but rather the patient's overall experience.

The clinician group recognised that there was a need to measure the client's hearing ability to perform their job, but other measures of global wellbeing, relationships and participation restrictions would also be helpful. The most used measure of hearing ability within Australia currently is the Client Orientated Scale of Improvement (COSI) [33], which the clinician group described as a talking tool to help facilitate conversation in an appointment and measure client progress. They explained that using a metric (such as the COSI) as a talking tool helped them to structure appointments and track progress, which was seen as a strength.

10.4.2 Stakeholder Feedback

During the second round of stakeholder involvement, the team presented the two constructed questionnaires and asked for feedback on how understandable the questions were, how well they reflected the experience of hearing-impaired people, and whether anything needed to be changed before being implemented in a clinical setting.

A key theme in feedback was accessibility. Participants (both patients and clinicians) discussed the need to have multiple data input methods to suit a variety of ages and abilities. For example, having a touch screen to complete a survey in reception may not be accessible to some people; therefore, paper options are also necessary. It was recommended that this be a consideration for all data being collected, whether before or after the appointment.

It was clear from the feedback that both clinicians and members of the hearing-impaired community valued measuring intervention outcomes beyond purely how the client can hear in different situations. This reflected the diverse categories and assigned themes identified in the workshops where a whole-person approach and the relevance of the feelings of the patients appeared strongly in the data.

10.4.2.1 Feedback on Tools in a Pilot Deployment

For the purposes of being integrated into the clinic life, the WPQ (measuring whole-person hearing impact) questionnaire was amalgamated with a general history questionnaire asking questions about their symptoms, referral pathways etc. The survey was sent to clients in advance of their clinical appointment via email and was also available as a paper version upon arrival at the clinic, to maximise accessibility as was requested in the stakeholder workshops. A question requesting the patient to attend an interview to give feedback on the WPQ was added to the survey: *As we develop the survey, we want to know that it is effective in measuring your whole-person experience. We value any feedback you can give us. After your appointment, with your permission, a member of our team will ask you a few questions about the survey and whether you think it captures what you are going through. This is completely voluntary and if you choose not to participate there are no consequences to you or the care you receive at Soundfair.*

Patient feedback revealed that the WPQ questionnaire was easy to understand and asked questions highly relevant and broad enough to encapsulate the main aspects of their whole-person experience and the impact arising from their hearing condition. Interestingly, they also disclosed that they were not expecting an audiology service to ask some of the questions contained within the WPQ given their presumed expectation or prior experience with an audiology service. This was despite the question topic being highly relevant to their experience. This is an important insight about the relevance of participatory design and real-life context as part of the Living Lab approach. The patients would usually not have brought this up because they thought that their experience was irrelevant to be spoken about in an audiology appointment context. The fact they were asked about all their whole-person desires for care in the workshop meant it was incorporated and Soundfair is now actively asking about these experiences and creating potential new avenues of care.

Feedback was also gained from the clinician and front-of-house staff. After small amendments were made, the survey was implemented into the regular Soundfair appointment protocol. After it was embedded into the protocol for 6 months, 25 patients had completed the survey and their responses were stored for input into the dashboard. Again, this was during the ongoing strict lockdowns in Victoria, Australia and consequently, patient numbers were very low.

The PCCQ survey was emailed to all clients attending the clinic in a 6-month period from February-July 2021. Ten responses were received in total. The anonymity of the PCCQ survey prevented immediate follow-up with patients, but also responses could not be matched to any other metrics (such as the WPQ score). Instead, the research team contacted clients who had attended the clinic and had the survey emailed to them, asking if they had completed the survey and if they would mind providing us with feedback over the phone. They were assured that their responses would remain anonymous. Only three clients were available to provide feedback demonstrating the importance of anonymity and the difficulty of collecting and matching data in health care settings.

Feedback received was generally positive and no major changes to the survey were recommended. The only suggestion for improvement came when a patient had seen two different clinicians and believed one provided better PCC than the other; however, the survey did not allow for differentiation between clinicians. This was also reflected in the feedback from clinicians; the data was of limited use to them without knowing which clinician the responses pertained to. The addition of clinician identification may be a consideration for future iterations of this survey. The final PCCQ after feedback with 13 questions can be seen in Table 10.2. The final questions are mapped to the themes emerging from the literature review and from the workshop results.

10.4.2.2 Challenges During Data Collection (Data Quality)

The following challenges were faced during the data collection which also might have implications when data are collected to be inserted and analysed in the dashboard:

- Questionnaire documents need to be easily accessible to front-of-house staff to send to patients efficiently. This was amended by creating a common folder for the survey material that was accessible to staff.
- Frequency of testing the WPQ with each client was unclear. At a project meeting, it was established that measuring the WPQ at follow-up appointments would be ideal, as this could track difficulty and changes over time. However, as many clients only attended the Soundfair Hearing Centre once during the period of the pandemic restrictions, the efficacy of testing the WPQ longitudinally was not possible.
- The questionnaire tools were not accessible to non-English speakers (as was seen during the first iteration of this test). Where possible, an interpreter was used, but this added to appointment length and possibly lost some nuance of the survey. Translating the survey into other languages may be an area of future research.

Table 10.2 Person-centred care questionnaire (PCCQ)

No	Question	Literature theme	Workshop motif
1	Generally, do you feel your care is well-coordinated? Consider how easy it is to navigate your health pathway, and how different health professionals integrate their care for you	Co-ordination of care	Journey/ecosystem
2	Did you feel well-understood by the clinician?	Understanding the person	Feeling heard
3	Did you feel the service was tailored to your individual situation?	Individualised management	Feeling heard
4	Were you involved as much as you wanted to be in decisions about your care?	Individualised management	Decision making
5	Did the staff communicate with you in a friendly and respectful way?	Communication	Communication
6	Was there an atmosphere of trust during the consultations?	Client/clinician relationship	Relationship
7	Did you feel at ease in dealing with the staff?	Client/clinician relationship	Relationship
8	Did you feel that you and the staff were partners throughout the process of your care?	Client/clinician relationship	Relationship
9	Did you feel emotionally supported by the clinician? (E.g. Showing empathy, allowing you to voice any anxieties or fears)	Client/clinician relationship	Menial health
10	Were your family/friends/carers involved as much as you wanted them to be in decision about your care?	Involvement of others	Community
11	Did your care team provide enough support to help you to manage your own health and wellbeing?	Self-management	Journey
12	Was any information that was provided clear and accessible to you?	Access/usability	Communication
13	Did the service meet your reason for attending today?	Expectations	Expectations

- The WPQ adds to the clinical time, but clinicians do find it useful as a talking tool to make sure all areas of hearing loss impact are covered.

The final WPQ is a clinical questionnaire that encompasses the impact of hearing loss over a range of life areas. If used longitudinally it can be used to track changes in impact resulting from the intervention. Clinicians find it a useful tool but must balance its usefulness with clinical time management given there are already other related metrics that funding providers contractually require.

The PCCQ is a measure that allows clients to give feedback on areas of PCC. To give honest feedback, clients prefer an anonymous survey, but the usefulness of this data in the absence of being able to track it to a clinician is limited from the clinic's perspective. Adding the option for clients to indicate who their clinician was, could remedy this and increase the tool's usefulness while protecting their anonymity.

10.4.3 Piloting the Dashboard

10.4.3.1 Economic Considerations

Clinic Sustainability was a topic not spoken about with the hearing-impaired group, as this is something that is much more relevant to clinicians. Even so, there was some reluctance in terms of talking about the economic measures amongst the clinician group. Some that were brought up included attrition, referral source satisfaction, dollar per hour, Average Selling Price (ASP) and diary efficiency. Helpful sustainability measures are likely to vary between clinics, indicating the need for flexible options on sustainability measures in any widely available dashboard in the future. However, for the purposes of creating and piloting the dashboard to suit the clinic, a meeting was conducted with the team at Soundfair to brainstorm metrics that may be useful to include in the dashboard such as appointment type, funding category and income from appointment.

10.4.3.2 Data Collection, Integration and Input

The project officer created a database that allowed data input for the WPQ, PCCQ and sustainability measures. Pivot charts were created to display the data in a meaningful way.

Figure 10.2 shows a bar graph of PCC score (PCCQ) broken into PCC categories, with optional data slicer for month and year.

The bar graph (Fig. 10.2) is showing PCC data across four months (February to June). The different PCC categories can be seen on the left and are derived from the mapped literature themes in Table 10.2. The numbers associated with each data point represent the average score for the questions in each PCC category (questions are rated on a scale of -2 to $+2$). In this first iteration, the data did not factor in a

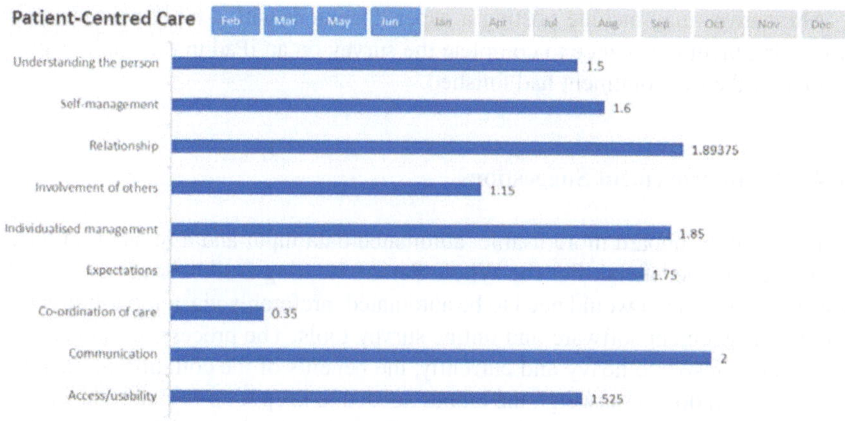

Fig. 10.2 The PCC bar graph showing data from February, March, May, June

score for items where 'not applicable' was selected (e.g. 'involvement of others' and 'coordination of care' were scored as '0' if the client selected 'not applicable') and subsequently skewed the data.

The dashboard was made available to Soundfair staff for the duration of the data collection period. However, it was deemed too cumbersome to manually input the data at regular intervals; therefore, the data were added en masse in September 2021, at the end of the data collection period. A meeting was then held with the clinical staff to discuss the usability and feasibility of the dashboard.

As the aim of this project was to create a minimal viable product (MVP) dashboard, the data entry was manual and required the staff to know how to use the dashboard to input the data correctly. This took a while to implement and presented several logistical obstacles, such as:

- Matching client data across the dashboard
- Obtaining and collating the metrics that were selected for use
- Lack of automation of data collection made the data input time-consuming.

These logistical problems could be alleviated if future dashboards were made to integrate with pre-existing patient management software that would input data to the dashboard automatically or collate data with the option to add it into the dashboard via means of plug-in software.

Other problems with usability included:

- PCC dashboard wording (e.g. 'relationship' and 'access/usability') was not easily understood as the categories used were considered jargon by clinicians. Simpler wording of categories that concisely captured the essence of the category without needing a glossary would make this section more understandable.
- The PCC survey was distributed via email to maintain anonymity, which meant that the older client demographic was less likely to fill in the survey.

Alternatives may include posting a paper document with a reply-paid envelope or offering them the chance to complete the survey on an iPad in the clinic waiting room after their appointment had finished.

10.4.3.3 Improvement Suggestions

To make the dashboard more usable, automated data input and a revision of terms used would be beneficial. For the Whole-Person Hearing Dashboard to be feasible in a clinical setting, it would need to be automated, preferably via compatibility with patient management software and online survey tools. The process of manual data extraction is resource-heavy and currently, the benefits of the collation of data into one dashboard do not outweigh the labour needed to keep it up-to-date. The current dashboard data output is not distinct enough from the clinic's standalone data output sources to warrant the extra effort required to constantly update all the data into one place on the dashboard. However, in addition to automation, the value of the dashboard would increase if current metrics could be analysed over time or allow correlations analyses between metrics. Metrics that should be improved are:

1. Income from the appointment: This metric is currently slightly restrictive, as it is likely to vary over the course of each patient's rehabilitation journey. Instead, using the total income from each patient over the course of their appointments would be more helpful for Soundfair's clinic as it takes out the fluctuation between initial and follow-up appointments.
2. Net Promoter Score (NPS—likelihood patients would recommend organisation): While this information, anonymised, is interesting to see how the clinic is performing overall, collecting this data anonymously prevents the clinic from following up any bad or moderate ratings. Thus, currently this measurement is not particularly helpful but is a commonly used industry metric allowing benchmarking of services. In the future, this could be improved by either asking the patient to rate the NPS non-anonymously or providing them the option to be contacted for follow-up.
3. WPQ longitudinal data collection: While it was always the plan to collect WPQ data and map it over time, COVID restrictions and the structure of the Soundfair clinical appointments at the time prevented repeat measurements from being taken during this trial. In the future, drawing correlations between provision of PCC and change in WPQ is likely to be beneficial.
4. Changes to PCC anonymity: Although it was a key request from the Hearing-Impaired group in the stakeholder workshop to keep measurements of PCC anonymous, the applicability and utility in the clinical setting becomes limited. It would be more helpful for the clinic if measures of PCC could be mapped to a clinician, and to changes in WPQ score over time. Correlations could also be made between delivery of PCC and income from appointment, if that is a desirable metric. PCC scores could also be used as a development tool for clinicians to identify the areas of PCC they need to work on, if the scores were able

to be mapped to the treating clinician. While this question could be added into the survey while keeping the overall survey anonymous, it may still impact the client's response.

5. Overall data integration: The benefit of a dashboard is that data is integrated and displayed in a way that would otherwise be not available or not meaningful. As PCC is a key, novel addition to this dashboard, having anonymised data limits the benefit that the dashboard may have over standalone data.

10.5 Discussion

10.5.1 Summary of Case Study

The PCCQ and WPQ have direct clinical applicability and are helpful, standalone, in a clinical setting; specifically, as feedback on how well a clinic practices PCC and to ensure all aspects of a person's experience with hearing loss are encapsulated into the goals and intervention decisions. Both questionnaires were well-received by clinical staff and clients and have been successfully integrated into the Soundfair Hearing Centre. The completion rate of the WPQ is much higher than that of the PCCQ, because the WPQ is completed in advance of the appointment and is used as a talking tool in the clinic. The PCCQ, being anonymous and sent after the appointment via email, has a lower response rate which is not unexpected for such a survey.

The Dashboard, while interesting to clinical staff, is in its current format not worth the effort required to manually collate all data into a single database and maintain it. The benefit from this dashboard would come from more intricate insights drawn between delivery of PCC, whole person outcomes and clinic sustainability as these correlations would reveal more insights than the stand-alone metrics available outside of the dashboard. However, while keeping the PCCQ anonymous, the utility of the dashboard is limited. The anonymity limits integration with other metrics. Flexibility with this issue (perhaps by giving clients the option to conduct the survey non-anonymously) is likely to improve this issue and add value to the dashboard.

We can conclude that a considerable improvement in collecting high-quality data was achieved through the participatory approach and the development of tools for patient outcomes and person-centred care. However, the realisation of a true AI infrastructure faced barriers which we discuss here and make suggestions to increase the utility and applicability of AI in health.

10.5.2 Discussion on Opportunities and Challenges for AI

As there were core emotions and qualities that were desirable across several aspects of person-centred care, these core measures could be sampled in time across a number of patients and through time per patient (Fig. 10.3). By sampling across a range of core emotions, qualities and functions we may not need to be able to measure all of them per patient. This would be helpful as organisations are often faced with survey fatigue [34]. Reducing the patient reporting burden while maintaining a current view of patient-centeredness within a practice might address this. The difficulty to obtain data could be attributed partially to COVID, but it is likely that it is also problematic beyond the pandemic.

Figure 10.3 shows that by combining AI informed sampling of core measures we may be able to ask fewer questions of patients but gather enough information to gain an overall view on PCC for a clinic within a given timeframe, e.g., a weekly view. By sampling different core measures for each patient over time, we can understand an individual patient's view of their PCC experience. The advantage is that different types of data can be used to build an overall picture rather than every patient answering all the PCCQ questions every time, avoiding survey fatigue. For example, not every patient must answer repeatedly the questions about how they felt about the service or if they were involved in decision making at every touchpoint during their service journey. This way providers can ascertain how individual clinics are doing without the need of having complete data sets from patients on every visit. The complexity of

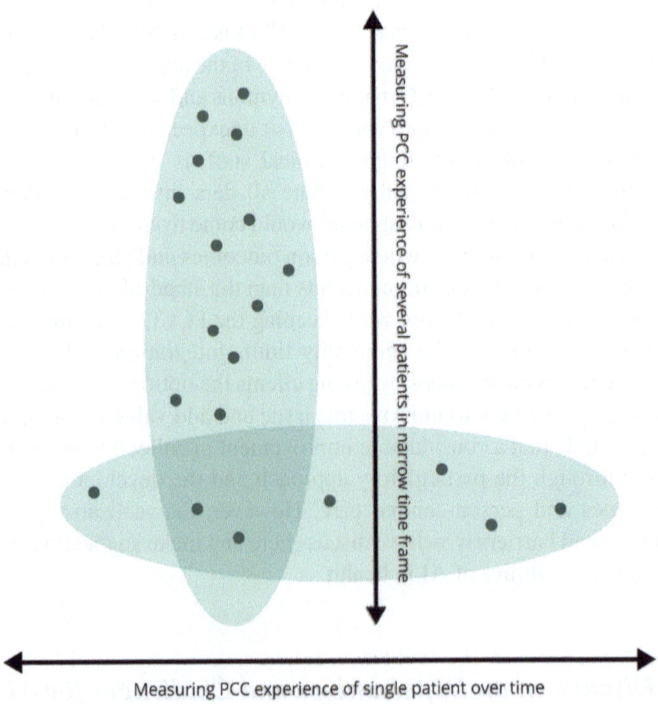

Fig. 10.3 AI informed sampling measures of PCC across patients for clinic performance and measures over time for individual's PCC journey

creating this dynamic survey while maintaining the integrity of both individual and overall views of PCC would be too complex for human intervention. This kind of data collection would rely on a validated AI model and an explainable approach that could be amended with human intervention, e.g. if a clinician wanted to get more data from a specific patient.

Person-centred care is supposed to provide better patient outcomes and many case studies point to this connection. Evaluating outcomes and making decisions based on the data, practitioners and practices can evolve to become more patient-centred and improve patient outcomes. However, there may be other approaches or only some critical aspects that really make a difference. In this case machine learning might challenge the notion of person-centred care through data-based evidence, i.e. that non-PCC practice would be more effective. Assuming that ML is consistent with other studies, a PCC and AI (ML) tool may still make recommendations that may not be in the traditional PCC model. However, the reasons why these aspects are chosen may not be readily obvious to us. Gunning and Aha [35] note that the best learning mechanism, deep learning neural nets, have the lowest explanatory factor (i.e. how the machine made that decision). This raises what Grant [36] calls a beneficence problem, balancing the desire for benefit maximisation with the duty of non-maleficence (not doing harm to others). Grant [36] notes an example where ML made recommendations that would do harm to one population on the basis that the overall good was maximised (p. 236). In Grant's case, they were able to uncover the problem because of the very clear distinction between just two groups, in other cases, these kinds of issues may be much more subtle and there could be no way of understanding how the ML arrived at its decision. Casacuberta and Vallverdú [37] point out that emotions are not universal and are contextual to culture and even context. They note that even with an approach that measures physiological data to derive bodily reactions they still need to:

- Ensure there is sufficient data from minority groups
- Have those groups interpret the data in their language to ensure meaningful accuracy
- Capture emotions in relevant contexts
- Perfectly anonymise the data to protect cultural privacy concerns.

A limitation in our study was that minority groups were not represented well because of the language difficulties and hence a lack of accessibility of the tools for clients who were non-English-speaking. This meant that clients could not fill out the surveys, or they would need to do so through use of an interpreter which added time to the appointment, impacting on clinical efficiency. Translation of the data collection tools into languages commonly spoken by the clinic clientele could be a way to improve accessibility in the future. The addition of emotions is a further hurdle for developing and capturing a universal notion of PCC and machine learning capabilities to match. Triberti el al. [27] also notes the interpretational difficulties of emotions. Looking for desired emotions can simplify this by defining a more limited range. However, there could be similar instances where patients might express that they are "uncomfortable" which could have many meanings in different contexts.

Table 10.3 Summary of required activity for ML readiness

Level	Quality	Description	Audiology data
Level AAA	Safe	Data are issue free, include integrity checks, have complete provenance information	Unresolved
Level AA	Auto-analyse	Data supports the automation of bias detection, feature selection, normalisation, and more	Known data bias–not resolved
Level A	Analyse	Known meta-data and meaningful values to the problem at hand	Some for established data, mostly economic data not PCC data
Level B	Believe	The data have known and correct data types, data pedigree known (data history), and documented missing values	Data types not agreed across sectors. Increased return rate by patients' needs to confirm the required data set
Level C	Conceive	Machine readable data, accessible	The prototype successfully loaded some data. Not all data can be integrated due to anonymity concerns

Hence recommendations based on such data need to be discussed with the patients and decisions made together.

10.5.3 *Quality of Data*

As noted above there are some aspects of data that are known to be missing at this point. Reviewing the quality of data indicate other issues that need to be considered for an AI application, outlined in Table 10.3.

While there are some measures that audiologists use that are standardised and have been in operation for a few years, which with work, could reach level B and possibly level A this is situated within the realm of business measures and basic satisfaction scales, rather than measures of PCC. As PCC measures are developed, these readiness levels will need to be kept in mind for any future AI development. Agreeing on fundamental aspects and meaning of data will be vital to capture aspects of PCC across different facets of care using AI approaches. While there will be increasing complexity across health sectors and even geographies, this is where AI will be most useful and can support decision-makers at a policy level. Figure 10.4 shows the potential for the data to be scaled by looking at the two dimensions of location and health domains. Once there are more standardised measures available, the objective is to compare PCC performance geographically or across health services. The smallest unit for the health domain is the hearing clinic which then can be compared in its PCC performance to other clinics. The performance of clinics can be compared to geographic locations of different sizes, such as cities, states or nations. But also,

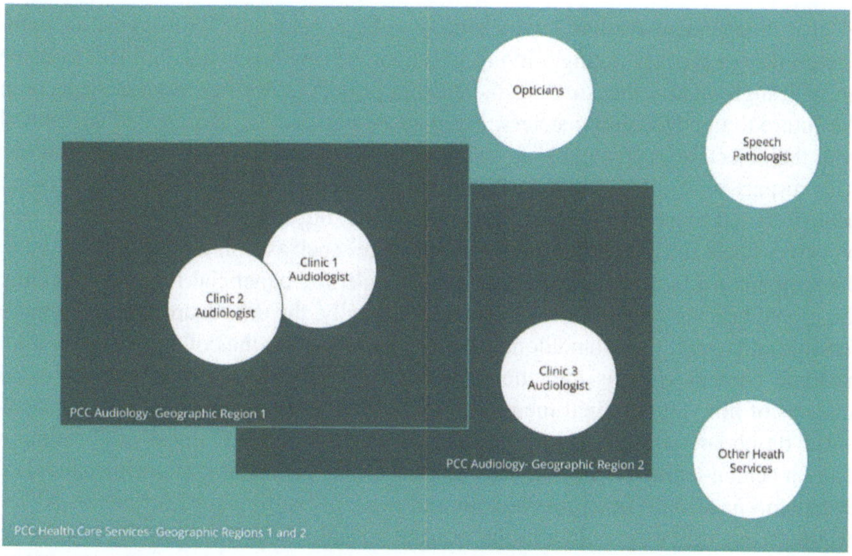

Fig. 10.4 Standardised PCC measures from many clinics have the potential to scale through AI across different locations and different health services

other health domains such as opticians can be compared with the hearing clinics when equivalent measures on PCC are used. Once PCC measures can be collected by clinics and across health services there is potential to link PCC to improved outcomes and increasing effectiveness within and across sectors. AI then has the potential to look for patterns that could inform policy and practice by location or sector.

Triberti et al. [27] suggest that explainable AI will be useful in health care practice as a mechanism to ensure that people can understand the recommendation and make a final decision based on their interactions with the patient. They note the importance of user experience and user-centred design to overcome some potential drawbacks of poor AI implementation. In the case of evaluation, the collection, stakeholders and users of the measures are more varied. We would argue that co-design can play a pivotal role in mediating the needs of this broader spectrum of stakeholders.

10.6 Conclusions

Primary outcomes of this project resulted in the creation of two beneficial clinical tools to measure patient outcomes and the provision of PCC. We showed that the complexity in health care needs to be reflected in tools collecting data that are representative of the context. Also data integration across measures can create barriers due to anonymity, a limited amount of data, data integration and ability of clients to give independent feedback which need to be considered. We suggest an iterative co-design process taking a living labs approach with key stakeholders to come up with high-quality measures in the current project as well as similar projects in the future to uncover such barriers. From an AI perspective, the created dashboard with the objective to create low-level AI capabilities currently has some limitations with respect to feasibility, but further fine-tuning could be used to change clinical behaviour and hone the clinical provision of PCC. Further investigation on the best way to evaluate the patient journey, with measures such as wait time to appointment, the temperature in the waiting room etc. may also be beneficial for understanding the global hearing rehabilitation experience. Finally, the dashboard would be more feasible and useful than standalone metrics by automating the collation of data from multiple clinical systems into the dashboard and providing a more sophisticated analysis of how longitudinal metrics from all three areas interact. Future iterations of the dashboard would need to consider automation and usefulness of correlation data on person-centred care practices. Ethical issues concerning minorities and data ownership have only been touched on and need to be discussed further in AI for health. To do this we would add the need to consider how the data can be used to inform the performance of hearing professionals in a positive way in regard to PCC. A living lab is ideal for managing this kind of complexity and creating solutions with stakeholders in a participatory manner over time.

References

1. McMillan, S.S., Kendall, E., Sav, A., King, M.A., Whitty, J.A., Kelly, F., Wheeler, A.J.: Patient-centered approaches to health care: a systematic review of randomized controlled trials. Med. Care Res. Rev. **70**, 567–596 (2013)
2. Santana, M.J., Manalili, K., Jolley, R.J., et al.: How to practice person-centred care: a conceptual framework. Heal Expect **21**, 429–440 (2018). https://doi.org/10.1111/hex.12640
3. Grenness, C., Hickson, L., Laplante-Lévesque, A., Davidson, B.: Patient-centred care: a review for rehabilitative audiologists. Int. J. Audiol. **53**(2014). https://doi.org/10.3109/14992027.2013.847286
4. Håkansson Eklund, J., Holmström, I.K., Kumlin, T., et al.: "Same same or different?" A review of reviews of person-centered and patient-centered care. Patient Educ. Couns. **102**, 3–11 (2019). https://doi.org/10.1016/j.pec.2018.08.029
5. Ekman, I., Swedberg, K., Taft, C.: Person-centered care—ready for prime time. Cardiovasc Nurs. **10**, 248–251 (2011)
6. Laplante-Lévesque, A., Hickson, L., Grenness, C.: An Australian survey of audiologists' preferences for patient-centredness. Int. J. Audiol. **53**(2014). https://doi.org/10.3109/14992027.2013.832418
7. Tai, S., Barr, C., Woodward-Kron, R.: Towards patient-centred communication: an observational study of supervised audiology student-patient hearing assessments. Int. J. Audiol. **58**, 97–106 (2019). https://doi.org/10.1080/14992027.2018.1538574
8. Visser, F.S., Stappers, P.J., van der Lugt, R., Sanders, E.B.-N.: Context mapping: experiences from practice. CoDesign **1**, 119–149 (2005). https://doi.org/10.1080/15710880500135987
9. Robertson, T., Simonsen, J.: Participatory design: an introduction. In: Simonsen, J, Robertson, T. (eds.) International Handbook of Participatory Design, pp. 1–18. Routledge, New York, NY (2012)

10. Suchman, L.: Human-Machine Reconfigurations: Plans and Situated Actions. Cambridge University Press (2006)
11. Sanders, E.B.N., Stappers, P.J.: Convivial toolbox: Generative research for the front end of design, 1st edn. BIS, Amsterdam (2012)
12. Brandt, E., Binder, T., Sanders, E.B.-N.: Ways to engage telling, making and enacting. In: Routledge International Handbook of Participatory Design, pp. 145–181. Routledge, New York (2012)
13. Freeman, L.: Test and evaluation for artificial intelligence. Insight **23**, 27–30 (2020). https://doi.org/10.1002/inst.12281
14. Lawrence, N.D.: Data Readiness Levels, pp. 1–10 (2017)
15. Ognjanović, L., Šendelj, R.: AI enhanced services in person-centred care in neurology. In: Karabegovi, I. (ed.) New Technologies, Development and Application III, pp. 522–529. Springer International Publishing, Cham (2020)
16. Gyldenkaerne, C.H., From, G., Mønsted, T., Simonsen, J.: PD and the challenge of AI in health-care. ACM Int. Conf. Proc. Ser. **2**, 26–29 (2020). https://doi.org/10.1145/3384772.3385138
17. Malmberg, L., Rodrigues, V., Lännerström, L., et al.: Service design as a transformational driver toward person-centered care in healthcare. Serv. Des. Serv. Think. Healthc. Hosp. Manag. 1–18. https://doi.org/10.1007/978-3-030-00749-2_1
18. Park, M., Giap, T.T.T., Jang, I., et al.: Listening to patients' voices: applying the design-thinking method for teaching person-centered care to nursing students. Nurs. Forum. **57**, 9–17 (2022). https://doi.org/10.1111/nuf.12641
19. Ferguson, M., Leighton, P., Brandreth, M., Wharrad, H.: Development of a multimedia educational programme for first-time hearing aid users: a participatory design. Int J Audiol **57**, 600–609 (2018). https://doi.org/10.1080/14992027.2018.1457803
20. Ehn, P.: Scandinavian design: on participation and skill. In: Participatory Design: Principles and Practices, pp. 41–77 (1993)
21. Carroll, J.M.: Dimensions of participation in simon's design. Des. Issues **22**, 3–18 (2006). https://doi.org/10.1162/desi.2006.22.2.3
22. Sanoff, H.: Community participation in riverfront development. CoDesign **1**, 61–78 (2005). https://doi.org/10.1080/15710880512331326022
23. Kusunoki, D.: Applying participatory design theory to designing evaluation methods. In: CHI '12 Extended Abstracts on Human Factors in Computing Systems, pp. 1895–1900. ACM, Austin, USA (2012)
24. Wright, M., Getta, A.D., Green, A.O., et al.: Co-designing health service evaluation tools that foreground first nation worldviews for better mental health and wellbeing outcomes. Int. J. Environ. Res. Publ. Heal. **18**, 8555 (2021). https://doi.org/10.3390/IJERPH18168555
25. Cooper, S., Cant, R., Waters, D., et al.: Measuring the quality of nursing clinical placements and the development of the placement evaluation tool (PET) in a mixed methods co-design project. BMC Nurs. **19**, 1–10 (2020). https://doi.org/10.1186/S12912-020-00491-1/TABLES/5
26. Bjerring, J.C., Busch, J.: Artificial intelligence and patient-centered decision-making, **34**, 349–371 (2021). https://doi.org/10.1007/s13347-019-00391-6
27. Triberti, S., La, D.T., Sebri, V., et al.: Artificial intelligence in healthcare practice: how to tackle the "Human" challenge. In: Lim, C.-P., Chen, Y.-W., Vaidya, A., et al (eds.) Handbook of Artificial Intelligence in Healthcare vol. 2: Practicalities and Prospects (2022)
28. Vilariño, F.: Unveiling the social impact of AI through living labs. In: Barth, J., Fotopoulou, E., Brauer, C. (eds.) (Forthcoming) Artificitial Intelligence and Innovation Management, p. 215/232. World Scientific (2022)
29. European Network of Open Living Labs: Social impact of artificial intelligence (AI)—action oriented task force. In: Digit. Living Lab Days 2020 Rep. (2020). https://issuu.com/enoll/docs/digital_living_lab_days_2020_report/s/11087058
30. Vollmer, S., Mateen, B.A., Bohner, G., et al.: Machine learning and artificial intelligence research for patient benefit: 20 critical questions on transparency, replicability, ethics, and effectiveness. BMJ **368**, 1–11 (2020). https://doi.org/10.1136/bmj.l6927

31. University of Gothenburg Centre for Person Centred Care.: Innovative standard for patient participation in person-centred care now available (2020). https://www.gu.se/en/gpcc/innovative-standard-for-patient-participation-in-person-centred-care-now-available. Accessed 7 Feb 2022
32. Sterling, L., Burrows, R., Barnet, B., et al.: Emotional factors for teleaudiology. In: Saunders, E. (ed.) Tele-Audiology and the Optimization of Hearing Healthcare Delivery, pp. 1–18. IGI Global, Hershey, Pennsylvania (2019)
33. Dillon, H., James, A., Ginis, J.: Client oriented scale of improvement (COSI) and its relationship to several other measures of benefit and satisfaction provided by hearing aids. J. Am. Acad. Audiol. **8**, 27–43 (1997)
34. de Koning, R., Egiz, A., Kotecha, J., et al.: Survey fatigue during the COVID-19 pandemic: an analysis of neurosurgery survey response rates. Front Surg **8**, 1–7 (2021). https://doi.org/10.3389/fsurg.2021.690680
35. Gunning, D., Aha, D.W.: DARPAs_Explainable_Artificial.PDF. AI Mag. 44–58 (2019)
36. Grant DG (2018) Ethics and artificial intelligence in public health social work. Artif. Intell. Soc. Work 231–249.https://doi.org/10.1017/9781108669016.015
37. Casacuberta, D., Vallverdú, J.: Biases in assigning emotions in patients due to multicultural. In: Lim, C.-P., Chen, Y.-W., Vaidya, A., et al. (eds.) Issues in Handbook of Artificial Intelligence in Healthcare vol. 2: Practicalities and Prospects (2022)

Gareth Priday is a Director and founder of the Australian Network of Living Labs and a member of the Future Self and Design Living Lab (FSDLL) at Swinburne University (Melbourne, Australia). Gareth is also a Futurist at Action Foresight. As a practitioner, he helps communities to create positive and engaging futures and enables their implementation through codesign.

Professor Sonja Pedell is Director of Swinburne University's Future Self and Design Living Lab. The FSD Living Lab has core development capabilities in developing innovative socio-technical systems and co-designing with older adults and communities for lifelong enjoyment and well-being. Prior to taking up this role at Swinburne, Dr Pedell completed a Master of Psychology from the Technical University of Berlin and was employed as an Interaction Designer, Usability Consultant and Product Manager in industry for several years.

Jessica Vitkovic is a leader, researcher, clinician and advocate in vestibular audiology, clinical audiology pedagogical design and person-centred practice. She is also a passionate creative with a drive to design with the end-user in mind and has a track record in creating new services to meet unmet needs of consumers.

Lauren Story is a clinical diagnostic audiologist and tertiary educator at the University of Melbourne. She dedicated her PhD to exploring the family experience of chronic balance problems and continues to strive for delivery of family-centred care in her clinical practice. Lauren joined Soundfair to aid in the development of the Whole-Person Hearing Dashboard to track person-centred experiences throughout the clinical journey. It is her hope that this, along with other research conducted by Soundfair, will aid in the widespread implementation of person-centred practices throughout the profession.

Chapter 11
BioGNN: How Graph Neural Networks Can Solve Biological Problems

Pietro Bongini, Niccolò Pancino, Franco Scarselli, and Monica Bianchini

Abstract Graph Neural Networks (GNNs) have known an important and fast development in the last decade, with many theoretical and practical innovations. Their main feature is the capability of processing graph structured data with minimal loss of structural information. This makes GNNs the ideal family of models for processing a wide variety of biological data: metabolic networks, structural formulas of molecules, and proteins are all examples of biological data that are naturally represented as graphs. As an example, GNNs were employed, with very good results, for the prediction of protein-protein interactions. This was achieved by applying a clique detection model on graphs representing the interaction of the secondary structures of pairs of proteins. The introduction of composite GNN models, designed for processing heterogeneous graphs, has allowed researchers to study even more complex networks. For instance, drug side-effects were predicted based on a graph describing the interactions between drugs and human genes. Another very important innovation was brought by generative models, that were introduced for graph data after the success of generative models for images. In particular, GNNs were used to build a sequential model for the generation of potential drug candidates, in the form of molecular graphs, with the purpose of enhancing existing drug discovery techniques. The increasing accuracy and efficacy of these models, as well as the development of more complex biological databases, ensure even more interesting future developments in the application of GNNs to biological data.

P. Bongini · N. Pancino · F. Scarselli · M. Bianchini
Department of Information Engineering and Mathematics, University of Siena, Via Roma 56, 53100 Siena, (SI), Italy

P. Bongini (✉) · N. Pancino
Department of Information Engineering, University of Florence, Via di Santa Marta 3, 50139 Florence, FI, Italy
e-mail: pietro.bongini@gmail.com

© The Author(s), under exclusive license to Springer Nature Switzerland AG 2023
C.-P. Lim et al. (eds.), *Artificial Intelligence and Machine Learning for Healthcare*, Intelligent Systems Reference Library 228,
https://doi.org/10.1007/978-3-031-11154-9_11

11.1 Overview of the Research Area

Graphs are a ubiquitous and very expressive form of data representation, providing information not only on entities but also on relationships between entities. In the biological domain, graphs are used to represent a wide variety of different data types, including proteins, structural formulas of molecules, pathways, metabolic networks, drug–protein interactions, Protein–Protein Interfaces (PPIs), and gene interaction networks. Deep learning techniques have known a great development recently, bringing solutions to problems of increasing complexity and variety. Deep learning solutions have been developed for various types of structured data, including graphs. More specifically, Graph Neural Networks (GNNs) [1] are capable of processing graphs with minimal loss of information [2], thus representing the ideal model to solve biological problems on graphs. In this Chapter, three applications of GNNs to biological problems taken from the real world are presented and discussed.
The rest of this Chapter is organized as follows. In this introductory Sect. 11.1.1 introduces the domain of biological problems on graphs, Sect. 11.1.2 provides an overview of the literature concerning GNN models and their application to biological data. Section 11.2 describes the GNN model, introducing the general mathematical formulation in Sect. 11.2.1, a composite variant for heterogeneous graphs in Sect. 11.2.2, a layered variant in Sect. 11.2.3, a discussion on the approximation power in Sect. 11.2.4, and the software implementation in Sect. 11.2.5. Finally, Sect. 11.3 provides a detailed description of the three relevant applications, introducing: a model for the prediction of PPIs in Sect. 11.3.1, a model for the prediction of Drug Side–Effects (DSEs) in Sect. 11.3.2, and a model for the generation of molecular graphs in Sect. 11.3.3. Finally, Sect. 11.4 draws some conclusions and describes GNN future prospects for biological problems.

11.1.1 Biological Problems on Graphs

Biological data are often naturally represented with graphs. Molecules have always been perceived as graphs, in which atoms correspond to nodes and chemical bonds correspond to edges. These structures can be made hierarchical, embedding molecule fragments into graph nodes, in order to represent polymers. Proteins can be represented at various scales, as graphs of atoms, residues, or secondary structure elements. Similar representations can be used for nucleic acids. Networks of biological interactions can be represented as single graphs containing many entities, also of different types (such as genes, proteins, drugs). Pathways, and knowledge networks on biological entities can be processed as graphs as well. In general, problems on graphs can be classified into three categories, which can be straightforwardly applied to the biological domain:

- Node-focused problems require a prediction on all or a subset of the graph nodes.
- Edge-focused problems require a prediction on all or a subset of the graph edges.
- Graph-focused problems require a prediction for each graph in a dataset.

In each of these three problem categories, predictions can be of two types: regression of real-valued functions or classification on a discrete set of possible labels. The prediction of DSEs or PPIs can be formulated as a node-focused classification problem. Calculating levels of activity or molecular properties, like free energy of solvation, is a graph-focused regression task. Link prediction, for instance for predicting polypharmacy effects or drug-protein interactions, can be set as an edge-focused classification task. Discriminating compounds with anti-HIV or anti-cancer activity from those without is a graph-focused classification task. Additionally, graph generation problems require generating new graphs which follow certain property distributions defined by the dataset under analysis. Molecular graph generation problems are particularly relevant in the field of Drug Discovery research, providing molecular graphs for possible new drug candidates.

11.1.2 Deep Learning Models for Biological Graphs

Since the seminal work, published in 2009 [1], GNNs have grown into a large family of models [3], divided into two main subfamilies. On the one hand, recurrent GNNs, based on the original model [1], exploit the concept of information diffusion between neighbor nodes, and encode structural information and features into node states, which are updated recurrently. Message Passing Neural Networks [4], Graph Isomorphism Networks [5], Graph Nets [6], and Gated Graph Sequence Neural Networks [7] belong to this category. On the other hand, convolutional GNNs exploit convolutions between neighbor nodes, in order to either calculate the message based on graph signals in the spectral domain [8, 9] or calculate node embeddings based on spatial neighbor aggregation [10]. These methods can be refined, for instance, by introducing multiple types of aggregation [11], graph attention mechanisms [12], self-explaining models [13], or identifying critical links in the input graphs [14].

GNNs have been employed in various biological settings [15], for instance to predict the mutagenicity [16] or anti-HIV activity of compounds [17, 18] or to predict protein functionalities [19] and taxonomic groups [20]. Drug discovery is a field in constant development which is increasingly influenced by the use of artificial intelligence techniques [21], and GNNs in particular [22]. These methods are growingly needed to cut the huge monetary and time costs to develop new drug compounds [23, 24]. In particular, deep learning models for drug discovery [25] focus on the computer aided drug design domain, where in silico experiments allow for a faster search and design of new candidate drugs [26]. In this scope, we have developed three applications of GNNs to molecular data. The first helps identify PPIs, in order to allow the development of fast in silico predictors of interactions between macromolecules. The second focuses on the prediction of DSEs, in order to screen out candidate drugs with too many potential side–effects before submitting them to long and expensive clinical trials. The third application builds a model for the automatic and fast generation of structural formulas for potential drug candidates. These three methods are based on the original GNN model [1], which will be described in the following Sect. 11.2.

11.2 Graph Neural Networks

Graph Neural Networks originate from the idea of a deep learning model that can process graphs in their natural form [1], transmitting information between their nodes [27]. Retaining structural information [2] is a great improvement with respect to euclidean models, that need data to be preprocessed and embedded into vectors. In the following, the mathematical formulation of GNNs is presented, corresponding to the original model [1]. This formulation was used in the three applications that are the focus of this Chapter.

11.2.1 The Graph Neural Network Model

Given a graph $G = (N, E)$, composed of a set of nodes N and a set of edges $E \subseteq N \times N$, we can define a label l_n describing each node $n \in N$ and a label $e_{n,m}$ for each $(n, m) \in E$. A GNN assigns a state x_n to each node $n \in N$, and updates it iteratively by sending messages through the edges connecting n to its neighbors $Ne(n)$. A GNN is fully described by two functions f_w and g_w that respectively regulate the state updating process, and the output calculation.
To define f_w, two other functions need to be specified. A message function $M(n, m, t)$, defined in Eq. (11.1), describes how messages are calculated based on the iteration t, labels and states of the source node m, the destination node n, and the edge (m, n):

$$M(n, m, t) = (x_m^{t-1}, l_m, e_{m,n}) \tag{11.1}$$

An aggregation function $A(n, t)$, defined in Eq. (11.2), decides how the messages coming from the neighborhood of a node are aggregated:

$$A(n, t) = \sum_{m \in Ne(n)} M(n, m, t) \tag{11.2}$$

In particular, two aggregations are possible: average or sum of the messages. The hyperparameter a allows to select the aggregation by assuming value 1 or $1/|Ne(n)|$. Finally, these two functions are used to define a state updating function f_w, as in Eq. (11.3):

$$x_n^t = f_w(x_n^{t-1}, l_n, a \sum_{m \in Ne(n)} (x_m^{t-1}, l_m, e_{m,n})) \tag{11.3}$$

Once the maximum number of iterations K is reached (this quantity is defined as a hyperparameter), the GNN calculates an output on nodes, edges, or whole graphs, depending on the problem under analysis.
In node focused problems, an output is defined on all or a subset of nodes $n \in N_{out} \subseteq N$. In this case, the output function g_w is defined by Eq. (11.4):

$$y_n = g_w(x_n^K,\ l_n) \tag{11.4}$$

In edge focused problems, an output is defined on all or a subset of edges $(m, n) \in E_{out} \subseteq E$. In this case, the output function g_w is defined by Eq. (11.5):

$$y_{m,n} = g_w(x_n^K,\ x_m^K,\ e_{m,n}) \tag{11.5}$$

In graph focused problems, an output is computed on each node $n \in N_{out}$ like in node focused problems and then averaged over the whole graph G. This process is defined in Eq. (11.6):

$$y_G = \frac{1}{|N_{out}|} \sum_{n \in N_{out}} g_w(x_n^K,\ l_n) \tag{11.6}$$

GNNs implement the state updating function f_w and the output function g_w with one MultiLayer Perceptron (MLP) each. These two MLPs are used as building blocks, replicating the structure of the graph in input in order to obtain an encoding network. In the encoding network, a copy of f_w is present on each node $n \in N$, while a copy of g_w is present on each output node $n \in N_{out}$. Ultimately, this network is unfolded also on the time axis, as many times as K, obtaining the unfolded encoding network. Weight sharing between copies of f_w and between copies of g_w allows the model parameters to be independent from the number of nodes, edges, and iterations. The depth of the GNN model can then be calculated by multiplying the number of layers in the state updating MLP by the number of iterations K and adding the number of layers in the output network. An example of an unfolded encoding network is represented in Fig. 11.1.

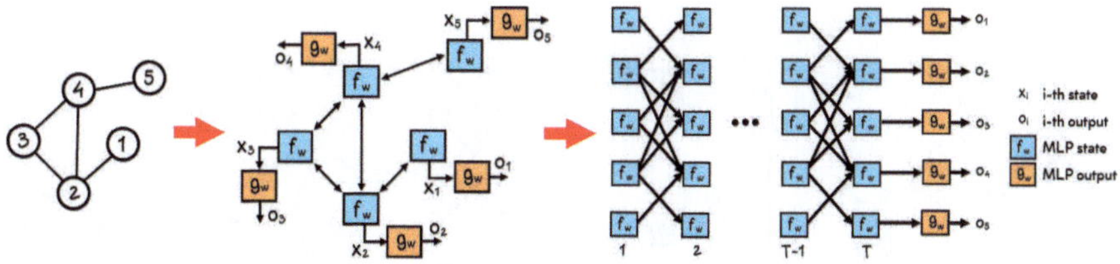

Fig. 11.1 Example of how the GNN builds its unfolded encoding network on an input graph, in a node-focused problem. Figure taken from [28]

11.2.2 Composite Graph Neural Networks

GNNs can be adapted to heterogeneous graphs, in which multiple types of nodes coexist. For instance, a knowledge graph with different entities and relationships can be seen as a heterogeneous graph in which each entity corresponds to a node type. Composite Graph Neural Networks (CGNNs) manage different types of edges (relationships) by assigning a one-hot encoding vector to each edge, accounting for the type of relationship represented. Instead, different node types are treated with different state updating functions. In particular, each node type i will correspond to a state updating MLP $f_{w,i}$. Message passing operations need to be adapted to the communication between nodes of different types, which might have labels accounting for different features, and of variable size. Therefore, given a function $T(n)$ that assigns a node type to each node $n \in N$, each state updating function follows the computation defined in Eq. (11.7):

$$x_n^t = f_{w,i}(x_n^{t-1},\ l_n,\ a \sum_{m \in Ne(n)} (x_m^{t-1},\ e_{m,n}))\ :\ i = T(n) \tag{11.7}$$

The output functions described in Sect. 11.2.1 are still valid. The only modification consists in not sending the node label in input to the output network g_w, because of the aforementioned dimensional and semantic differences between labels of nodes of different types. The unfolded encoding network of a CGNN takes the form sketched in Fig. 11.2.

11.2.3 Layered Graph Neural Networks

Multiple GNNs can be stacked together, yielding an even deeper model, called Layered Graph Neural Network (LGNN) [29]. The first layer acts like a regular GNN, calculating its output based only on the input graph. Each of the subsequent layers is instead fed with additional information, coming from the previous layer. This additional information is attached to each node $n \in N$ in the graph, and can be the output

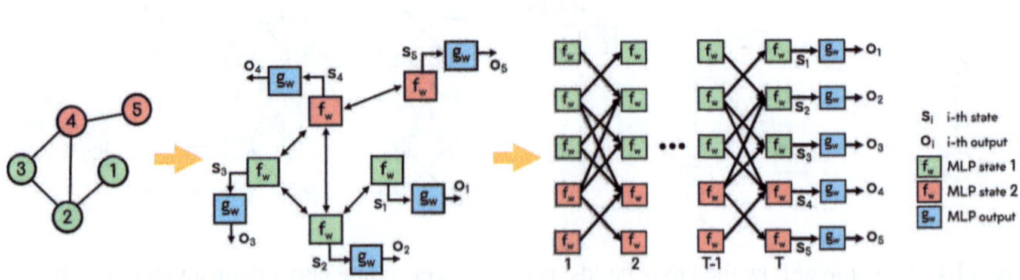

Fig. 11.2 Example of how the CGNN builds its unfolded encoding network on an input graph, in a node-focused problem. Two node types (green and red) are present in the example graph. Figure adapted from [28]

of the previous layer at node n: y_n, the final state x_n^K, or both. As a consequence, each layer refines the calculations of the previous one, basing its decision on elaborated knowledge of the input. Formally, the label of node n in the i–th layer, $i > 1$, can be rewritten as $l_n^i = [l_n, x_n^{i-1}]$, or $l_n^i = [l_n, y_n^{i-1}]$, or $l_n^i = [l_n, x_n^{i-1}, y_n^{i-1}]$, where x_n^{i-1} and y_n^{i-1} are, respectively, the state and the output of node n at layer $i-1$ of the cascaded architecture. In this case, x_n^i always indicates the state after all the iterations (x_n^K) of state updating at layer i.

11.2.4 Approximation Power of Graph Neural Networks

Measuring the approximation capabilities of GNNs has always been an interesting line of theoretical research. The first work of this type was published in parallel with the original model [2]: it is based on the concept of unfolding tree. Given a graph $G = (N, E)$, the unfolding tree T_n of a generic node $n \in N$ is built by taking n as the root, adding its neighbors as child nodes, and then recursively adding the neighbors of each child node as its children, as described in Eq. (11.8):

$$
\begin{aligned}
T_n^k &= \text{Tree}(x_n, \{T_m^{k-1}, \forall m \in Ne(n)\}) \ \text{ if } k > 1 \\
T_n^1 &= \text{Tree}(x_n)
\end{aligned}
\tag{11.8}
$$

The unfolding tree T_n^k represents all the information on node n available to the GNN after k iterations. Therefore, two nodes n and m with identical unfolding trees $T_n^k = T_m^k$ are indistinguishable to the network and are said to be unfolding equivalent, for k greater than or equal to the diameter of G. GNNs have been demonstrated to be universal approximators on graphs for all functions that preserve the unfolding equivalence (i.e. functions that produce the same result on any pair of unfolding equivalent nodes) [2].

Moreover, the approximation power of GNNs can be measured also by their capability of simulating the Weisfeiler–Lehman graph isomorphism test [5]. This test associates a canonical form to each graph and marks a pair of graphs as isomorphic if they have identical canonical form [30]. Since the one dimensional Weisfeiler–Lehman test (1-WL) cannot distinguish all the possible pairs of graphs, higher order tests are defined: the D-dimensional Weisfeiler–Lehman test (D–WL) is based on tuples of nodes of dimension D. The higher D, the more non-isomorphic graphs can be distinguished by the test. GNN models can be classified as D-WL if they can replicate the D-WL test. Interestingly, the 1-WL test is analogous to an iteration of neighborhood aggregation in recurrent GNNs, proving that all recurrent GNNs are of class 1-WL when they are equipped with injective neighborhood aggregation and output functions [5]. Currently, while some convolutional GNNs cannot replicate the 1-WL test, most GNNs are of class 1-WL, and no model has been classified as 2-WL or greater [5]. Significant efforts have been made in the direction of 2-WL

GNNs, building non-local models that exploit information on higher order neighborhoods [31]. Moreover, the equivalence between the unfolding tree method and the Weisfeiler–Lehman test as evaluators of the approximation power of GNNs has been recently demonstrated [32].

11.2.5 Software Implementation

This formulation is implemented in a Python framework for the development and deployment of GNNs: GNNkeras. [33] This framework, designed as an easily usable Python package, allows to program, configure, and deploy GNNs as Tensorflow Keras models. Classes and utilities to train and evaluate GNN models are available for node, edge, and graph focused problems, both in regression or classification setups, as well as in graph generation problems. Standard GNNs for homogeneous graphs as well as Composite GNNs, Layered GNNs, and Layered Composite GNNs can be implemented in a few lines of code. The optimization guaranteed by Tensorflow and Keras allows the models developed with GNNkeras to be scalable and efficient.

11.3 Biological Applications

This Section describes our studies on biological applications of GNNs. Problems such as PPI detection, DSE prediction, and molecular graph generation, constitute a good testing ground for demonstrating the capabilities of these networks to process graph structured biological datasets. These applications show the behavior of the model in the heterogeneous case, in a mixed inductive–transductive learning setup, with a layered architecture, and in the always challenging framework of graph generative learning.

11.3.1 Prediction of Protein-Protein Interfaces

Predicting PPIs is fundamental in order to detect interactions between proteins and predict the quaternary structures of protein complexes [34, 35]. A variety of approaches exist, based on sequence homology [36], Bayesian methods [37], docking [38] or SVMs [39]. Though GNNs have been applied to molecular interaction prediction [40, 41], we are not aware of specific applications to PPI detection before our method [42].

The prediction of PPIs can be addressed as a maximum clique problem [43], by constructing a correspondence graph from the graphs of secondary structures of the two peptides [44]. The interface will then correspond to the maximum clique in the correspondence graph [43]. Clique detection problems have already been addressed with GNNs [45], and with LGNNs [29]. The maximum clique search is a NP–complete problem, and solving it with traditional algorithms from the operations research field has a prohibitive computational cost, except for very small graphs [46].

As a first step, we built a dataset of correspondence graphs between pairs of monomers. In particular, we focused on pairs of peptides forming heterodimers, without disulfide bridges, and with a minimum surface of 200 Å^2. We obtained a set of 12,455 interfaces and built the two protein secondary structure graphs for each. These were then merged into a correspondence graph following the method described in [43, 44].

In order to train and test GNNs on this problem, the supervisions, labeling each node as part of the maximum clique or not, were generated with the Bron–Kerbosch algorithm [47]. Cliques with a minimum size of three nodes were labeled as biologically significant by checking if the secondary structures belonging to them were part of PPIs according to PDBePISA [48]. Finally, we obtained 512 correspondence graphs, each containing at least one biologically significant clique. After splitting disconnected components into multiple graphs, we got 1044 connected graphs, 537 of which contain a positive clique, while the remaining 507 contain only negative cliques.

A standard GNN architecture was trained and tested on the dataset described above. The problem is addressed as a node focused classification task. The model performance cannot be measured based on the accuracy, as the dataset is highly unbalanced, with negative nodes (not belonging to an interface) representing almost the 99% of examples. To provide a balanced metric, we use the F1-score, which combines precision and recall. The architecture of the MLP module dedicated to the output function g_w was kept fixed, using a one-layered MLP and a softmax activation function. In order to search for the best hyperparameters for f_w, we performed a 10-fold cross-validation, that determined the best architecture to be a one-layered MLP with sigmoid activation. This setup was used also to test a 5-layered LGNN network, where each GNN layer shares the same architecture.

For the evaluation of the LGNN performance, another 10-fold cross-validation was carried out. The LGNN is composed of 5 GNN layers, each with state dimension equal to 3. Moreover, to manage the unbalanced supervisions, positive examples are weighted more than negative examples. The models are trained with the Adam optimizer [49] and a cross–entropy loss function.

LGNNs that integrate only the node states in the labels of the following layer obtain the best performance. As illustrated in Fig. 11.3, a clear improvement in recall, and a slight improvement in precision can be observed through the LGNN layers. Moreover, the F1-score increases by more than five percentage points from the first GNN layer to the fifth. Integrating only the output or both the state and the output in the node labels, the F1-score decreases through the LGNN layers. The other parameters remain almost stable, except for recall, which slightly increases through the LGNN layers. However, the standard deviation of the recall tends to grow, suffering from a marked dependence on the initial conditions of the experiment. The results confirm the expectations based on biological data and show good performance in determining

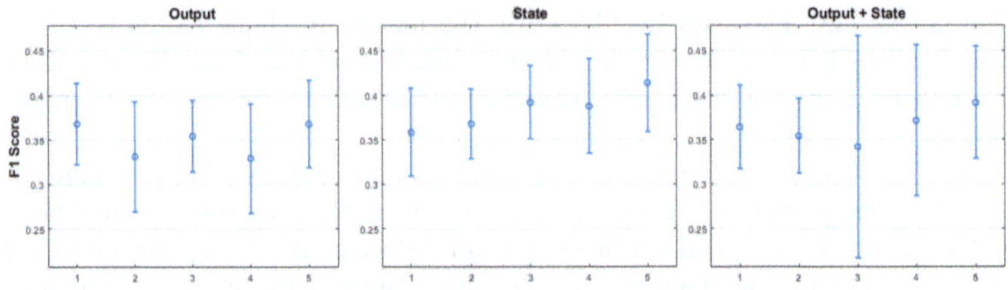

Fig. 11.3 5 levels LGNN 10-fold cross validation results: F1-score. Figure taken from [42]

the interaction sites, recognizing on average about 60% of the interacting nodes. These results allow us to draw the conclusion that this approach is really promising for the task under analysis, showing the inherent capability of GNNs in solving biological problems on graph-structured data.

11.3.2 Drug Side-Effect Prediction

DSEs represent a common health risk, and a huge cost for public care systems and pharmaceutical companies [50]. Moreover, their occurrence is increasing worldwide [51]. They often determine failures in clinical trials of candidate drugs, slowing down the drug discovery processes and increasing their costs [52]. An accurate prediction of DSEs in silico would allow discarding the drug candidates with too many potentially dangerous DSEs before submitting them to clinical trials, saving money, time, and health of the participants [53]. DSE predictors have evolved from statistical methods based on euclidean data [53, 54] to techniques based on clustering [55] or random forests [56], and finally to methods based on deep (yet euclidean) MLPs [57]. Although GNNs have been employed for a similar task, which consists in predicting polypharmacy side-effects [58, 59], we are not aware of other GNN approaches for the prediction of side–effects of single drugs before our method: DruGNN [28]. The main novelty of our method is represented by processing a heterogeneous relational dataset in its native graph structured form, exploiting the unique capabilities of GNNs [1, 2, 5].

DruGNN is a method for the prediction of DSEs based on GNNs that exploits heterogeneous data coming from multiple sources. Therefore, integrating these data in a relational graph structured dataset was the first step of our work in this direction. Using relational information is fundamental, yet DSE prediction has been based on euclidean data so far: even when topological information about the metabolic network or the molecule structure was used, this was encoded into euclidean vectors before being processed [54, 57]. Instead, DSEs are caused by complex biological phenomena, involving different types of entities and their relations, including drug targets [53] and metabolic data [55]. As a consequence, our dataset merges data coming from multiple sources and representing different entities, such as drugs and

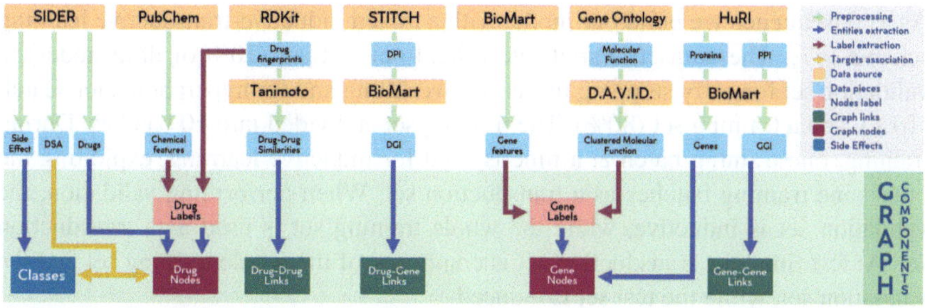

Fig. 11.4 Sketch of the dataset construction. Each data source is represented by an orange rectangle. Cyan rectangles represent data pieces. Preprocessing steps are represented by green arrows, which can include feeding data in input to other sources to obtain refined data. Graph node subsets are represented by purple rectangles, with their labels sketched as pink rectangles. Green rectangles are subsets of graph edges, while the blue rectangle represents the classes (side-effects). Red arrows represent the composition of feature labels from data pieces, while blue arrows show the composition of graph entities (nodes, edges, classes). The yellow arrow represents the association of drug nodes to side-effect classes. This Figure is taken from the DruGNN paper [28]

genes. The dataset consists of a single graph, in which each drug, and each gene, are mapped to a node. Both drug nodes and gene nodes are described by feature vectors. Edges represent drug-drug relationships, drug-gene interactions, and gene-gene interactions. Side-effect labels are associated to each drug node. These labels will be used, according to the inductive-transductive scheme, as either transductive features for known drugs, or class supervisions for new drugs [28]. The DSE targets were retrieved from SIDER [60], PPIs from the Human Reference Interactome [61], and Drug-Protein Interactions (DPIs) from STITCH [62]. Each protein was mapped to the gene it is a product of using Biomart [63]. Drug features were obtained on PubChem [64]. Drug structural information was extracted from the SMILES representation of each molecule and encoded in a fingerprint with RdKit .[1] Fingerprints allowed also to calculate the Tanimoto similarity, which allowed to build links between pairs of similar drugs. Gene features were obtained from Biomart [63], and integrated with molecular function ontology information from Gene Ontology [65], clustered to high level terms using DAVID [66]. After filtering side-effects with a minimum number of 100 occurrences, discarding those with few occurrences and all the related information, we obtained a dataset composed of 1341 drugs mapped to 360 DSEs, and interacting with 7881 genes. Edges are composed of: 12,002 gene-gene interaction links, 314,369 DPIs, and 5252 drug-drug similarity links. The dataset construction process is sketched in Fig. 11.4.

DruGNN addresses the problem as a multi–class multi–label node classification task (obviously, only drug nodes are classified, meaning that V_{out} will correspond to the subset of drug nodes). Since two types of nodes (drugs and genes) need to be processed, we use a CGNN (see Subsect. 11.2.2). Moreover, the expected use of this technique is to predict DSEs of new drugs given the DSEs of known drugs.

[1] RDKit: Open–Source Cheminformatics Software, by Greg Landrum. https://www.rdkit.org/.

As a consequence we build our model with a mixed inductive-transductive learning scheme [67]. The dataset is split into a held-out test set (10% of drug nodes), a validation set for early stopping in case of overfitting and for hyperparameter search (10%), and a training set (80%). The training set is divided into 10 batches. During training, one training batch at a time is used for inductive learning, exploiting the other nine training batches as a transduction set. When performing validation, the validation set is inductive, while the whole training set is used as a transduction set. At test time, the transduction set is composed of the whole training set and the validation set, while the test set is induced.

The best network hyperparameters were found with a grid-search over the validation set, which allowed to determine the following architecture: two one-layer MLPs, implementing f_w for the two node types, with 50 units each; one-layer g_w with 200 units, average neighborhood aggregation $a = 1/|Ne(n)|$; ReLU activation for all the hidden layers; Adam optimizer [49] with initial learning rate equal to 10^{-3}; no dropout. This architecture was kept fixed in all the subsequent experimentation. Two ablation studies were performed. The first one, over the set of side–effects, allowed to determine the model performance variation when narrowing the search to a variable number of most common DSEs. The results showed that the model applies a scheme similar to transfer learning between the different classes (which can be seen as independent and parallel problems to solve), improving its performance for larger sets of DSEs. An inversion of this behavior occurs for very small sets of side-effects, where transfer learning is not possible. The second ablation study was aimed at determining the importance of each feature/edge group in the dataset, by observing the performance drop implied by its removal. The results showed that all the data sources are important for this task, yet the model shows high robustness to feature/edge ablation thanks to the GNN capabilities and to the dataset structure.

DruGNN was also compared with other GNN models, and with a simple euclidean MLP predictor, in order to assess the performance gap brought by the use of the original GNN model [1]. In particular, we compared to GraphSAGE [11], GCNs [10], and with a MLP (providing a non graph-structured baseline). The graph-based models were trained and tested with the same inductive-transductive scheme of DruGNN. The hyperparameters of all the models were tuned with a grid search analogous to that performed for DruGNN. The results are reported in Table 11.1, and show that the MLP has a performance gap of approximately five percentage points with respect to the worst graph-based model. DruGNN has an advantage of approximately three percentage points, in line with theoretical expectations derived from using a recurrent GNN [2, 5, 32].

These results show that exploiting relational graph structured information is crucial for predicting DSEs accurately. Moreover, integrating data from multiple heterogeneous sources is fundamental, as DSEs are complex processes involving various biological entities and their relations. CGNNs are the ideal model for processing this heterogeneous graph dataset. Exploiting a mixed inductive-transductive learning scheme, which simulates the expected behavior of the model in a real-world scenario, allowed us to deploy a usable method: to predict the side-effects of a new

Table 11.1 Comparison between different models of the GNN family. Model configuration is reported; all of the models were optimized with a small hyperparameter search. K: maximum number of state update iterations for DruGNN; SD: state dimension for DruGNN; DL: number of dense layers and units in each dense layer; CL: number of convolutional layers and units in each convolutional layer. For GCN and GraphSage, the dense layer is the last one before the output layer. Table taken from [28]

Model	Configuration	Avg. Acc. %
DruGNN	$K = 6, SD = 50, DL = 1 \times 200$	86.30
GCN	$CL = 2 \times 36, DL = 116$	82.94
GraphSAGE	$CL = 2 \times 72, DL = 1 \times 168$	83.11
MLP	$DL = 3 \times 25$	77.98

drug, it is sufficient to add the compound to the dataset, using information on the known DSEs for the prediction.

11.3.3 Molecular Graph Generation

The generation of molecular graphs is of particular interest for drug discovery, as it could provide a technique for designing large amounts of possible drug candidates. Moreover, traditional drug design techniques proceed by modifying existing drug molecules, rather than generating new structures from scratch. Therefore, graph generators based on deep learning could bring substantial innovation to the field. Graph generation is a complex problem for ML models, which can be tackled with two families of approaches. On the one hand, generators based on Variational AutoEncoders (VAEs) build the graph in one single step, generating the adjacency matrix, the node feature matrix when nodes are labeled, and the edge feature matrix when edges are labeled. These approaches can generate molecules based on SMILES strings [68, 69], the molecular graphs themselves [70], or even graphs of molecule fragments [71]. On the other hand, sequential generators build the graph one step at a time, adding one node or a group of nodes at each step. GraphRNN [72] is a typical example of this process, though not applied to molecule generation. These approaches can be based on recurrent neural networks, adversarial mechanisms [73], or reinforcement learning [74], and they analyze the sequence of steps or decisions needed to generate the graph, rather than the graph itself. GNNs have the great advantage of processing the graph itself, with minimal loss of information [2], thus representing an ideal model for a sequential graph generator.

Our method, called Molecular Generative Graph Neural Network (MG^2N^2) for drug discovery [75], consists of a sequential generator that generates one atom at a time, following an algorithm of node expansion: each generated node is put in an expansion queue. The head node is analyzed in order to generate its neighbors

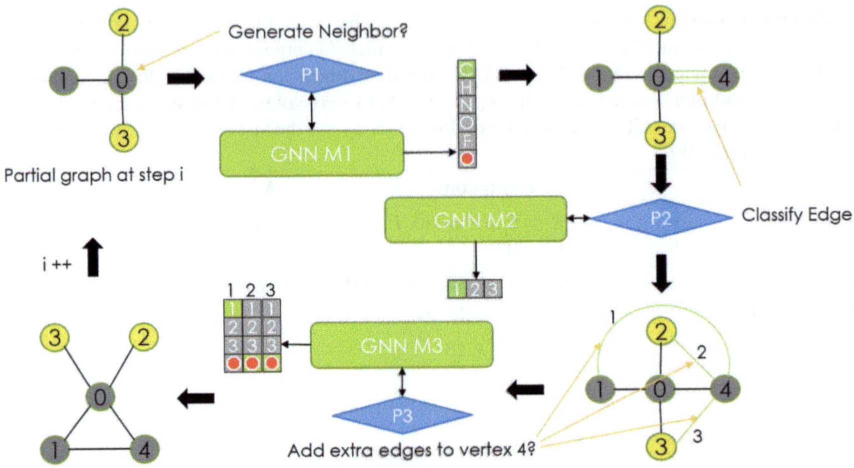

Fig. 11.5 Flowchart of the generation algorithm. An example step is summarized, with the three GNN modules (M1, M2, M3), the three problems they are assigned to (P1, P2, P3), their inputs, and their outputs. Grey nodes represent carbon atoms, while yellow nodes represent hydrogen atoms. Green edges stand for candidate edges, while black edges represent single bonds. C,H,N,O,F are the element symbols. Classes 1,2,3 represent single, double, and triple bonds, respectively. The red octagons represent the decision *stop* (M1) or *do not generate this edge* (M3). This image is taken from [75]

and then popped out of the queue. The process stops when a maximum number of nodes is reached, or the queue becomes empty. MG^2N^2 is composed of three GNN modules: the first one generates the neighbor node or decides to "stop" (pop the head node out of the queue). The other two modules are called when the decision is different from "stop". The second decides the type of edge connecting the generated node to the head node. The third module decides for possible extra connections between the generated node and the rest of the graph (this is necessary to generate molecules that are represented by graphs with cycles). GNN modules are trained on a separate basis, assuming each of the other two modules to behave perfectly. This strong assumption is justified by a much lower computational cost, and the possibility to independently retrain each of the modules, making modifications and adjustments easier. An example step of this algorithm is visually summarized as a flowchart in Fig. 11.5.

Graph generation is a discrete stochastic process. Neural networks are deterministic models once trained, and therefore not easily adaptable to this kind of task. Special types of activation functions can be used to make their behavior stochastic. In our case, we have two GNN edge classifier modules, and one GNN node classifier module. These models, if equipped with regular softmax output layers, would always generate the same decisions. The solution consists in equipping them with Gumbel softmax output layers. A Gumbel softmax is a regular softmax with the addition of white noise with a Gumbel distribution. This layer provides a stochastic output, with

Table 11.2 Validity, Uniqueness, and Novelty of generated compounds assessing the quality of our models and the baselines on the QM9 dataset. Table cited from [75]

Model	Valid	Unique	Novel	VUN	Avg. QED	Avg. logP	Avg. Mol. Wt.
ChemVAE	0.103	0.675	0.900	0.063	–	–	–
MPGVAE	0.910	0.680	0.540	0.334	–	–	–
GrammarVAE	0.602	0.093	0.809	0.045	–	–	–
GraphVAE	0.557	0.760	0.616	0.261	–	–	–
MolGAN	**0.981**	0.104	0.942	0.096	–	–	–
Ours(C2)	0.511	**0.888**	**1.000**	**0.454**	0.461 (0.116)	0.272 (1.336)	134.8 (45.7)
Ours(C3)	0.668	0.340	**1.000**	0.227	0.404 (0.088)	0.238 (1.093)	75.3 (52.8)
Test	–	–	–	–	0.482 (0.096)	0.270 (1.325)	127.3 (7.6)

each class having probability of being selected equal to the probability estimated by the softmax [76].

Experiments were performed on the QM9 [77] and Zinc [78] datasets of molecules. Initially, a hyperparameter search allowed to tune the models to the task under analysis. After this step, generative experiments were issued in order to compare the model to other similar approaches. In each experiment, 10,000 molecular graphs are generated. The chemical characteristics of these molecules, including QED, logP, and molecular weight, are measured with RdKit and compared with the dataset standard, measured over the held-out test set. Then, the metrics defined in [70] are used to estimate the quality of the compounds. In particular, Validity accounts for the fraction of valid compounds over the generated molecules; Uniqueness measures the fraction of unique molecules among the generated ones; Novelty represents the fraction of novel compounds (i.e. not found in the original dataset) among the unique ones. A new metric is introduced, summarizing these three quantities in one score, called VUN, and obtained by multiplying them together.

The comparison on QM9 was carried out with ChemVAE [68], GrammarVAE [69], MolGAN [74], the state of the art approach for unconditional generation GraphVAE [70], and the MPNN-based MPGVAE [79]. The results, summarized in Table 11.2 show that our approach outperforms all the selected baselines.

MolGAN has the highest validity among these methods, thanks to its RL–based decision process, which is optimal for learning chemical rules. Its uniqueness and novelty are low, though. This is because VAEs generate the graph from a latent representation, which makes them more effective in modeling the stochastic distributions composing the chemical space of compounds. While retaining a validity lower than MolGAN but higher than VAEs, our approach is capable of generating more unique and novel compounds than the other methods, thanks to the higher amount of infor-

Table 11.3 Validity, Uniqueness, and Novelty of generated compounds assessing the quality of our model and the baselines on the Zinc dataset. Table cited from [75]

Model	Valid	Unique	Novel	VUN
GrammarVAE[69]	0.310	0.108	**1.000**	0.033
ChemVAE[68]	0.170	0.310	0.980	0.052
GraphVAE[70]	0.140	0.316	**1.000**	0.044
CGVAE[80]	**1.000**	**0.998**	**1.000**	**0.998**
Ours	0.753	0.107	**1.000**	0.081

mation conveyed by the graph representation in input to the GNN modules, and to the stochastic sequential decision process implemented.

The comparison on Zinc was carried out with ChemVAE [68], GrammarVAE [69], and the state of the art approach CGVAE [80]. The results are shown in Table 11.3. The great difference in performance between CGVAE and the other methods is largely justified by the different approach to the problem. In CGVAE, molecules are kekulized during the preprocessing stage, thus aromatic bonds are reduced to either single or double bonds. The other hard chemical laws, like valence rules, that would invalidate the generated molecule if violated, are enforced as hard constraints, preventing the possibility of generating invalid molecules [80]. In all the other reported methods, including ours, these rules are learned by the model [75].

These results lead to the conclusion that GNNs allow to build very powerful sequential graph generators. Modularity is an important feature of the model, making it easier to train and to modify. As other sequential generators, our model is easily interpretable, as the step in which a particular decision is taken, and even the responsible module, are straightforwardly identifiable.

11.4 Conclusions and Future Perspectives

The results of the methods described in Sect. 11.3 clearly demonstrate the capabilities of GNNs in extracting and elaborating relevant information from graph structured data, solving interesting biological problems, such as PPI identification, DSE prediction, and molecular graph generation. These findings are in line with theoretical expectations on the expressive capabilities of GNNs and show many possible future directions for research and application of new and existing models.

A very interesting idea for improving the PPI prediction technique described in Sect. 11.3.1 is to build monomeric and correspondence graphs at the amino–acid scale, rather than using the coarser secondary structure element scale. Moreover, though increasing computational costs, this representation would allow to avoiding the loss of information implied by compressing a group of amino–acids into a single node representing the secondary structure. Predictions would also become more accurate, describing the interfaces at the amino–acid level.

Interesting future directions for DruGNN (see Sect. 11.3.2) include the possibility of developing a DSE predictor based on the graphs representing the structural formulas of molecules. This predictor would also allow to analyze the output of molecular graph generators in real time. In particular, combining this method with MG^2N^2 [75] would allow to build a very powerful generator of potential drug candidates with low expected side-effect profiles [28].

Regarding MG^2N^2 (see Subsect. 11.3.3), another interesting matter of future work is represented by an analogous model for conditional generation, that takes in input particular conditions the generated compounds should satisfy. This feature is particularly important for drug discovery studies. Another important direction would be to create a hierarchical or fragment based version of MG^2N^2, capable of generating larger molecules while also retaining higher Validity.

From a general perspective, these three applications show, together with the rapidly growing literature on this matter, that GNNs can be applied to a wide variety of biological problems inspired by real-world applications. Their capabilities of processing graph structured information and the increasing amount of relational data available on biological phenomena will lead to an even more important role for GNNs and their biological applications.

References

1. Scarselli, F., Gori, M., Tsoi, A.C., Hagenbuchner, M., Monfardini, G.: The graph neural network model. IEEE Trans. Neural Netw. **20**(1), 61–80 (2009)
2. Scarselli, F., Gori, M., Tsoi, A.C., Hagenbuchner, M., Monfardini, G.: Computational capabilities of graph neural networks. IEEE Trans. Neural Netw. **20**(1), 81–102 (2009)
3. Wu, Z., Pan, S., Chen, F., Long, G., Zhang, C., Yu, P.S.: A comprehensive survey on graph neural networks. IEEE Trans. Neural Netw. Learn. Syst. (2020)
4. Gilmer, J., Schoenholz, S.S., Riley, P.F., Vinyals, O., Dahl, G.E.: Neural message passing for quantum chemistry. In: Proceedings of the 34th International Conference on Machine Learning, vol. 70, pp. 1263–1272 (2017)
5. Xu, K., Hu, W., Leskovec, J., Jegelka, S.: How powerful are graph neural networks? In: International Conference on Learning Representations (2018)
6. Battaglia, P.W., Hamrick, J.B., Bapst, V., Sanchez-Gonzalez, A., Zambaldi, V., Malinowski, M., Tacchetti, A., Raposo, D., Santoro, A., Faulkner, R., Gulcehre, C., Song, F., Ballard, A., Gilmer, J., Dahl, G., Vaswani, A., Allen, K., Nash, C., Langston, V., Dyer, C., Heess, N., Wierstra, D., Kohli, P., Botvinick, M., Vinyals, O., Li, Y., Pascanu, R.: Relational inductive biases, deep learning, and graph networks (2018)
7. Li, Y., Tarlow, D., Brockschmidt, M., Zemel, R.: Gated graph sequence neural networks (2015)
8. Bruna, J., Zaremba, W., Szlam, A., LeCun, Y.: Spectral networks and deep locally connected networks on graphs. In: 2nd International Conference on Learning Representations, ICLR 2014 (2014)
9. Defferrard, M., Bresson, X., Vandergheynst, P.: Convolutional neural networks on graphs with fast localized spectral filtering. In: Advances in Neural Information Processing Systems, pp. 3844–3852 (2016)

10. Kipf, T.N., Welling, M.: Semi-supervised classification with graph convolutional networks. In: 5th International Conference on Learning Representations, ICLR 2017 (2017)
11. Hamilton, W.L., Ying, Z., Leskovec, J.: Inductive representation learning on large graphs. In: Advances in Neural Information Processing Systems, pp. 1024–1034 (2017)
12. Veličković, P., Cucurull, G., Casanova, A., Romero, A., Liò, P., Bengio, Y.: Graph attention networks (2017)
13. Dai, E., Wang, S.: Towards self-explainable graph neural network. In: Proceedings of the 30th ACM International Conference on Information and Knowledge Management, pp. 302–311 (2021)
14. Munikoti, S., Das, L., Natarajan, B.: Scalable graph neural network-based framework for identifying critical nodes and links in complex networks. Neurocomputing **468**, 211–221 (2022)
15. Zhou, J., Cui, G., Hu, S., Zhang, Z., Yang, C., Liu, Z., Wang, L., Li, C., Sun, M.: Graph neural networks: a review of methods and applications. AI Open **1**, 57–81 (2020)
16. Bianchi, F.M., Grattarola, D., Livi, L., Alippi, C.: Hierarchical representation learning in graph neural networks with node decimation pooling. IEEE Trans. Neural Netw. Learn, Syst (2020)
17. Wu, B., Liu, Y., Lang, B., Huang, L.: Dgcnn: Disordered graph convolutional neural network based on the gaussian mixture model. Neurocomputing **321**, 346–356 (2018)
18. Lee, J.B., Rossi, R., Kong, X.: Graph classification using structural attention. In: Proceedings of the 24th ACM SIGKDD International Conference on Knowledge Discovery and Data Mining, pp. 1666–1674 (2018)
19. Li, G., Müller, M., Ghanem, B., Koltun, V.: Training graph neural networks with 1000 layers. In: International Conference on Machine Learning, pp. 6437–6449, PMLR (2021)
20. Kong, K., Li, G., Ding, M., Wu, Z., Zhu, C., Ghanem, B., Taylor, G., Goldstein, T.: Flag: adversarial data augmentation for graph neural networks. *arXiv preprint* arXiv:2010.09891 (2020)
21. Smith, J.S., Roitberg, A.E., Isayev, O.: Transforming computational drug discovery with machine learning and AI. ACS Med. Chem. Lett. **9**(11), 1065–1069 (2018)
22. Kim, J., Park, S., Min, D., Kim, W.: Comprehensive survey of recent drug discovery using deep learning. Int. J. Mol. Sci. **22**(18), 9983 (2021)
23. Wouters, O.J., McKee, M., Luyten, J.: Estimated research and development investment needed to bring a new medicine to market, 2009–2018. JAMA **323**(9), 844–853 (2020)
24. Dickson, M., Gagnon, J.P.: Key factors in the rising cost of new drug discovery and development. Nat. Rev. Drug Discov. **3**(5), 417–429 (2004)
25. Lipinski, C.F., Maltarollo, V.G., Oliveira, P.R., da Silva, A.B., Honorio, K.M.: Advances and perspectives in applying deep learning for drug design and discovery. Front. Robot. AI **6**, 108 (2019)
26. Macalino, S.J.Y., Gosu, V., Hong, S., Choi, S.: Role of computer-aided drug design in modern drug discovery. Arch. Pharmacal Res. **38**(9), 1686–1701 (2015)
27. Scarselli, F., Yong, S.L., Gori, M., Hagenbuchner, M., Tsoi, A.C., Maggini, M.: Graph neural networks for ranking web pages. In: The 2005 IEEE/WIC/ACM International Conference on Web Intelligence (WI'05), pp. 666–672, IEEE (2005)
28. Bongini, P., Pancino, N., Dimitri, G. M., Bianchini, M., Scarselli, F., Lio, P.: Modular multi–source prediction of drug side–effects with DruGNN. IEEE/ACM Trans. Comput. Biol. Bioinform. (2022)
29. Bandinelli, N., Bianchini, M., Scarselli, F.: Learning long-term dependencies using layered graph neural networks. In: The 2010 International Joint Conference on Neural Networks (IJCNN), pp. 1–8, IEEE (2010)
30. Weisfeiler, B., Leman, A.: The reduction of a graph to canonical form and the algebra which appears therein. NTI Ser. **2**(9), 12–16 (1968)
31. Morris, C., Ritzert, M., Fey, M., Hamilton, W.L., Lenssen, J.E., Rattan, G., Grohe, M.: Weisfeiler and leman go neural: higher-order graph neural networks. In: Proceedings of the AAAI Conference on Artificial Intelligence **33**, 4602–4609 (2019)
32. D'Inverno, G.A., Bianchini, M., Sampoli, M.L., Scarselli, F.: An unifying point of view on expressive power of gnns (2021)

33. Pancino, N., Bongini, P., Scarselli, F., Bianchini, M.: Gnnkeras: a keras-based library for graph neural networks and homogeneous and heterogeneous graph processing. SoftwareX **18**, 101061 (2022)
34. Janin, J., Bahadur, R.P., Chakrabarti, P.: Protein-protein interaction and quaternary structure. Q. Rev. Biophy. **41**(2), 133–180 (2008)
35. Lane, T.J., Shukla, D., Beauchamp, K.A., Pande, V.S.: To milliseconds and beyond: challenges in the simulation of protein folding. Current opinion in structural biology **23**(1), 58–65 (2013)
36. Xue, L.C., Dobbs, D., Honavar, V.: Homppi: a class of sequence homology based protein-protein interface prediction methods. BMC Mioinformatics **12**(1), 1–24 (2011)
37. Hwang, H., Petrey, D., Honig, B.: A hybrid method for protein-protein interface prediction. Protein Sci. **25**(1), 159–165 (2016)
38. Hwang, H., Vreven, T., Weng, Z.: "Binding interface prediction by combining protein-protein docking results, proteins: structure. Funct. Bioinf. **82**(1), 57–66 (2014)
39. Bradford, J.R., Westhead, D.R.: Improved prediction of protein-protein binding sites using a support vector machines approach. Bioinformatics **21**(8), 1487–1494 (2005)
40. Huang, K., Xiao, C., Glass, L.M., Zitnik, M., Sun, J.: Skipgnn: predicting molecular interactions with skip-graph networks. Sci. Rep. **10**(1), 1–16 (2020)
41. Liu, Y., Yuan, H., Cai, L., Ji, S.: Deep learning of high-order interactions for protein interface prediction. In: Proceedings of the 26th ACM SIGKDD International Conference on Knowledge Discovery and Data Mining, pp. 679–687 (2020)
42. Pancino, N., Rossi, A., Ciano, G., Giacomini, , Bonechi, S., Andreini, P., Scarselli, F., Bianchini, M., Bongini, P.: Graph neural networks for the prediction of protein-protein interfaces. In: ESANN, pp. 127–132 (2020)
43. Gardiner, E.J., Artymiuk, P.J., Willett, P.: Clique-detection algorithms for matching three-dimensional molecular structures. J. Mol. Graph. Modell. **15**(4), 245–253 (1997)
44. Grindley, H.M., Artymiuk, P.J., Rice, D.W., Willett, P.: Identification of tertiary structure resemblance in proteins using a maximal common subgraph isomorphism algorithm. J. Mol. Biol. **229**(3), 707–721 (1993)
45. Gori, M., Monfardini, G., Scarselli, F.: A new model for learning in graph domains. In: Proceedings. 2005 IEEE International Joint Conference on Neural Networks, 2005., vol. 2, pp. 729–734, IEEE (2005)
46. Bomze, I.M., Budinich, M., Pardalos, P.M., Pelillo, M.: The maximum clique problem. In: Handbook of Combinatorial Optimization, pp. 1–74, Springer (1999)
47. Bron, C., Kerbosch, J.: Algorithm 457: finding all cliques of an undirected graph. Commun. ACM **16**(9), 575–577 (1973)
48. Krissinel, E.: Crystal contacts as nature's docking solutions. J. Comput. Chem. **31**(1), 133–143 (2010)
49. Kingma, D.P., Ba, J.: Adam: a method for stochastic optimization (2014)
50. Ernst, F.R., Grizzle, A.J.: Drug-related morbidity and mortality: updating the cost-of-illness model. J. Am. Pharmac. Assoc. **41**(2), 192–199 (2001)
51. Kantor, E.D., Rehm, C.D., Haas, J.S., Chan, A.T., Giovannucci, E.L.: Trends in prescription drug use among adults in the United States from 1999–2012. Jama **314**(17), 1818–1830 (2015)
52. Billingsley, M.L.: Druggable targets and targeted drugs: enhancing the development of new therapeutics. Pharmacology **82**(4), 239–244 (2008)
53. Mizutani, S., Pauwels, E., Stoven, V., Goto, S., Yamanishi, Y.: Relating drug-protein interaction network with drug side effects. Bioinformatics **28**(18), i522–i528 (2012)
54. Yamanishi, Y., Kotera, M., Kanehisa, M., Goto, S.: Drug-target interaction prediction from chemical, genomic and pharmacological data in an integrated framework. Bioinformatics **26**(12), i246–i254 (2010)
55. Dimitri, G.M., Liò, P.: DrugClust: a machine learning approach for drugs side effects prediction. Comput. Biol. Chem. **68**, 204–210 (2017)
56. Cakir, A., Tuncer, M., Taymaz-Nikerel, H., Ulucan, O.: Side effect prediction based on drug-induced gene expression profiles and random forest with iterative feature selection. Pharmacogenomics J. 1–9 (2021)

57. Uner, O.C., Cinbis, R.G., Tastan, O., Cicek, A.E.: DeepSide: a deep learning framework for drug side effect prediction (2019)
58. Deac, A., Huang, Y.-H., Veličković, P., Liò, P., Tang, J.: Drug-drug adverse effect prediction with graph co-attention (2019)
59. Zitnik, M., Agrawal, M., Leskovec, J.: Modeling polypharmacy side effects with graph convolutional networks. Bioinformatics **34**(13), i457–i466 (2018)
60. Kuhn, M., Letunic, I., Jensen, L.J., Bork, P.: The SIDER database of drugs and side effects. Nucleic Acids Res. **44**(D1), D1075–D1079 (2016)
61. Luck, K., Kim, D.-K., Lambourne, L., Spirohn, K., Begg, B.E., Bian, W., Brignall, R., Cafarelli, T., Campos-Laborie, F.J., Charloteaux, B., et al.: A reference map of the human binary protein interactome. Nature **580**(7803), 402–408 (2020)
62. Szklarczyk, D., Santos, A., Von Mering, C., Jensen, L.J., Bork, P., Kuhn, M.: STITCH 5: augmenting protein-chemical interaction networks with tissue and affinity data. Nucleic Acids Res. **44**(D1), D380–D384 (2016)
63. Smedley, D., Haider, S., Durinck, S., Pandini, L., Provero, P., Allen, J., Arnaiz, O., Awedh, M.H., Baldock, R., Barbiera, G., et al.: The BioMart community portal: an innovative alternative to large, centralized data repositories. Nucleic Acids Res. **43**(W1), W589–W598 (2015)
64. Kim, S., Chen, J., Cheng, T., Gindulyte, A., He, J., He, S., Li, Q., Shoemaker, B.A., Thiessen, P.A., Yu, B., et al.: PubChem in 2021: new data content and improved web interfaces. Nucleic Acid Res. **49**(D1), D1388–D1395 (2021)
65. Ashburner, M., Ball, C.A., Blake, J.A., Botstein, D., Butler, H., Cherry, J.M., Davis, A.P., Dolinski, K., Dwight, S.S., Eppig, J.T., et al.: Gene ontology: tool for the unification of biology. Nat. Genet. **25**(1), 25–29 (2000)
66. Huang, D.W., Sherman, B.T., Lempicki, R.A.: Systematic and integrative analysis of large gene lists using DAVID bioinformatics resources. Nat. Protoc. **4**(1), 44–57 (2009)
67. Ciano, G., Rossi, A., Bianchini, M., Scarselli, F.: On inductive-transductive learning with graph neural networks. IEEE Trans. Pattern Anal. Mach, Intell (2021)
68. Gómez-Bombarelli, R., Wei, J.N., Duvenaud, D., Hernández-Lobato, J.M., Sánchez-Lengeling, B., Sheberla, D., Aguilera-Iparraguirre, J., Hirzel, T.D., Adams, R.P., Aspuru-Guzik, A.: Automatic chemical design using a data-driven continuous representation of molecules. ACS Central Sci. **4**(2), 268–276 (2018)
69. Kusner, M.J., Paige, B., Hernández-Lobato, J.M.: Grammar variational autoencoder. In: International Conference on Machine Learning, pp. 1945–1954, PMLR (2017)
70. Simonovsky, M., Komodakis, N.: GraphVAE: towards generation of small graphs using variational autoencoders. In: International Conference on Artificial Neural Networks, pp. 412–422, Springer (2018)
71. Jin, W., Barzilay, R., Jaakkola, T.: Junction tree variational autoencoder for molecular graph generation. In: International Conference on Machine Learning, pp. 2323–2332, PMLR (2018)
72. You, J., Ying, R., Ren, X., Hamilton, W.L., Leskovec, J.: GraphRNN: generating realistic graphs with deep auto-regressive models. In: International Conference on Machine Learning, pp. 5708–5717 (2018)
73. Wang, H., Wang, J., Wang, J., Zhao, M., Zhang, W., Zhang, F., Xie, X., Guo, M.: GraphGAN: graph representation learning with generative adversarial nets. In: Thirty-Second AAAI Conference on Artificial Intelligence, pp. 2508–2515 (2018)
74. De Cao, N., Kipf, T.: MolGAN: an implicit generative model for small molecular graphs (2018)
75. Bongini, P., Bianchini, M., Scarselli, F.: Molecular generative graph neural networks for drug discovery. Neurocomputing **450**, 242–252 (2021)
76. Jang, E., Gu, S., Poole, B.: Categorical reparameterization with gumbel-softmax. In: 5th International Conference on Learning Representations (ICLR), 2017
77. Ramakrishnan, R., Dral, P.O., Rupp, M., von Lilienfeld, O.A.: Quantum chemistry structures and properties of 134 kilo molecules. In: Scientific Data, vol. 1 (2014)
78. Irwin, J.J., Shoichet, B.K.: Zinc–a free database of commercially available compounds for virtual screening. J. Chem. Inf. Model. **45**(1), 177–182 (2005)
79. Flam-Shepherd, D., Wu, T., Aspuru-Guzik, A.: Graph deconvolutional generation (2020)

80. Liu, Q., Allamanis, M., Brockschmidt, M., Gaunt, A.: Constrained graph variational autoencoders for molecule design. Adv. Neural Inf. Process. Syst. **31**, 7795–7804 (2018)

MIX
Papier aus verantwortungsvollen Quellen
Paper from responsible sources
FSC® C105338

If you have any concerns about our products,
you can contact us on
ProductSafety@springernature.com

In case Publisher is established outside the EU,
the EU authorized representative is:
Springer Nature Customer Service Center GmbH
Europaplatz 3, 69115 Heidelberg, Germany

Printed by Libri Plureos GmbH
in Hamburg, Germany